Sudden Cardiac Death

Edited by Peter Magnusson
and Jo Ann LeQuang

Published in London, United Kingdom

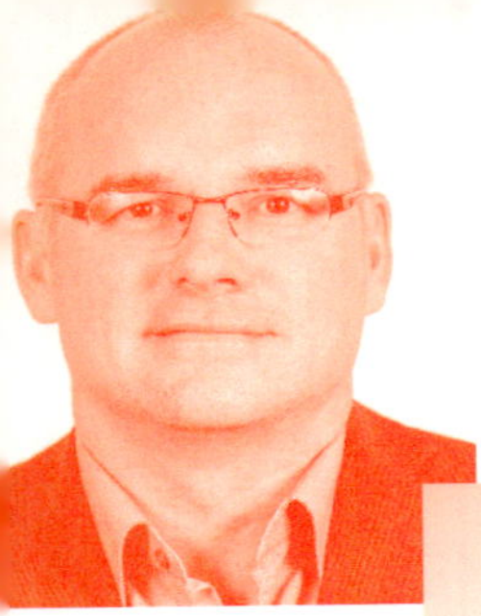
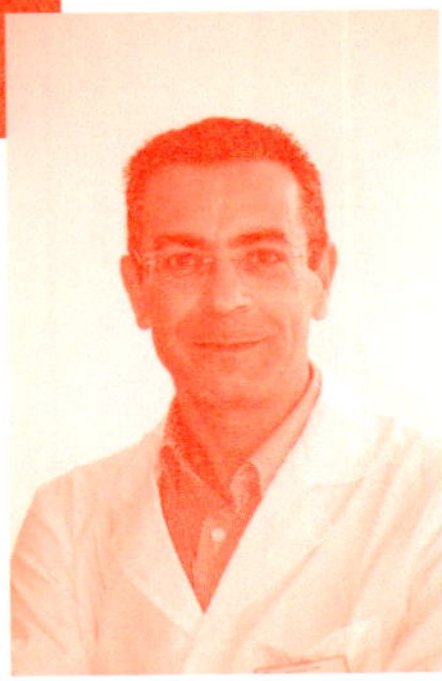
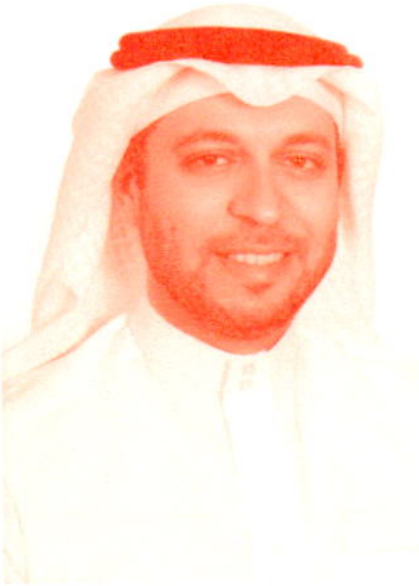
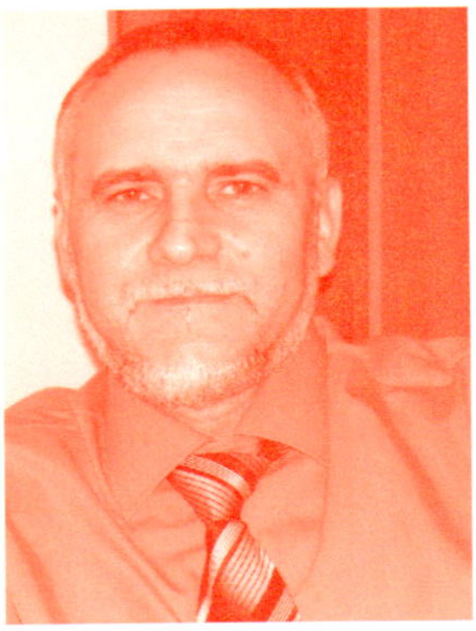
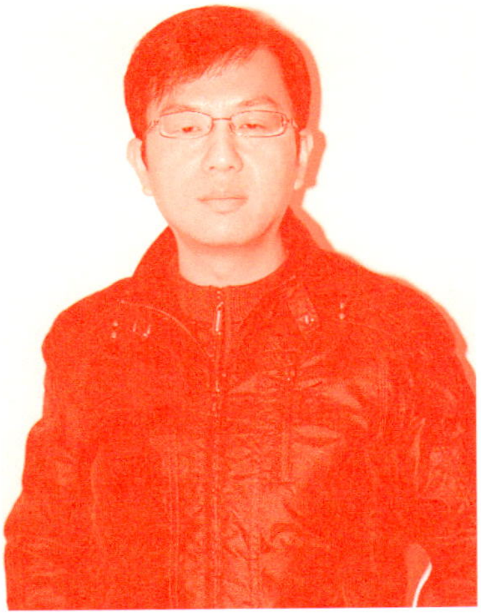
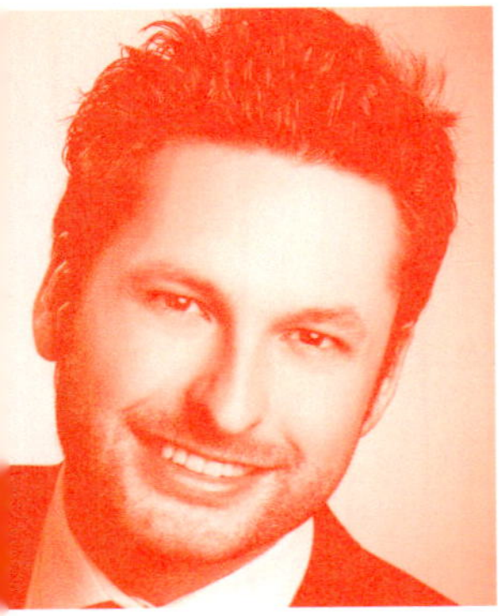
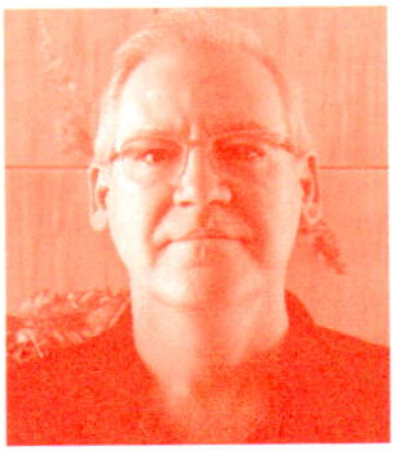

IntechOpen

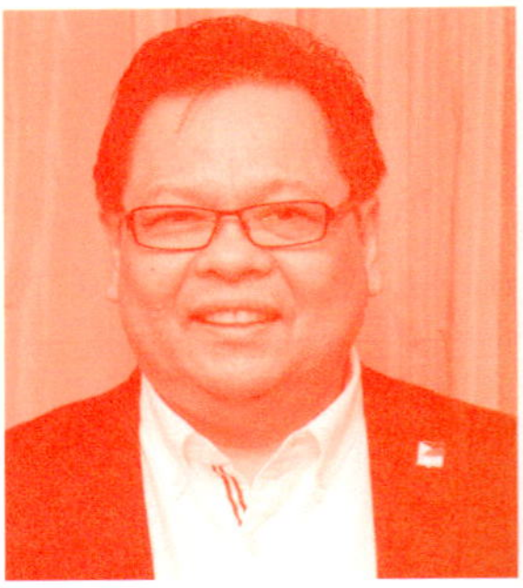
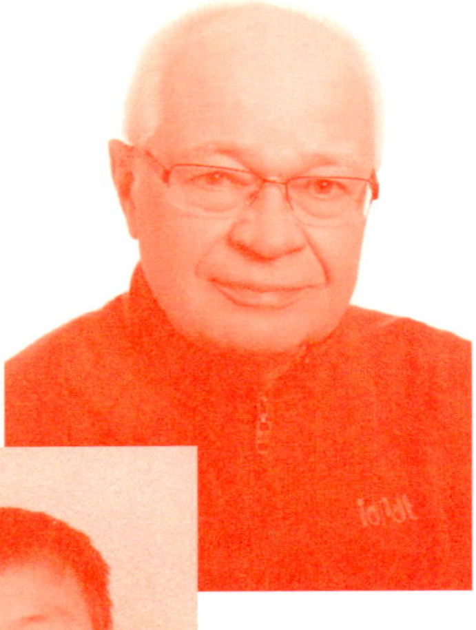
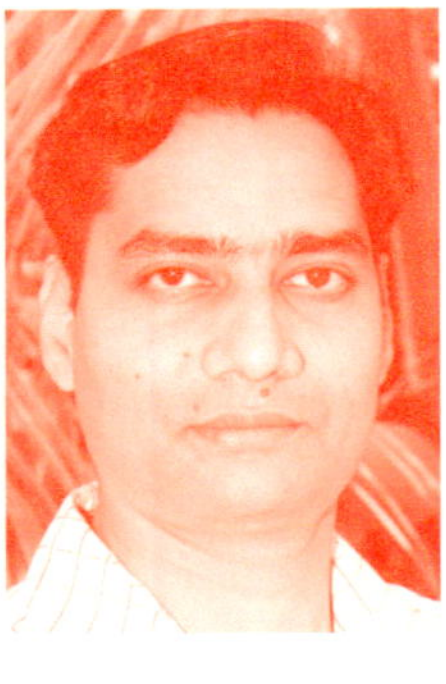
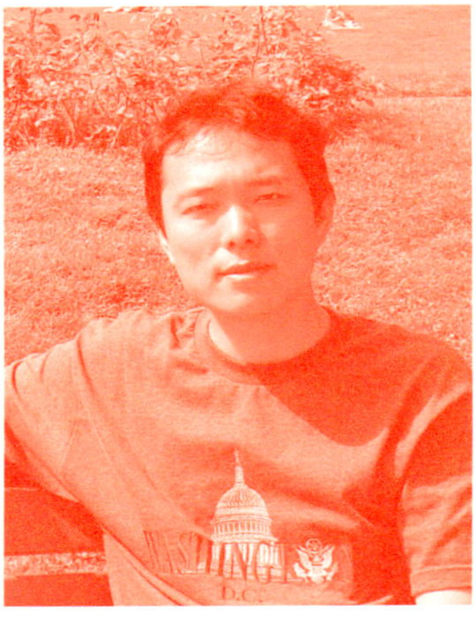
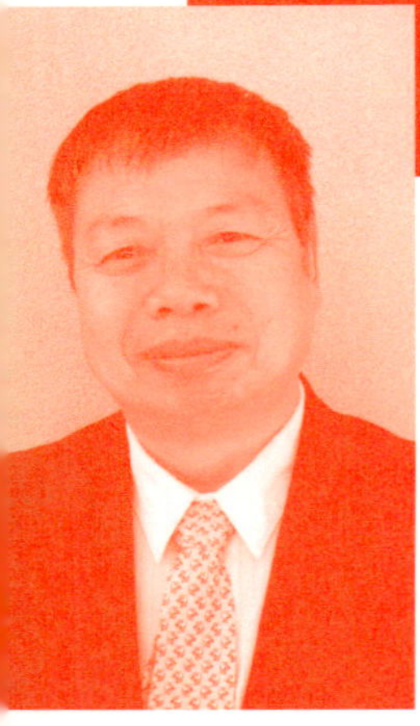
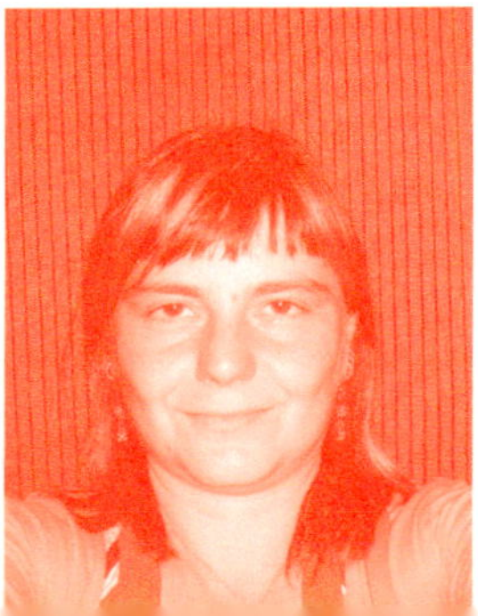

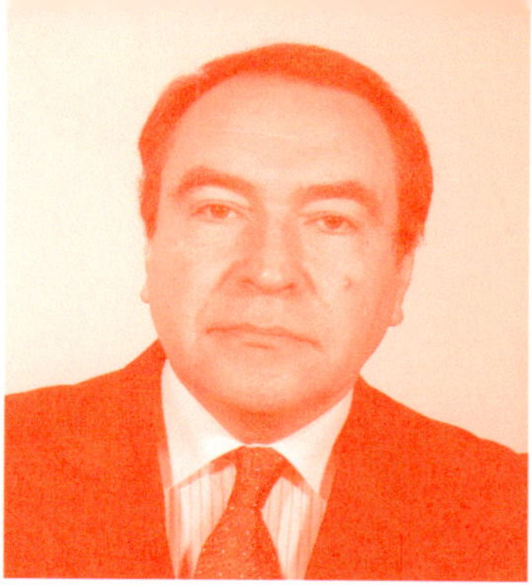

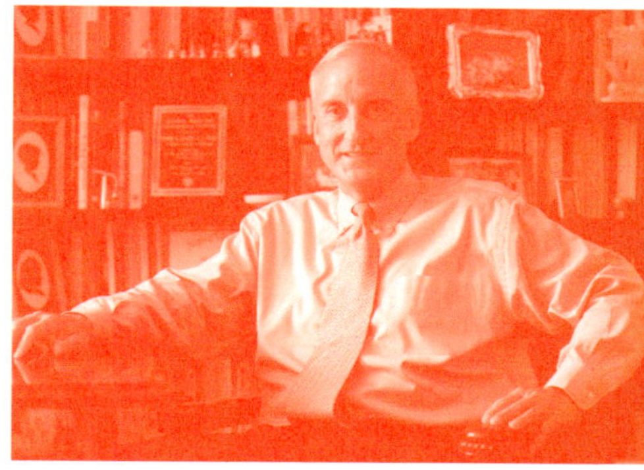

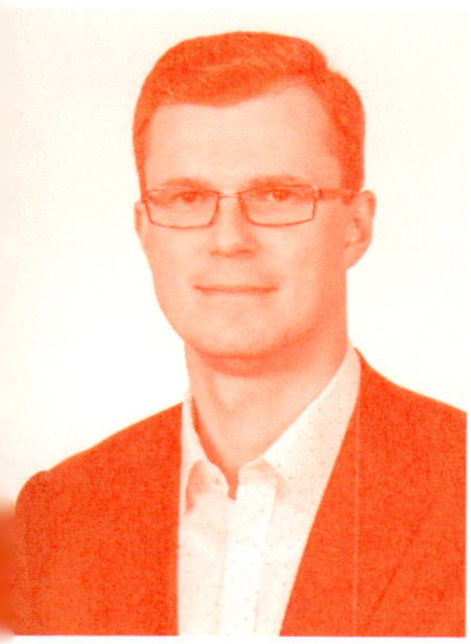

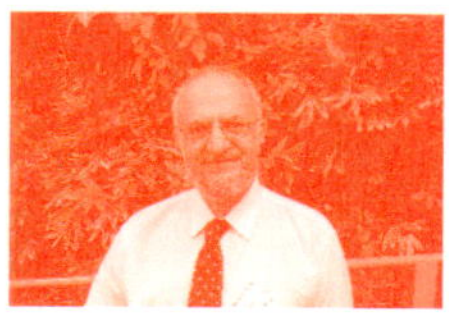

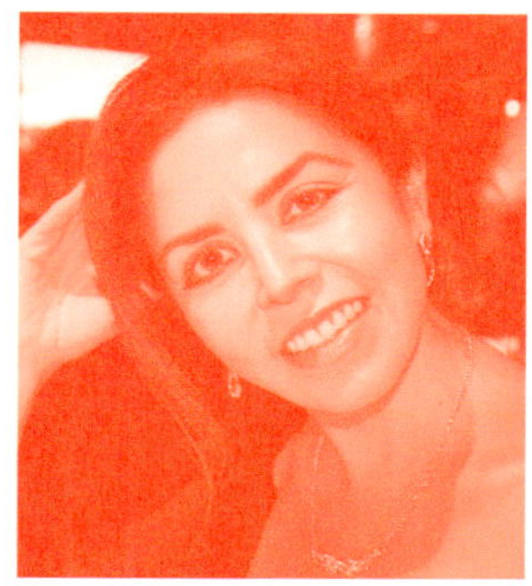

Supporting open minds since 2005

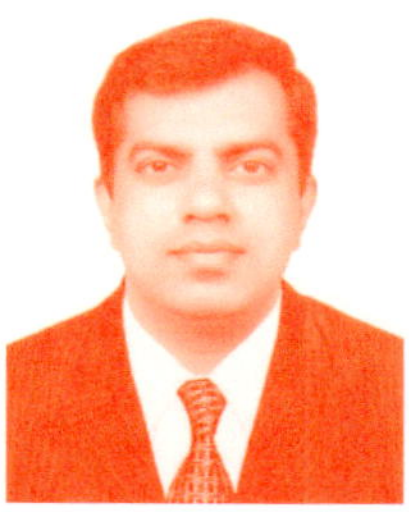

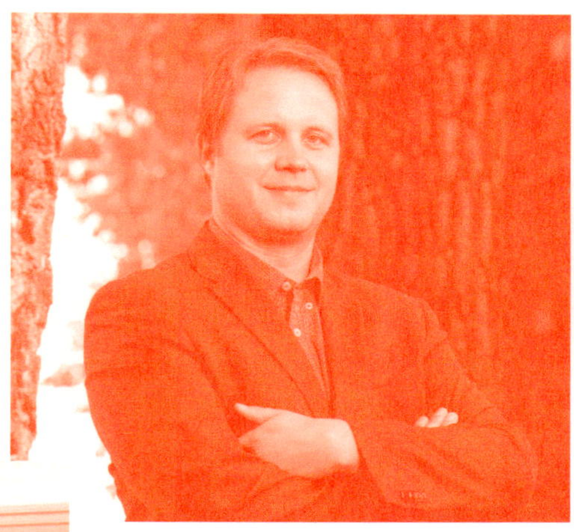

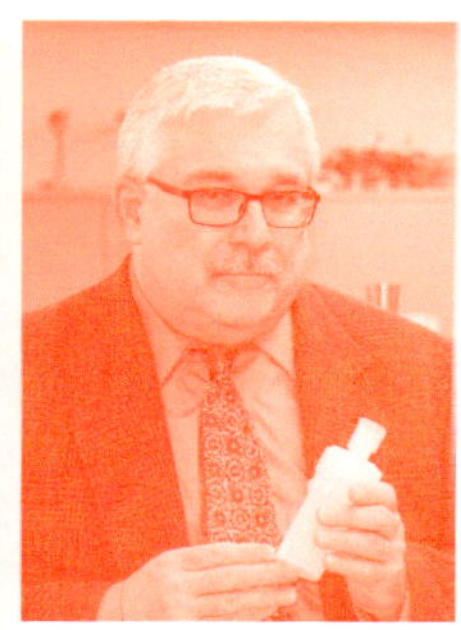

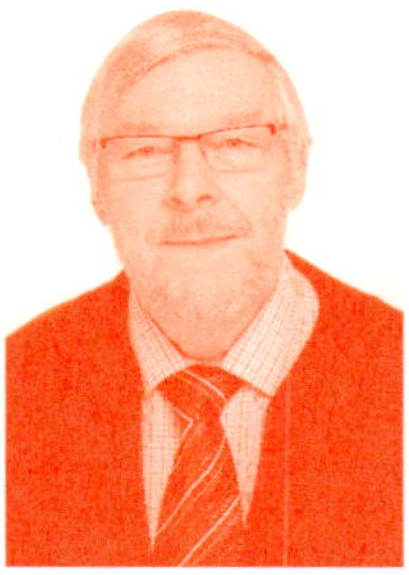

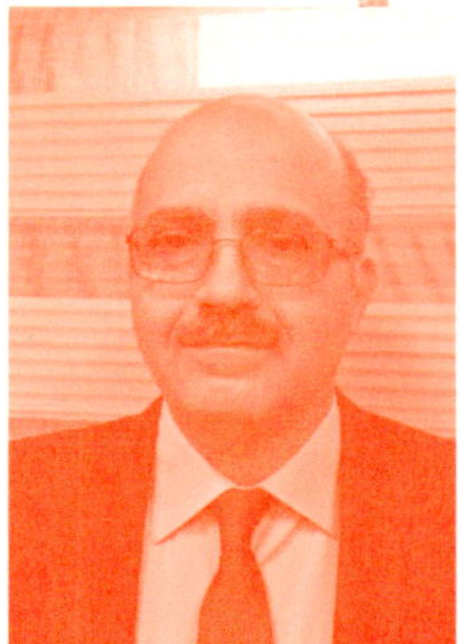

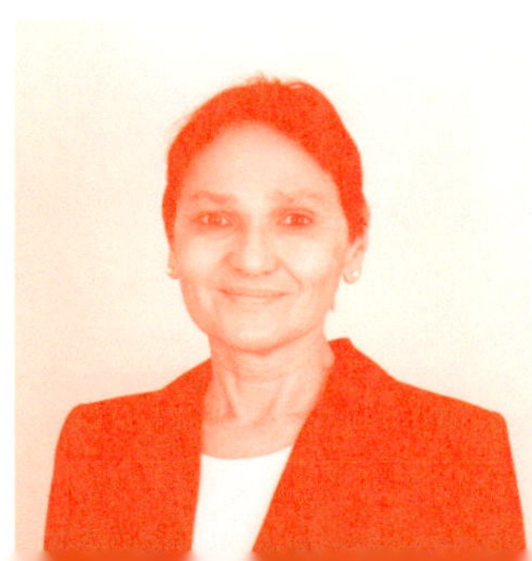

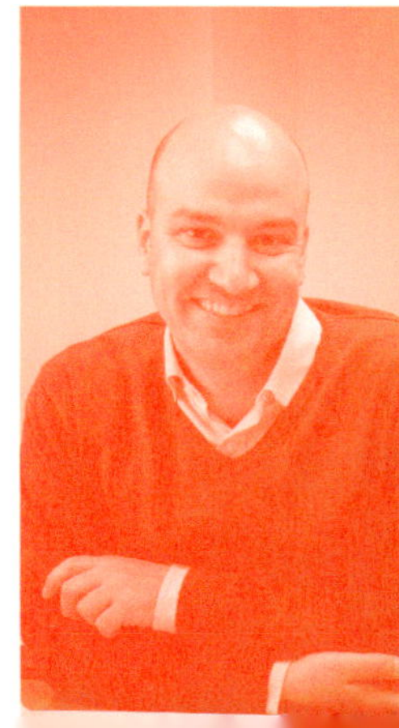

Sudden Cardiac Death
http://dx.doi.org/10.5772/intechopen.89286
Edited by Peter Magnusson and Jo Ann LeQuang

Contributors
Abdullah Abdulrhman Al Abdulgader, Peter Magnusson, Jo Ann LeQuang, Joseph V. Pergolizzi, Jaipaul Singh, Carlin Hanoman, Sunil Rupee, Khemraj Rupee, Farah Ahmed Sleiman, Manal M. A. Smail, Frank C. Howarth, Keshore Bidasee, Samar Abdulkhalek, Abla Mohammed Ismail, Marianna Leopoulou, Rakesh Garg, Pratishta Yadav, Abhishek Kumar, Leonid Makarov, Cindy Darnell Bowens, Priscilla Yu, Ivie D. Esangbedo, Lakshmi Raman, Gustav Mattsson

First published in London, United Kingdom, 2020 by IntechOpen
IntechOpen is the global imprint of INTECHOPEN LIMITED, registered in England and Wales, registration number: 11086078, 5 Princes Gate Court, London, SW7 2QJ, United Kingdom
Printed in Croatia

British Library Cataloguing-in-Publication Data
A catalogue record for this book is available from the British Library

Additional hard and PDF copies can be obtained from orders@intechopen.com

Sudden Cardiac Death
Edited by Peter Magnusson and Jo Ann LeQuang
p. cm.
Print ISBN 978-1-83880-069-7
Online ISBN 978-1-83880-070-3
eBook (PDF) ISBN 978-1-83962-854-2

For EU product safety concerns:
IN TECH d.o.o., Prolaz Marije Krucifikse Kozulić 3, 51000 Rijeka, Croatia, info@intechopen.com or visit our website at intechopen.com.

Meet the editors

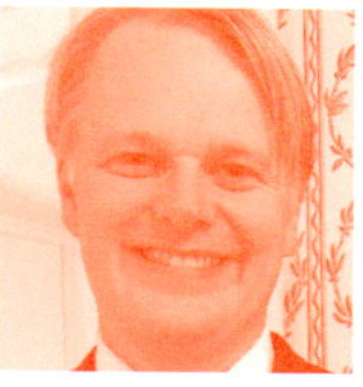

Peter Magnusson is a senior consultant in cardiology and active in diverse research projects including topics such as arrhythmia, cardiomyopathy, heart failure, valvular disease, and digital medicine. He is affiliated to Karolinska Institute, Sweden and Center for Research and Development Region Gävleborg, Uppsala University, Sweden. In November he will finish his PhD studies at Karolinska Institute with the thesis "Implantable Cardioverter Defibrillator Treatment in Patients with Hypertrophic Cardiomyopathy." Dr. Magnusson's research involves epidemiological studies, qualitative methods, observational studies, and randomized controlled trials. He is passionate about teaching and supervision, especially in academic projects. Currently, he is striving for implementation of research findings in order to improve health care.

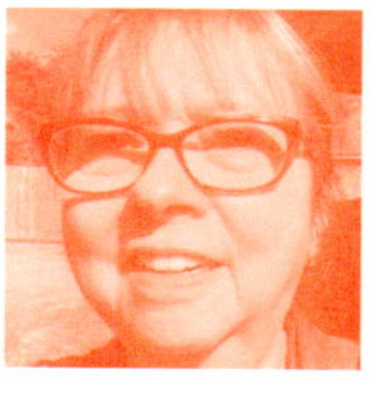

Jo Ann LeQuang is a medical writer who got her start working in the pacemaker industry when she was hired to work for Intermedics to assist in setting up a translation department for software localization for implantable devices. She worked at the Cardiac Rhythm Management Division of St. Jude Medical (now Abbott) and together with Tom Kenny worked on *The Nuts & Bolts of Cardiac Pacing* series of books. She has worked independently since 2003 and has been an author on more than forty peer-reviewed medical articles. In 2017, she won the Unsung Heroes Award for advocacy for chronic pain patients. She is Director of Scientific Communication at NEMA Research, Inc., and serves on the Board of Directors of No Baby Blisters, a nonprofit organization dedicated to finding the cure for epidermolysis bullosa, an orphan disease that affects newborns.

Contents

Preface

Sudden cardiac death is typically related to arrhythmia that results in circulatory collapse. As the name suggests, sudden cardiac death may occur without warning in a patient without symptoms. Most cases of sudden cardiac death can be attributed to ventricular tachycardia or fibrillation. The underlying mechanisms need to be elucidated, which may be challenging in the individual case. This book covers several aspects of pathophysiological pathways and etiologies.

The implantable cardioverter defibrillator is a cornerstone in the prevention of sudden cardiac death. In addition, the wearable cardioverter defibrillator may be an alternative in selected cases. As such, this book presents information on defibrillator technology and clinical applications. It also highlights risk-stratification in ion channel diseases and structural heart disease such as dilated cardiomyopathy. Overall, this book serves as a guide to the prevention of sudden cardiac death. Together, we will fight the global threat of sudden cardiac death among diverse disease conditions.

We hope you will enjoy this informative book!

Peter Magnusson
Centre for Research and Development,
Region Gävleborg / Uppsala University,
Sweden

Department of Medicine,
Cardiology Research Unit,
Karolinska Institute,
Sweden

Jo Ann LeQuang
NEMA Research, Inc.,
USA

Chapter 1

Cardiopulmonary Resuscitation: Recent Advances

Abhishek Kumar, Pratishtha Yadav and Rakesh Garg

Abstract

Cardiac arrest is the most significant reason for mortality and morbidities worldwide. With a better understanding of the pathophysiology of cardiac arrest, simple adaptations in basic life support to upcoming modifications in post-resuscitation care have been proposed by various resuscitation councils throughout the globe. Role of point of care cardiac ultrasound during cardiopulmonary resuscitation (CPR) has been explored and its contribution for identifying reversible causes and its real time management has been explored. A higher blood and tissue oxygenation levels contributed to an increased rate of return of spontaneous circulation (ROSC) which has to lead us to explore more options to increase the oxygenation. Starting from the CPR training, the use of sensors for spirometric feedback in ventilation maneuvers can help improve the quality of CPR. High flow nasal oxygenation during CPR has shown promising results. Extracorporeal CPR is another entity that has shown survival benefits in a selected group of patients. The aim of the newer advances has always been to decrease the morbidity and improve survival outcomes in terms of neurological deficit as well. These guidelines are reviewed and updated regularly to improve knowledge and training based on the current evidence. This chapter shall focus on recent advances in cardiopulmonary resuscitation.

Keywords: airway management, arrhythmias, cardiac arrest, cardiopulmonary resuscitation, epinephrine, extracorporeal circulation, post-resuscitation care, recent advances

1. Introduction

The recent era of cardiopulmonary resuscitation (CPR) began in 1960 by Kouvenhoven et al. [1], when the first time closed-chest compressions were brought into the clinical scenario. It was found that rhythmic chest compression can help in restoring spontaneous circulation of defibrillating heart after cardiac arrest. It was found that this technique was able to give the success rate of as high as 70% in anesthesia-induced arrest in operation theater [1]. This non-invasive technique replaced the conventional open-chest compression technique.

Since the introduction of closed-chest compression technique, various research has been continuously conducted to find techniques and interventions for overall improvement of cardiac arrested patients after CPR. Various communities are working on innovative techniques to improve the outcome of CPR. Resuscitation councils have a common basic goal of improving circulation and improving the outcome of the victim. The common feature was the willingness to bundle different

 IntechOpen

tried and tested ideas together, applying them for treatment for cardiac arrest. This chapter focuses on ideas and the innovative techniques, analyze their efficacy, and bring forward the latest updates to improve the CPR outcome.

2. Basic life support

2.1 Bystander CPR

During an event of cardiac arrest, sooner the temporary circulation is reestablished via chest compression, better are the chances of survival with good neurological function [2]. Clinical studies have shown an increase in survival if the victim receives early resuscitation including defibrillation. The analysis showed a four times increase in chance of survival in victims who received an early bystander CPR [3], which can be achieved if the bystander starts CPR by the time the professional rescuer team arrives at the site. Hence, it is encouraged to promote this critical aspect in our basic cardiopulmonary life support management to cardiac arrest victims through public awareness campaigns. Surveys among medical and public groups have shown the declining rates of bystander CPR. The primary reason was the apprehension of contracting the contagious disease and causing harm during the process [4, 5].

Since 1990, a simpler version of "chest compression-only" CPR is being explored for bystanders. A new concept came into the picture: cardiocerebral resuscitation. It emphasizes that circulation is more important than ventilation during the early efforts of resuscitation. One survey showed that it is more acceptable among the common public [6]. It has been reported that "chest compression-only" CPR or compression-only life support (COLS) is a viable option for providing immediate resuscitation by bystanders with an improved overall outcome as compared to no CPR [7].

2.2 CPR (dispatcher-assisted)

Emergency medical dispatcher services are crucial links in emergency health services [8, 9]. They are the first responders of an emergency call. Their role involves identifying the emergency, guiding the bystander and simultaneously dispatching an emergency medical service (EMS). Internationally, various strategies have been explored to increase the rate of bystander CPR. One of such strategies is to enhance the role of the emergency medical dispatchers and comprises services like giving CPR instructions to assist bystanders: dispatcher-assisted CPR (DA-CPR). For this system to work effectively, there is a need for optimal training of the dispatchers for providing instructions to bystanders to deliver CPR. EMS system needs to be configured to support DA-CPR. This strategy can have a positive impact on point of care instructions. It increases the feasibility of bystander CPR and improves the outcome of cardiac arrest outside the hospital.

If we combine the above-mentioned strategies of early bystander CPR and DA-CPR, the results can be promising. This will result is the early restoration of circulation and better neurological outcomes. It will be more acceptable by the bystanders to provide only chest compression as mouth to mouth breathing is either not acceptable or not performed appropriately delaying chest compression. A recent meta-analysis has demonstrated the beneficial survival outcome DA-CPR [10]. The recent international consensus strongly recommends that emergency medical dispatch service centers have a proper system to support DA-CPR services [11].

2.3 Cardiocerebral resuscitation (CCR)

The concept was cardiocerebral resuscitation was first developed by the University of Arizona Saver Heart Center Resuscitation Group [3, 12–15]. The original idea had three components which include continuous chest compression by bystanders, EMS advanced cardiac life support, and aggressive post-resuscitation care. The notion of CCR involves chest compressions only and avoiding mouth to mouth ventilation in cases of witnessed cardiac arrest. The basis of this model was a three-phase time-sensitive model of cardiac arrest for ventricular fibrillation by Weisfeldt and Becker [16]. The first phase is the electric phase that lasts less than 4 min and the appropriate intervention is defibrillation followed by ventilation. The second phase is the circulatory phase (4–15 min) when the fibrillating heart has consumed all of the energy stores. During this phase, it is preferable to start with chest compression followed by defibrillation to perfuse the myocardium and reduce metabolic acidosis which in turn increases the success of defibrillation. There is a high possibility of developing asystole or pulseless electrical activity if defibrillation is done before chest compression in such cases [17].

Considering the above discussion, the main question arises if the rescue breaths are a misnomer? Recent data has shown a decrease in survival among patients with bystander initiated rescue effort with assisted-ventilation, especially in a subset of patients who are at a greater chance of survival like witnessed cardiac arrest and shockable rhythm [18, 19]. There are many drawbacks of mouth to mouth resuscitation like the decreased willingness of bystander, inability to deliver optimal rescue breaths by lay-person along with long interruptions to chest compressions during cardiac arrest [20]. Even if interruptions are minimal, positive pressure ventilation increases the intrathoracic pressure, decreasing the venous return, eventually worsening the perfusion of vital organs [21].

There are two subsets of cardiac arrest: primary cardiac arrest with arterial blood-rich in oxygen and other being secondary to respiratory arrest with deoxygenated arterial blood [3]. Above approach may not be very useful in the later.

3. Ventricular fibrillation (VF) and pulseless ventricular tachycardia (pVT): debrillation

3.1 Early vs. late rhythm analysis

Rhythm analysis is an important component of the CPR algorithm. It helps us to determine further course of action based upon the type of rhythm: shockable or non-shockable. No specific time frame is given to check the rhythm by the currently available literature. A randomized control trial was conducted to compare the impact of brief interval 30–60 s versus long interval of 120 s of chest compression before rhythm analysis in OHCA [22]. It was concluded that the duration for rhythm analysis is to be decided by the EMS team based on local circumstances. It is usually preferable to have an early rhythm analysis in cases where bystander CPR was given before EMS arrival. The authors also emphasized on delivering high-quality chest compressions before defibrillation.

3.2 Analysis during compressions with fast reconfirmation

There is a need for rhythm analysis intermittently while performing CPR. Chest compressions can create artifacts that make it difficult to analyze the rhythm. [23]. Thus, interruptions of chest compressions (CCs) are mandatory during

CPR. Ineffective and interrupted chest compressions can lead to poor outcomes post-CPR [24, 25]. While using an AED, the duration of interruption includes time for rhythm analysis, charging, and a warning to stand clear of the patient before a shock is delivered.

The analysis during compressions with fast reconfirmation (ADC-FR) is a new technology that can significantly reduce the CC interruptions. It comprises of special accelerometers embedded in the defibrillator pads that can sense the CCs. During the CCs, high pass digital filters are applied to analyze the ECG. This filtered rhythm is then compared with the previously validated data to determine whether the rhythm is shockable or not. This rhythm is further cross-checked with the compression-free ECG picked up during the interruption of CCs. In case of shockable rhythm, the defibrillator gets charged just 4 s before 2 min CPR interval. This ensures minimal interruption during CPR.

In a retrospective study, the sensitivity and specificity were found to be >95% and 99%, respectively, for identifying shockable/non-shockable rhythm which exceeds the AHA recommendations for standard artifact-free ECG analysis. Recent studies have demonstrated higher CC fractions have a higher likelihood of ROSC and survival after OHCAs [25–32]. We can conclude that ADC-FR is a new alternative that can accurately differentiate shockable from non-shockable rhythm [33]. More clinical studies need to be conducted to provide supportive evidence for ADC-FR.

3.3 Defibrillation strategy

Defibrillation is one of the most important strategies that can improve post-cardiac arrest patients' outcome. Over the last two decades, various studies have demonstrated the relevance of early defibrillation in shockable rhythms [34]. With every minute of delay in defibrillation, there is a decrease in survival by 7–10%. Combined crucial basic life support strategy of early CPR and early defibrillation can improve the overall survival of the patient [35]. The development of an automated external defibrillator (AEDs) was an important breakthrough. Efforts are being made to encourage targeted lay-person early defibrillation. These devices can record the rhythm, analyze it, and deliver a shock. A recent study has demonstrated better neurological outcomes with the application of public access AED to patients of OHCA regardless of the first documented rhythm [36].

There is an evidence of high first shock success rate with biphasic waveform with less incidence of post-shock myocardial dysfunction for both atrial and ventricular arrhythmias, as compared to monophasic waveform [37, 38]. It is recommended to start with the biphasic shock energy of 150 or 360 J in case of the monophasic waveform. There is a strong recommendation to follow defibrillators' manufacturer's instructions for initial and subsequent shocks [23]. Single shock is always preferred over stacked shocks to minimize interruptions in chest compressions [37, 38]. Secondly, it is seen that if a biphasic waveform is unable to defibrillate, then chest compressions are the next best step. It is recommended to escalate the defibrillation energy with subsequent biphasic shocks. This escalation may be useful in preventing the risk of fibrillation [39].

3.4 Hands-on defibrillation

"All clear" is a routine warning given before the delivery of defibrillation. Due to potential side effects, it is important not to be in touch with the patient while delivering a shock. There have been some case reports in the literature of rescuer being thrown away [40, 41] to as severe as death [42]. In all these cases, the rescuers were barehanded. The main aim of defibrillation is to deliver the appropriate dose (100–360 J) of energy to defibrillate the patient without causing any harm to the rescuer [43]. The energy used is same for cardiac arrest with ventricular fibrillation and pulseless ventricular tachycardia. Lloyd et al. first demonstrated the safety of gloves while defibrillation [44]. This triggered the idea of "hands-on defibrillation" minimizing the CC interruptions during shock delivery. In previous studies, the relationship between the success rate of defibrillation and the time delay between chest compression and shock delivery has already demonstrated [45, 46]. Subsequently, studies have been conducted to determine the efficacy of different types of gloves. One study concluded nitrile glove, neoprene gloves, and fire-fighter gloves can prevent the detection of defibrillation in 99% of cadaver cases [47]. A polythene sheet as thin as 0.002 inches can reduce the current delivered [48]. With the use of these new safety measures, hands-on defibrillation can be made safer.

4. Airway, oxygenation, and ventilation

Oxygen supplementation during CPR has been an acceptable practice. But the concentration of oxygen delivery during CPR can benefit or harm the overall survival depending on the clinical situations. Similarly, various devices have been used in various clinical settings for securing the airway. Ventilation strategies during CPR have been also proposed by various guidelines but the optimal ventilation protocol remains uncertain.

4.1 Oxygen dose during CPR

The optimum tissue and blood oxygenation during CPR are unknown and no study has been done to define the oxygenation goals during CPR. The common practice of giving 100% oxygen during CPR has been challenged in some clinical situations. Most of the current guidelines suggest the use of maximal possible oxygen concentration during CPR. There are numerous limitations to these recommendations. Lack of current clinical evidence to suggest optimal tissue/blood oxygenation during CPR and unavailability of techniques measuring tissue oxygenation during CPR are important limitations in deciding optimum dosing of oxygen.

4.2 Airway management during CPR

Airway management during CPR includes basic airway management by the bag and mask ventilation with or without oropharyngeal airways and advanced airway management like supraglottic airway devices (SAD) and endotracheal intubation. The optimal management of airway during CPR is an unclear and traditional belief of superiority of advanced airway over basic airway management has been challenged by some of the recent observational studies. Most of the studies comparing various advanced airway devices like an endotracheal tube, combitube, supraglottic airway devices and bag and mask device during CPR were observational studies and were done in OHCA patients. The data were extrapolated for IHCA settings. Most of the newer guidelines in developing and low resource countries also recommend the use of any advanced airway or bag and mask to secure airway to achieve adequate ventilation. Type of airway device in use depends on the skills of rescuer [49]. Tracheal intubation mandates training of health care provider and may be unsuccessful in emergencies with high chances of unrecognized-esophageal intubation. Comparatively, insertion of supraglottic devices is easier. A stepwise approach to airway management including bag and mask, supraglottic devices, and the endotracheal tube is commonly followed during CPR. This stepwise approach has never been validated in any human studies or RCT.

One of the serious complication in airway management during CPR is unrecognized esophageal intubation. There are few methods of confirming the correct placement of endotracheal tube which have been applied and tested in various settings. Waveform capnography is the most reliable method used to ensure the correct placement of an advanced airway device. This non-invasive monitoring has high sensitivity and specificity with very low false-positive rates [50]. Waveform capnography is an indicator of pulmonary blood flow and guides the quality of CPR. The use of esophageal detection devices and airway ultrasound during CPR is limited due to the lack of RCT and have considered inferior to waveform capnography.

5. Circulation support

5.1 Inspiratory impedance threshold device (ITD)

The efficacy of CPR chiefly depends upon the negative intrathoracic pressure which drives the venous return and cardiac output. Inspiratory impedance threshold device was put forward for the first time in the mid-1990s by Lurie. With the help of a pressure-sensitive unidirectional valve between the patient and the ventilation tool, it augments the negative intrathoracic pressure created during chest recoil which in turn increases venous return and hence improves cardiac output. As per 2010 guidelines by American Heart Association guidelines for CPR, it was put underclass 2b recommendation [51]. Two randomized studies have been conducted until now. In the first study, non-blinded randomized control study active compression and decompression device was used along with the ITD, the results showed a statistically significant survival benefit of 3% with this intervention [52]. In the second blinded study, ITD was used along with CPR; however, it was discontinued due to the futility of the intervention [53]. Due to these discrepancies in the outcome, ITD, when used with CPR, may offer no advantage but it may offer some survival benefit when used with a compression-decompression device. To date, no studies have been conducted on the use of ITD during in-hospital cardiac arrest.

5.2 Mechanical CPR devices

There is a constant emphasis on the term "high quality" used along with CPR. For a resuscitation to be successful with good neurological outcome, chest compressions need to be adequate. Clinical studies have demonstrated that the CCs quality is often poor and variable [54, 55]. These limitations lead to the invention of mechanical CPR devices, that can provide automated, high-quality CCs without any risk of fatigue. Two trials, CIRC and LINC trials, have failed to demonstrate any added advantage of using this device [56, 57].

Various studies have been conducted to compare the mechanical device to the manual CC so far, none of them demonstrated any significant difference between the two methods. It is suggested to use mechanical CPR devices in situations where sustained high-quality CC are not possible like where safety is at risk, conditions where fatigue may impair the delivery of high-quality CPR (Hypothermic arrest) or in certain procedures (coronary angiography, preparation for ECPR).

5.3 Extracorporeal CPR (ECPR)

Extracorporeal membrane oxygenation is also known as extracorporeal life support. It provides mechanical support to circulation as well as an extracorporeal gas exchange when the conventional resuscitation techniques fail [58]. Since its introduction in 1972, its role has been explored in various fields including cardiac arrest [59, 60]. ECMO can be a ray of hope for the patients who fail to respond to conventional CPR and helps extend the recovery period for treatable causes of cardiac arrest. It is necessary to familiarize oneself with the hemometabolic effects and limitations of ECMO to extract maximum benefit for a selected group of patients. It is expected to be more successful in IHCA and OHCA where early and effective CPR was started on time. The major challenge is gaining vascular access which can be difficult in an emergency scenario as well as time-consuming. Time is very crucial in cardiac resuscitation, ECPR time may be divided into two parts: time taken to start ECMO and time to achieve temperature management. The ideal time suggested by previous studies is between 30 and 60 min [61–63]. Successful ECPR demands coronary angiography/PCI along with temperature management. The CHEER trial covered 26 patients (11 OHCA and 15 IHCA) with refractory cardiac arrest who were given ECPR. The results were dramatic with a successful resuscitation of 92% and survival to hospital discharge was achieved in 54% cases [64].

Although evidence is limited, ECPR is recommended in cases of refractory CPR. The major limitation of this technique is a lack of resources and training to deliver ECPR.

6. Pharmacological advances

Various drugs have been used during cardiopulmonary resuscitations in OHCA and IHCA with different efficacy in terms of patients' survival, survival to discharge, and survival to neurological outcomes. Task forces have given their recommendations based on available literature with preferences given to RCTs and systemic reviews than observational studies. The pharmacological drugs used have been different in different cardiac arrest clinical situations depending on the patient profile, presence of intravenous access, and institutional protocols.

6.1 Epinephrine

International Consensus on CPR in 2015 suggested the use of epinephrine with weak recommendations considering short term benefits like ROSCs and uncertainty in long term benefits like improvement in neurological outcomes. The standard dose considered is 1 mg epinephrine. There is a weak recommendation of using high dose epinephrine (0.2 mg/kg) compared to standard-dose epinephrine (1 mg bolus). ACLS also recommend the use of intravenous epinephrine as the first choice of the drug during cardiac resuscitation. Epinephrine increases the perfusion to brain and heart by its alpha-1 mediated vasoconstriction and increases heart rate and myocardial contractility by its beta-1 mediated properties. Early administration of epinephrine is suggested in non-shockable rhythm compared to shockable VF/pulseless VT rhythm. The appropriate timing of administration has not been suggested by international resuscitation guidelines.

6.2 Vasopressin

Use of vasopressin in place of standard-dose epinephrine has not been suggested by any task forces or resuscitation guidelines due to lack of any evidence suggesting no improvement in short term benefits like ROSC and admission to discharge criteria or any long term benefits in quality of life/neurological outcomes. The combination of epinephrine and vasopressin has also been non-superior to epinephrine alone in improving clinical outcomes in patients [65–67].

6.3 Antiarrhythmic drugs

Antiarrhythmic drugs are used in refractory ventricular dysrhythmias during cardiac arrest. Refractory ventricular arrhythmias are defined as the "persistent or recurrent VT/pulseless VT after 1 shock."

6.3.1 Amiodarone

Amiodarone is a mainly a class III antiarrhythmic drug but also shows class I, II, and IV antiarrhythmic properties which showed benefits in ROSC. Although, no long term benefits were observed in survival to discharge benefits by the drug administration compared to placebo [68]. Amiodarone should only be used in the case when cardioversion/defibrillation and epinephrine administration have failed to revert the fatal arrhythmias to sinus rhythm. The dosing regimen during CPR is 300 mg intravenous/intraosseous bolus followed by the second dose of 150 mg failing the initial bolus dose to convert the rhythm. After successful cardioversion, amiodarone infusion should be continued for 6 h at the rate of 1 mg/min followed by 0.5 mg/min for the next 18 h.

6.3.2 Lidocaine

Lidocaine is a local anesthetic which has been used as a substitute of amiodarone during a cardiac arrest for refractory VF/pulseless VT in cases of unavailability of the later. The initial dose is 1–1.5 mg/kg by the intravenous or intraosseous route. The evidence for the use of lidocaine during cardiac arrest is lacking and no survival benefits have been shown with its use [69].

6.3.3 Magnesium sulfate

Magnesium sulfates have been used in torsade's de points caused by low serum magnesium levels. There is no survival benefit with the routine use of magnesium sulfate during cardiac arrest and routine use of magnesium sulfate during cardiac arrest is discouraged [70].

7. Recent advances in post-resuscitation care

There has been considerate literature available in post-resuscitation care from 2010 in various domains of resuscitation. All the post-resuscitation care interventions are aimed to increase the survival to discharge ratio and decrease the neurological morbidities and mortalities.

7.1 Oxygen supplementation after ROSC

Hypoxia during a cardiac arrest has been the cause of neurological injury and post-cardiac arrest morbidity. The optimum level of blood oxygenation for improving the neurological outcome has been studied but no RCTs and systemic reviews are available to support or refute normoxia or hyperoxia. Hypoxia has been well known to cause irreversible brain damage and hyperoxia has been implicated in neurological injury due to increased free radicals. With the availability of current literature, emphasis should be given to prevent further hypoxia after cardiac arrest [71].

7.2 Post-resuscitation ventilation

Cardiac arrest has been associated with brain injury as well as injury to other organs including lungs. The optimal PCO2 to prevent further injury to the brain is critically important and need to optimize our ventilator strategy. Normocarbia is preferred in post-cardiac arrest to maintain the physiological homeostasis and acid-base balance. Ventilatory strategies should be individualized to patients. Hypercapnia and hypocapnia should be avoided.

7.3 Hemodynamic support

Hemodynamic support is necessary to maintain organ perfusions. Vital organs like brain, kidneys, and heart are most vulnerable to get affected by low perfusion states. A state of post-cardiac arrest shock is mostly due to cardiogenic shock and needs inotropic support. Vasopressors are also supplemented to achieve hemodynamic goals like maintaining the mean arterial pressure (MAP). The cutoff value for mean arterial pressure has not been suggested by any large RCTs or systemic reviews but most of the observational studies and data from other critical patients suggest maintaining a MAP > 65 mm Hg. Other goals like urine output have also been targeted. Hemodynamic goals should be individualized based on comorbidities and complexities of individual physiology [72, 73].

7.4 Temperature management

Targeted temperature management (TTM) has been the keystone of post-cardiac arrest care to prevent neurological injury and improving the outcome of the patients. The current evidence suggests maintenance of optimum core body temperature of 32–36°C for 24 h after cardiac arrest in initial shockable rhythm in which patients remained unresponsive after ROSC. TTM has also been suggested in OHCA for non-shockable rhythm. There is no role of inducing hypothermia by cold intravenous infusion in OHCA cardiac arrest [74].

7.5 Post-cardiac arrest seizures prophylaxis and treatment

Post-cardiac arrest seizures and status epilepticus have been linked with poor neurological outcomes. Post-cardiac arrest seizures can be due to brain damage during cardiac arrest. Seizures can further exacerbate the neurological injury. There is no sufficient literature to comment on the routine use of seizures prophylaxis after cardiac arrest. Based on the available current literature, the task force suggests against the routine use of seizures prophylaxis in IHCA and OHCA situations. There is a strong recommendation to treat post-cardiac arrest seizures. Various antiepileptic drugs have been used solely or in combinations in different dosing regimens to treat seizures to prevent further neurological injury and improve survival [75].

8. Physiological monitoring during CPR

Current CPR guidelines suggest a common approach to all the patients irrespective of the varied underlying physiological differences among patients and clinical situations. This mandates the development of newer strategies to target physiological parameters to guide resuscitation. Recent literature has reviewed the applications of various basic and advance physiological monitoring to improve precision during CPR and improve survival of the patients. Various strategies of monitoring include ETCO2 monitoring, coronary perfusion pressure monitoring, cardiac ultrasound and regional cerebral oxygen monitoring.

8.1 End-tidal carbon dioxide monitoring

ETCO2 is an indirect measure of the cardiac output and pulmonary blood flow. The right side of the heart receives CO_2 containing venous blood which is pumped to lungs for exhalation. Over 35 clinical studies have been conducted to explore the association and prognostication of end-tidal carbon dioxide with ROSC and survival of the patients [76, 77]. Low values of ETCO2 reflect low cardiac output state during chest compressions. Clinical significance of end-tidal carbon dioxide during CPR is varied with wide applications. It is well known that a low ETCO2 values (<10 mm Hg) have been associated with very high mortality [78]. It has been observed that a higher ETCO2 value during CPR has been associated with higher chances of ROSC. The American Heart Association also recommends ETCO2 level of greater than 20 mm Hg as an indicator of good chest compressions. There are some limitations of ETCO2 monitoring during CPR. There can be a significantly higher level of ETCO2 in asphyxia related cardiac arrest during the initial few minutes of CPR [79]. Similarly, epinephrine administration can reduce ETCO2 levels due to pulmonary vasoconstriction. Despite these limitations, ETCO2 remains one of the most important physiological parameters guiding resuscitation due to its availability, simplicity, and non-invasive technique.

8.2 Cerebral oximetry

Neurological injuries are common during cardiac arrest. Maintaining cerebral perfusion during CPR is crucial for survival and good neurological outcome. Cerebral oximetry is a newer technique to measure regional cerebral oxygenation using near-infrared spectroscopy (NIRS) devices. The device emits continuous near-infrared light from a source probe and received by a detector probe on the forehead. The light penetrates the cranial cavity (few centimeters) depending on the water and lipid content [80]. Change in light intensities due to differential absorption by oxygenated and deoxygenated blood in the cranial cavity detects rSO2. There is no RCT comparing the use of commercially available NIRS devices during CPR. A multicenter observational prospective study with cerebral oximetry during cardiac arrest in an adult cohort population showed a lower percentage of IHCA patients with ROSC who had lower values of rSO2 [81]. There are certain limitations to this technological advancement of the non-invasive method of measuring regional cerebral oxygenation. There are no defined values of rSO2 derived from RCTs and meta-analysis during CPR. There is a logistics issue in placing of NIRS monitors during CPR with commercially available monitors. Prospective studies are required to validate these devices and define values of rSO2 for target approach during CPR.

8.3 Focused cardiac ultrasound

Use of point of care cardiac ultrasound during a cardiac arrest has been implemented to find the cause of cardiac arrest (5Hs and 5Ts) rather than guiding the resuscitations. However, some imaging studies have revealed the intrathoracic structures beneath the described rescuer's hand position (lower half of sternum) during chest compression may be aorta or left ventricle outflow tract (LVOT) which would obstruct the blood outflow [82, 83]. A prospective study by Hwang et al. using transesophageal cardiac ultrasound identified compressions of aorta and LVOT in all the cases of chest compressions during CPR with variable degrees. The authors suggested that LV stroke volume increased by improving the precisions of compressions proximal to left ventricle guided by cardiac ultrasound [84]. However, no RCT has been done to explore the use of cardiac ultrasound during CPR. Moreover, there may be a risk of the potential harm of distracting the rescuers from high-quality CPR while focusing on cardiac ultrasound [85]. Simulation-based programs can be used to mitigate this problem.

9. Cardiac arrest in special circumstances

9.1 Traumatic cardiac arrest

The traumatic arrest is one of the etiologies of cardiac arrest with a very poor outcome [86–92]. To improve its outcome, there is a need to draw our attention to the possible reversible causes of traumatic cardiac arrest [93].

Recent data has clarified that traumatic cardiac arrest patients have no worse outcome than that of the medical causes of cardiac arrest [94]. Some of the reversible causes of cardiac arrest in traumatic patients are hypovolemia, tension pneumothorax, and cardiac tamponade.

9.1.1 Hypovolemia and rapid fluid resuscitation

In-depth analysis of traumatic cardiac arrest patients has demonstrated that the majority of the survivable traumatic cardiac arrest patients have pulseless electrical activity (PEA) [95]. This implies that the heart is beating, but the peripheral pulse is not palpable. It is often seen that this is a low output state rather than a true cardiac arrest. This is supported by the fact that such patients often have multiple wounds and suffer significant blood loss. Chest compressions are more effective in euvolemic patients as compared to suspected hypovolemic patients of traumatic cardiac arrest, rather they can worsen coronary perfusion [96]. Considering the etiology, the treatment algorithm must also be modified in these cases. Treatment must involve external compression to stop further loss, gaining access to wide-bore cannula, and initiate rapid transfusion of blood and blood products along with the attempts of CPR. In contrast to the traditional teaching, blood and blood products are preferred over the crystalloid transfusion [97, 98]. Although supportive evidence has demonstrated improved survival in patients receiving more fluid resuscitation (crystalloids) [99].

9.1.2 Tension pneumothorax

Tension pneumothorax may be suspected when there is decreased air entry even after checking the position of the endotracheal tube. It is one of the reversible causes of cardiac arrest, it is stated that chest compression should not delay the treatment of the reversible cause. It can either be achieved by immediate needle decompression or thoracotomy. In the case of positive pressure ventilation, thoracostomy is a preferred technique as it is more effective than needle decompression and less time-consuming that chest tube insertion [86]. Whereas, in the case of needle decompression, there can be technical difficulties like kinking, dislodgment, insufficient length of needle leading to insufficient decompression [100]. Decompression demonstrated the return of ROSC in these patients [101]. On the scene, decompression is recommended for all patients of traumatic cardiac arrest with tension pneumothorax [102].

9.1.3 Cardiac tamponade

Low energy penetrating wounds can cause myocardial injury leading to an accumulation of blood in pericardial space. Cardiac tamponade can be a cause of arrest in 10% of cardiac arrests in trauma. Cardiac tamponade needs to be evacuated immediately to achieve successful resuscitation post-CPR. Retrospective data collected from a military hospital has demonstrated survival as high as 21.5% in post-traumatic cardiac arrest patients post thoracotomy [95].

Ultrasound can help in timely diagnosis PEA, cardiac tamponade, tension pneumothorax, and even hypovolemia by IVC diameter [103].

9.2 Cardiac arrest after cardiac surgery

Cardiac arrests after cardiac surgeries are unique entities that need to be addressed uniquely. It usually takes place within the hospital facility which thereby increases the chances of early diagnosis. Timely resuscitation is possible in the presence of expertise with easy access to defibrillator or pacing facility, early CPR, and rapid sternotomy. About 8% of the cardiac surgery patients suffer from perioperative cardiac arrest, with a shockable rhythm in 30–50% and mechanical causes like cardiac tamponade or graft failure in 28% of the cases [104]. The incidence of different arrhythmias varies in different studies. A recent study reported the incidence of VF and pVT in 70%, asystole in 17%, and PEA in 13% of cardiac arrests [105].

During the cardiac arrest, various monitoring waveforms like arterial pressure, central venous pressure, and pulmonary artery pressure are non-pulsatile. If the ECG tracing reveals VF/ p VT, three stalked shocks must be delivered if available within 1 min. Brief CPR in patients shortly after cardiac surgery can induce lacerations and hemorrhage due to serrated sternal edges and projecting steel wires and hence not preferred [106, 107]. Numerous studies have demonstrated improved outcomes with early defibrillation for witnessed arrest [108, 109]. In the scenario of OHCA, single shock protocol is preferred but the same may not be applicable for witnessed IHCA and procedural settings. Subsequent shocks given within 1 min showed statistically significant survival benefits over the deferred second shock in VF/pVT [110]. Thus, considering the risks and benefits it is recommended to give three sequential shocks without intervening external cardiac massage in patients of VF/pVT if available within 1 min. A bolus of 300 mg intravenous amiodarone should be given via central line after failed defibrillation and CPR should be initiated [111]. Studies have demonstrated the advantage of internal cardiac massage as compared to external in establishing adequate cerebral and coronary perfusion (CPP) [112, 113]. Maximal CPP is a direct indicator of ROSC [114]. It is recommended to perform cardiac massage at the rate of 100–120 per minute with a target systolic pressure of at least 60 mm of Hg.

If the CPR is performed correctly, and still the target pressure is not achieved, it suggests a surgical problem like cardiac tamponade. PEA is commonly seen in cardiac tamponade or hemorrhage. Rapid sternotomy is the treatment of choice and once compression is released; internal massaging can be continued allowing initial stabilization while the patient is shifted back to the operating room. Direct visualization allows the diagnosis of the mechanical cause of the arrest and early intervention. Pottle and colleagues have demonstrated survival benefit when the sternotomy was done within 5 min of arrest supporting internal cardiac massage over external [115].

In asystole, epicardial pacing (DOO mode, maximal atrial, and ventricular output, 80–100/min) should be initiated within 1 min if available before CPR and resternotomy otherwise transcutaneous pacing may be used. Transcutaneous pacing involves delivery of electrical impulses through the patient chest by applying pads on thoracic wall stimulating the heart. It is mainly indicated during hemodynamic instability due to refractory bradycardia, sick sinus syndrome, and asystolic cardiac arrest. Transcutaneous pacing during cardiac arrest is more successful in witnessed cardiac arrest.

In cases of PEA, the pacemaker should be temporarily turned off to check the rhythm as it can mask the VF. Atropine is not recommended as a part of the resuscitation protocol for cardiac surgery patients [111].

Epinephrine is not routinely recommended as a part of the resuscitation protocol in post-cardiac surgery patients. Studies have demonstrated it can cause more harm than help. Although successful in restoring the circulation, it can raise the blood pressure to such high levels that can damage the anastomosis sutures leading to hemorrhage. Many research trials have shown the success of epinephrine in starting the initial rhythm but poor overall survival rates and increase brain damage [116]. If required, it can be used in impending arrest at a lower dose (50–300 mcg) only if ordered by an experienced clinician.

Usually, the post-cardiac surgical patients are intubated, there is a risk of endobronchial intubation, pneumothorax, and hemothorax. Management of airway and ventilation involves increasing the FiO_2 to 100% and excluding the positive end expiration pressure, checking the position of the endotracheal tube and excluding tension pneumothorax or hemothorax [39]. In case of tension pneumothorax or hemothorax, a wide-bore needle should be inserted in second intercostal's space, the midclavicular line to decompress immediately.

Cardiac arrests in post-cardiac surgery patients is a unique entity that mandates necessary changes in conventional resuscitation protocols to improve their outcome [104, 117].

9.3 Cardiac arrest in pregnancy

Cardiac arrest in pregnant patients is dealt with as a separate entity. Recent data has shown most etiology due to reversible cause with a high survival rate of >50% [118]. This challenges the historical concept of poor survival and futility of resuscitation [119]. This special group of young people responds well to resuscitation efforts, encouraging us to streamline resuscitation guidelines [118].

First and foremost is the need to identify common causes of arrest in pregnant patients, which must be reversed while resuscitating the patients to improve the chances of ROSC. Anesthetic complications like inadvertent spinal injection and airway complications are the most common cause followed by hemorrhage (intrapartum or postpartum) [120]. Other causes can be attributed to cardiovascular causes like peripartum cardiomyopathy, heart failure owing to pre-existing valve disease, drugs errors, anaphylaxis, and thromboembolic complications.

Resuscitation in pregnant patients requires sequential coordinated simultaneous interventions. A multidisciplinary team of health care providers including an obstetrician, neonatologist, anesthesiologist, intensivist, a cardiologist, and cardiovascular surgeon should be involved during resuscitation. High-quality chest compressions of 5–6 cm depth at the rate of 100–120 per minute at the mid sternal position with adequate recoil will provide a good circulatory function. The gravid uterus can lead to aortocaval compression, impairing venous return. Tilting the patient to a lateral position relieves the compression but does not allow chest compression. A study on mannequin demonstrated that a tilt of 27° was enough during chest compression to stop mannequin from falling but with the limitation of achieving 80% of force for CCs as compared to supine position [121]. A virtual gastroscopy demonstrated lateral displacement of the heart on lateral tilt offsetting the pumping action of chest compression [122]. A study utilized MRI to demonstrate compression of inferior vena cava and partial release on the lateral tilt of 30° in pregnant patients as compared to non-pregnant patients [123]. Considering this, manual displacement of the uterus can relieve the compression without affecting the vector force during chest compression, although delivery of the fetus is the ultimate and most comprehensive way of relieving the aortocaval compression. CPR is performed at a ratio of 30 compressions and 2 breaths. Oxygenation is the ultimate goal, the airway must be secured as soon as possible. It prevents aspiration and provides treatment for the respiratory cause of arrest. Considering the physiological changes of pregnancy and experienced laryngoscopist must perform intubation with an endotracheal tube of a smaller diameter. Recent studies have shown no advantage of the advanced airway during CPR in-hospital resuscitation, but this may not hold in pregnant patients keeping in view the physiological changes of pregnancy [124].

Rhythm analysis, defibrillation, and drugs used are similar to non-pregnant patients. Intravenous cannulation must be established above the diaphragm, to prevent the cut off of drugs due to gravid uterus causing aortocaval compression.

It is reasonable to perform perimortem caesarian delivery within 5 min of resuscitation maternal cardiac arrest. It maximizes the neonatal outcome as well as improves the maternal outcome [118].

10. Conclusion

Managing cardiac arrest can be very challenging considering its complexity and time sensitivity. However, over the last couple of years, lot of research has been done in this field and implementation of these research-proven interventions has led to improvement of the overall outcome. For example, we know that early identification of cardiac arrest, early implementation of bystander CPR, compression-only CPR, early activation of the EMS system, early defibrillation by AED, and aggressive post-arrest care that includes therapeutic hypothermia, early cardiac catheterization, seizure control, and goal-directed care improve outcomes.

Nomenclature

ADC-FR	analysis during compressions with fast reconfirmation
AED	automated electronic defibrillator
CA	cardiac arrest
CC	chest compression
CCP	cerebral and coronary perfusion
CCR	cardiocerebral resuscitation
CPR	cardiopulmonary resuscitation
DA-CPR	dispatcher assist CPR
ECMO	extracorporeal membrane oxygenation
ECPR	extracorporeal CPR
EMS	emergency medical service
IHCA	in-hospital cardiac arrest

ITD	inspiratory impedance threshold device
LVOT	left ventricle outflow tract
NIRS	near-infrared spectroscopy
OHCA	out of hospital cardiac arrest
PEA	pulseless electrical activity
pVT	pulseless ventricular tachycardia
ROSC	Return of spontaneous circulation
SAD	supraglottic airway devices
TTM	targeted temperature management
VF	ventricular fibrillation

Author details

Abhishek Kumar, Pratishtha Yadav and Rakesh Garg*
Department of Onco-Anaesthesia and Palliative Medicine, BRAIRCH, All India Institute of Medical Sciences (AIIMS), New Delhi, India

*Address all correspondence to: drrgarg@hotmail.com

References

[1] Kouwenhoven WB, Jude JR, Knickerbocker GG. Closed-chest cardiac massage. JAMA. 1960;**173**:1064-1067

[2] Halperin HR, Tsitlik JE, Guerci AD, Mellits ED, Levin HR, Shi A-Y, et al. Determinants of blood flow to vital organs during cardiopulmonary resuscitation in dogs. Circulation. 1986;**73**:539-550

[3] Ewy G. Cardiocerebral resuscitation: The new cardiopulmonary resuscitation. Circulation. 2005;**111**:2134-2142

[4] Ornato JP, Hallagan LF, McMahan SB, Peeples EH, Rostafinski AG. Attitudes of BLS instructors about mouth-to-mouth resuscitation during the AIDS epidemic. Annals of Emergency Medicine. 1990;**19**:151-156

[5] Brenner BE, Kauffman J. Reluctance of internists and medical nurses to perform mouth-to-mouth resuscitation. Archives of Internal Medicine. 1993;**153**:1763-1769

[6] Locke CJ, Berg RA, Sanders AB, Davis MF, Milander MH, Kern KB, et al. Bystander cardiopulmonary resuscitation: Concerns about mouth-to-mouth contact. Archives of Internal Medicine. 1995;**155**:938-943

[7] Ahmed SM, Garg R, Divatia JV, Rao SC, Mishra BB, Kalandoor MV, et al. Compression-only life support (COLS) for cardiopulmonary resuscitation by layperson outside the hospital. Indian Journal of Anaesthesia. 2017;**61**:867-873

[8] Perkins GD, Travers AH, Berg RA, et al. Part 3: Adult basic life support and automated external defibrillation: 2015 International Consensus on Cardiopulmonary Resuscitation and Emergency Cardiovascular Care Science with Treatment Recommendations. Resuscitation. 2015;**95**:e43-e69. DOI: 10.1016/j.resuscitation.2015.07.041

[9] Travers AH, Perkins GD, Berg RA, et al. Part 3: Adult basic life support and automated external defibrillation: 2015 International Consensus on Cardiopulmonary Resuscitation and Emergency Cardiovascular Care Science With Treatment Recommendations. Circulation. 2015;**132**:S51-S83. DOI: 10.1161/CIR.0000000000000272

[10] Hupfl M, Selig HF, Nagele P. Chest compression-only versus standard cardiopulmonary resuscitation: A meta-analysis. Lancet. 2010;**376**:1552-1557

[11] Soar J et al. 2019 International Consensus on Cardiopulmonary Resuscitation and Emergency Cardiovascular Care Science With Treatment Recommendations. Resuscitation. 2019;**145**:95-150

[12] Kern KB, Valenzuela TD, Clark LL, et al. An alternative approach to advancing resuscitation science. Resuscitation. 2005;**64**:261-268

[13] Kellum MJ, Kennedy KW, Ewy GA. Cardiocerebral resuscitation improves survival of patients with out-of-hospital cardiac arrest. The American Journal of Medicine. 2006;**119**:335-340

[14] Bobrow BJ, Clark LL, Ewy GA, et al. Minimally interrupted cardiac resuscitation by emergency medical services providers for out-of hospital cardiac arrest. JAMA. 2008;**229**:1158-1165

[15] Kellum MJ, Kennedy KW, Barney R, et al. Cardiocerebral resuscitation improves neurologically intact survival of patients with out-of hospital cardiac arrest. Annals of Emergency Medicine. 2008;**52**:244-252

[16] Weisfeldt M, Becker L. Resuscitation after cardiac arrest: A 3-phase time-sensitive model. JAMA. 2002;**288**:3035-3038

[17] Cobb L, Fahrenbruch C, Walsh T, Compass M, Olsufka M. Influence of cardiopulmonary resuscitation prior to defibrillation in patients with out-of-hospital ventricular fibrillation. JAMA. 1999;**281**:1182-1188

[18] SOS-KANTO Study Group. Cardiopulmonary resuscitation by bystanders with chest compression only (SOS-KANTO): An observational study. Lancet. 2007;**369**:920-926

[19] Ewy GA. Cardiac arrest—Guideline changes urgently needed. Lancet. 2007;**369**:882-884

[20] Assar D, Chamberlain D, Colquhoun M, et al. Randomized controlled trials of staged teaching for basic life support. 1. Skill acquisition at bronze stage. Resuscitation. 2000;**45**:7-15

[21] Aufderheide TP, Sigurdsson G, Pirrallo RG, et al. Hyperventilation induced hypotension during cardiopulmonary resuscitation. Circulation. 2004;**109**:1960-1965

[22] Stiell IG, Nichol G, Leroux BG, Rea TD, Ornato JP, Powell J, et al. Early versus late rhythm analysis in patients with out-of-hospital cardiac arrest. The New England Journal of Medicine. 2011;**365**:787-797

[23] Perkins GD, Handley AJ, Koster RW, Castrén M, Smyth MA, Olasveengen T, et al. European Resuscitation Council Guidelines for Resuscitation 2015: Section 2. Adult basic life support and automated external defibrillation. Resuscitation. 2015;**95**:81-99

[24] Berdowski J, Berg RA, Tijssen JGP, Koster RW. Global incidences of out-of hospital cardiac arrest and survival rates: Systematic review of 67 prospective studies. Resuscitation. 2010;**81**:1479-1487

[25] Brouwer TF, Walker RG, Chapman FW, Koster RW. Association between chest compression interruptions and clinical outcomes of ventricular fibrillation out-of hospital cardiac arrest. Circulation. 2015;**132**:1030-1037

[26] Soar J, Nolan JP, Beottiger BW, Perkins GD, Lott C, Carli P, et al. European Resuscitation Council Guidelines for Resuscitation 2015: Section 3. Adult advanced life support. Resuscitation. 2015;**95**:100-147

[27] Yu T, Weil MH, Tang W, Sun S, Klouche K, Povoas H, et al. Adverse outcomes of interrupted precordial compression during automated defibrillation. Circulation. 2002;**106**:368-372

[28] Cheskes S, Schmicker RH, Christenson J, et al. Perishock pause: An independent predictor of survival from out-of-hospital shockable cardiac arrest. Circulation. 2011;**124**:58-66

[29] Cheskes S, Schmicker RH, Verbeek PR, et al. The impact of peri-shock pause on survival from out-of-hospital shockable cardiac arrest during the Resuscitation Outcomes Consortium PRIMED Trial. Resuscitation. 2014;**85**:336-342

[30] Vaillancourt C, Everson-Stewart S, Christenson J, Andrusiek D, Powell J, Nichol G, et al. The impact of increased chest compression fraction on return of spontaneous circulation for out-of hospital cardiac arrest patients not in ventricular fibrillation. Resuscitation. 2011;**82**:1501-1507

[31] Sell RE, Sarno R, Lawrence B, Castillo EM, Fisher R, Brainard C, et al. Minimizing pre- and post-defibrillation pauses increases the likelihood of return of spontaneous circulation (ROSC). Resuscitation. 2010;**81**:822-825

[32] Christenson J, Andrusiek D, Everson-Stewart S, et al. Chest compression fraction determines

survival in patients with out-of-hospital ventricular fibrillation. Circulation. 2009;**120**:1241-1247

[33] Fumagalli F, Silver AE, Tan Q, Zaidi N, Ristagno G. Cardiac rhythm analysis during ongoing cardiopulmonary resuscitation using the analysis during compressions with fast reconfirmation technology. Heart Rhythm. 2018;**15**(2):248-255

[34] Larsen MP, Eisenberg MS, Cummins RO, Hallstrom AP. Predicting survival from out-of-hospital cardiac arrest: A graphic model. Annals of Emergency Medicine. 1993;**22**:1652-1658

[35] Valenzuela TD, Roe DJ, Cretin S, Spaite DW, Larsen MP. Estimating effectiveness of cardiac arrest interventions—A logistic regression survival model. Circulation. 1997;**96**:3308-3313

[36] Kishimori T et al. Public-access automated external defibrillator pad application and favorable neurological outcome after out-of-hospital cardiac arrest in public locations: A prospective population-based propensity score-matched study. International Journal of Cardiology. 2020;**299**:140-146

[37] Jacobs I, Sunde K, Deakin CD, Hazinski MF, Kerber RE, Koster RW, et al. Part 6: Defibrillation: 2010 International Consensus on Cardiopulmonary Resuscitation and Emergency Cardiovascular Care Science With Treatment Recommendations. Circulation. 2010;**122**(Suppl 2): S325-S337. DOI: 10.1161/CIRCULATIONAHA.110.971010

[38] Sunde K, Jacobs I, Deakin CD, Hazinski MF, Kerber RE, Koster RW, et al. Part 6: Defibrillation: 2010 International Consensus on Cardiopulmonary Resuscitation and Emergency Cardiovascular Care Science with Treatment Recommendations. Resuscitation. 2010;**81**(Suppl 1):e71-e85. DOI: 10.1016/j.resuscitation.2010.08.025

[39] Ley SJ. Cardiac surgical resuscitation: State of the Science. Critical Care Nursing Clinics of North America. 2019;**31**(3):437-452. DOI: 10.1016/j.cnc.2019.05.010

[40] Siniorakis E et al. Accidental shock to rescuer from an implantable cardioverter defibrillator. Resuscitation. 2009;**80**:293-294

[41] Stockwell B et al. Electrical injury during hands on defibrillation—A potential risk of internal cardioverter defibrillators? Resuscitation. 2009;**80**:832-834

[42] Montauk L. Lethal defibrillator mishap. Annals of Emergency Medicine. 1997;**29**:825

[43] Petley GW, Cotton AM, Deakin CD. Hands-on defibrillation: Theoretical and practical aspects of patient and rescuer safety. Resuscitation. 2012;**83**:551-556

[44] Lloyd MS et al. Hands-on defibrillation: An analysis of electrical current flow through rescuers in direct contact with patients during biphasic external defibrillation. Circulation. 2008;**117**:2510-2514

[45] Sato Y, Weil MH, Sun S, et al. Adverse effects of interrupting precordial compression during cardiopulmonary resuscitation. Critical Care Medicine. 1997;**25**:733-736

[46] Steen S, Liao Q, Pierre L, Paskevicius A, Sjoberg T. The critical importance of minimal delay between chest compressions and subsequent defibrillation: A haemodynamic explanation. Resuscitation. 2003;**58**:249-258

[47] Wampler D, Kharod C, Bolleter S, Burkett A, Gabehart C,

Manifold C. A randomized control hands-on defibrillation study-Barrier use evaluation. Resuscitation. 2016;**103**:37-40

[48] Wight JA et al. Hands-on defibrillation with a safety barrier: An analysis of potential risk to rescuers. Resuscitation. 2019;**138**:110. DOI: 10.1016/j.resuscitation.2019.02.043

[49] Garg R, Ahmed SM, Kapoor MC, Rao SC, Mishra BB, Kalandoor MV, et al. Comprehensive cardiopulmonary life support (CCLS) for cardiopulmonary resuscitation by trained paramedics and medics inside the hospital. Indian Journal of Anaesthesia. 2017;**61**:883-894

[50] Takeda T, Tanigawa K, Tanaka H, Hayashi Y, Goto E, Tanaka K. The assessment of three methods to verify tracheal tube placement in the emergency setting. Resuscitation. 2003;**56**:153-157

[51] Cave DM, Gazmuri RJ, Otto CW, Nadkarni VM, Cheng A, Brooks SC, et al. Part 7: CPR techniques and devices: 2010 American Heart Association guidelines for cardiopulmonary resuscitation and emergency cardiovascular care. Circulation. 2010;**122**:S720-S728

[52] Aufderheide TP, Frascone RJ, Wayne MA, Mahoney BD, Swor RA, Domeier RM, et al. Standard cardiopulmonary resuscitation versus active compression-decompression cardiopulmonary resuscitation with augmentation of negative intrathoracic pressure for out-of-hospital cardiac arrest: A randomised trial. Lancet. 2011;**377**:301-311

[53] Aufderheide TP, Nichol G, Rea TD, Brown SP, Leroux BG, Pepe PE, et al. A trial of an impedance threshold device in out-of-hospital cardiac arrest. The New England Journal of Medicine. 2011;**365**:798-806

[54] Wik L, Kramer-Johansen J, Myklebust H, Sorebo H, Svensson L, Fellows B, et al. Quality of cardiopulmonary resuscitation during out-of-hospital cardiac arrest. Journal of the American Medical Association. 2005;**293**(3):299-304

[55] Valenzuela TD, Kern KB, Clark LL, Berg RA, Berg M, Berg D, et al. Interruptions of chest compressions during emergency medical systems resuscitation. Circulation. 2005;**112**:1259-1265

[56] Wik L, Olsen J, Persse D, Sterz F, Lozano M, Brouwer MA, et al. Manual vs. integrated automatic load-distributing band CPR with equal survival after out of hospital cardiac arrest. The randomized CIRC trial. Resuscitation. 2014;**85**:741-748

[57] Rubertsson S, Lindgren E, Smekal D, Ostlund O, Silfverstolpe J, Lichtveld RA, et al. Mechanical chest compressions and simultaneous defibrillation vs conventional cardiopulmonary resuscitation in out-of-hospital cardiac arrest. The LINC Randomized Trial. JAMA. 2014;**311**(1):53-61

[58] Conrad SA, Broman LM, Taccone FS, et al. The extracorporeal life support organization Maastricht treaty for nomenclature in extracorporeal life support: A position paper of the extracorporeal life support organization. American Journal of Respiratory and Critical Care Medicine. 2018;**198**:447-451. DOI: 10.1164/rccm.201710-2130CP

[59] Keebler ME, Haddad EV, Choi CW, McGrane S, Zalawadiya S, Schlendorf KH, et al. Venoarterial extracorporeal membrane oxygenation in cardiogenic shock. JACC: Heart Failure. 2018;**6**:503-516. DOI: 10.1016/j.jchf.2017.11.017

[60] McRae K, de Perrot M. Principles and indications of extracorporeal life support in general thoracic surgery. Journal of Thoracic Disease. 2018;**10**(suppl 8):S931-S946. DOI: 10.21037/jtd.2018.03.116

[61] Chen Y-S, Chao A, Yu H-Y, Ko W-J, Wu I-H, Chen R-J, et al. Analysis and results of prolonged resuscitation in cardiac arrest patients rescued by extracorporeal membrane oxygenation. Journal of the American College of Cardiology. 2003;**41**:197-203

[62] Chen Y-S, Lin J-W, Yu H-Y, Ko W-J, Jerng J-S, Chang W-T, et al. Cardiopulmonary resuscitation with assisted extracorporeal life-support versus conventional cardiopulmonary resuscitation in adults with in-hospital cardiac arrest: An observational study and propensity analysis. Lancet. 2008;**372**:554-561

[63] Nagao K, Kikushima K, Watanabe K, Tachibana E, Tominaga Y, Tada K, et al. Early induction of hypothermia during cardiac arrest improves neurological outcomes in patients with out-of-hospital cardiac arrest who undergo emergency cardiopulmonary bypass and percutaneous coronary intervention. Circulation Journal. 2010;**74**:77-85

[64] Stub D, Bernard S, Pellegrino V, Smith K, Walker T, Sheldrake J, et al. Refractory cardiac arrest treated with mechanical CPR, hypothermia, ECMO and early reperfusion (the CHEER trial). Resuscitation. 2015;**86**:88-94

[65] Gueugniaud PY, David JS, Chanzy E, Hubert H, Dubien PY, Mauriaucourt P, et al. Vasopressin and epinephrine vs. epinephrine alone in cardiopulmonary resuscitation. The New England Journal of Medicine. 2008;**359**:21-30. DOI: 10.1056/NEJMoa0706873

[66] Ong ME, Tiah L, Leong BS, Tan EC, Ong VY, Tan EA, et al. A randomised, double-blind, multi-centre trial comparing vasopressin and adrenaline in patients with cardiac arrest presenting to or in the Emergency Department. Resuscitation. 2012;**83**:953-960. DOI: 10.1016/j.resuscitation.2012.02.005

[67] Wenzel V, Krismer AC, Arntz HR, Sitter H, Stadlbauer KH, Lindner KH, et al. A comparison of vasopressin and epinephrine for out-of-hospital cardiopulmonary resuscitation. The New England Journal of Medicine. 2004;**350**:105-113. DOI: 10.1056/NEJMoa025431

[68] Kudenchuk PJ, Cobb LA, Copass MK, Cummins RO, Doherty AM, Fahrenbruch CE, et al. Amiodarone for resuscitation after out-of-hospital cardiac arrest due to ventricular fibrillation. The New England Journal of Medicine. 1999;**341**:871-878. DOI: 10.1056/NEJM199909163411203

[69] Harrison EE. Lidocaine in prehospital counter shock refractory ventricular fibrillation. Annals of Emergency Medicine. 1981;**10**:420-423

[70] Hassan TB, Jagger C, Barnett DB. A randomised trial to investigate the efficacy of magnesium sulphate for refractory ventricular fibrillation. Emergency Medicine Journal. 2002;**19**:57-62

[71] Ihle JF, Bernard S, Bailey MJ, Pilcher DV, Smith K, Scheinkestel CD. Hyperoxia in the intensive care unit and outcome after out-of-hospital ventricular fibrillation cardiac arrest. Critical Care and Resuscitation. 2013;**15**:186-190

[72] Trzeciak S, Jones AE, Kilgannon JH, Milcarek B, Hunter K, Shapiro NI, et al. Significance of arterial hypotension after resuscitation from cardiac arrest. Critical Care Medicine. 2009;**37**:2895-2903. quiz 2904

[73] Bray JE, Bernard S, Cantwell K, Stephenson M, Smith K, VACAR Steering Committee. The association between systolic blood pressure on arrival at hospital and outcome in adults surviving from out-of-hospital cardiac arrests of presumed cardiac aetiology. Resuscitation. 2014;**85**:509-515. DOI: 10.1016/j.resuscitation.2013.12.005

[74] Walker AC, Johnson NJ. Targeted temperature management and postcardiac arrest care. Emergency Medicine Clinics of North America. 2019;**37**(3):381-393. DOI: 10.1016/j.emc.2019.03.002

[75] Knight WA, Hart KW, Adeoye OM, Bonomo JB, Keegan SP, Ficker DM, et al. The incidence of seizures in patients undergoing therapeutic hypothermia after resuscitation from cardiac arrest. Epilepsy Research. 2013;**106**:396-402. DOI: 10.1016/j. eplepsyres.2013.06.018

[76] Hartmann SM, Farris RWD, Di Gennaro JL, Roberts JS. Systematic review and meta-analysis of end-tidal carbon dioxide values associated with return of spontaneous circulation during cardiopulmonary resuscitation. Journal of Intensive Care Medicine. 2015;**30**:426-435

[77] Touma O, Davies M. The prognostic value of end tidal carbon dioxide during cardiac arrest: A systematic review. Resuscitation. 2013;**84**:1470-1479

[78] Sanders AB, Kern KB, Otto CW, et al. End-tidal carbon dioxide monitoring during cardiopulmonary resuscitation. A prognostic indicator for survival. JAMA. 1989;**262**:1347-1351

[79] Lah K, Krizmaric M, Grmec S. The dynamic pattern of end-tidal carbon dioxide during cardiopulmonary resuscitation: Difference between asphyxial cardiac arrest and ventricular fibrillation/pulseless ventricular tachycardia cardiac arrest. Critical Care. 2011;**15**:R13

[80] Tobias JD. Cerebral oxygenation monitoring: Near-infrared spectroscopy. Expert Review of Medical Devices. 2006;**3**:235-243

[81] Parnia S, Yang J, Nguyen R, et al. Cerebral oximetry during cardiac arrest: A multicenter study of neurologic outcomes and survival. Critical Care Medicine. 2016;**44**:1663-1674

[82] Shin J, Rhee JE, Kim K. Is the inter-nipple line the correct hand position for effective chest compression in adult cardiopulmonary resuscitation? Resuscitation. 2007;**75**:305-310

[83] Park YS, Park I, Kim YJ, et al. Estimation of anatomical structures underneath the chest compression landmarks in children by using computed tomography. Resuscitation. 2011;**82**:1030-1035

[84] Hwang SO, Zhao PG, Choi HJ, et al. Compression of the left ventricular & outflow tract during cardiopulmonary resuscitation. Academic Emergency Medicine. 2009;**16**:928-933

[85] Huisin't Veld MA, Allison MG, Bostick DS, et al. Ultrasound use during & cardiopulmonary resuscitation is associated with delays in chest compressions. Resuscitation. 2017;**119**:95-98

[86] Cimpoesu DC, Popa TO. Cardiopulmonary resuscitation in special circumstances. In: Resuscitation Aspects Theodoros Aslanidis. Zagreb: Intech Open Publishing House; 2017. pp. 13-28

[87] Cimpoesu D, Rotaru L, Petris A, et al. Current Protocols and Guidelines in Emergency Medicine. Iasi: "Gr. T. Popa" UMF Iasi Publishing House; 2011

[88] Tintinalli JE, Stapczynski JS, Ma OJ, et al. Tintinalli's Emergency Medicine a Comprehensive Study

Guide. 8th ed. New York: McGraw-Hill Publishing House; 2016. ISBN: 007179476X

[89] Nolan JP, Soar J, Wenzel V, et al. Cardiopulmonary resuscitation and management of cardiac arrest. Nature Reviews. Cardiology. 2012;**9**:499-511

[90] Simpson CR, Sheikh A. Adrenaline is first line treatment for the emergency treatment of anaphylaxis. Resuscitation. 2010;**81**:641-642

[91] Warner KJ, Copass MK, Bulger EM. Paramedic use of needle thoracostomy in the prehospital environment. Prehospital Emergency Care. 2008;**12**:162-168

[92] Escott ME, Gleisberg GR, Kimmel K, et al. Simple thoracostomy. Moving beyond needle decompression in traumatic cardiac arrest. JEMS: A Journal of Emergency Medical Services. 2014;**39**:26-32

[93] Russell RJ, Hodgetts TJ, McLeod J, Starkey K, Mahoney P, Harrison K, et al. The role of trauma scoring in developing trauma clinical governance in the Defence Medical Services. Philosophical Transactions of the Royal Society B. 2011;**366**:171-191

[94] Lockey D, Crewdson K, Davies G. Traumatic cardiac arrest: Who are the survivors? Annals of Emergency Medicine. 2006;**48**:240-244

[95] Morrison JJ, Poon H, Rasmussen TE, Khan MA, Midwinter MJ, Blackbourne LH, et al. Resuscitative thoracotomy following wartime injury. The Journal of Trauma. 2013;**74**:825-829

[96] Luna GK, Pavlin EG, Kirkman T, Copass MK, Rice CL. Hemodynamic effects of external cardiac massage in trauma shock. The Journal of Trauma. 1989;**29**:1430-1433

[97] Miller TE. New evidence in trauma resuscitation—Is 1:1:1 the answer? Perioperative Medicine. 2013;**2**:13

[98] Neal MD, Hoffman MK, Cuschieri J, Minei JP, Maier RV, Harbrecht RG, et al. Crystalloid to packed red blood cell transfusion ratio in the massively transfused patient: When a little goes a long way. The Journal of Trauma. 2012;**72**:892-898

[99] Leis CC, Hernandez CC, Blanco MJ, Paterna PC, Hernandez-de E, Torres EC. Traumatic cardiac arrest: Should advanced life support be initiated? The Journal of Trauma. 2013;**74**:634-638

[100] Martin M, Satterly S, Inaba K, Blair K. Does needle thoracostomy provide adequate and effective decompression of tension pneumothorax? The Journal of Trauma. 2012;**73**:1412-1417

[101] Mistry N, Bleetman A, Roberts KJ. Chest decompression during the resuscitation of patients in prehospital traumatic cardiac arrest. Emergency Medicine Journal. 2009;**26**:738-740

[102] Huber-Wagner S, Lefering R, Qvick M, Kay MV, Paffrath T, Mutschler W, et al. Outcome in 757 severely injured patients with traumatic cardiorespiratory arrest. Resuscitation. 2007;**75**:276-285

[103] Cureton EL, Yeung LY, Kwan RO, Miraflor EJ, Sadjadi J, Price DD, et al. The heart of the matter: Utility of ultrasound of cardiac activity during traumatic arrest. The Journal of Trauma. 2012;**73**:102-110

[104] Dunning J, Levine A, Ley SJ, et al. The Society of Thoracic Surgeons expert consensus statement for the resuscitation of patients who arrest after cardiac surgery. The Annals of Thoracic Surgery. 2017;**103**:1005

[105] Ngaage DL, Cowen ME. Survival of cardiorespiratory arrest after coronary artery bypass grafting or aortic valve surgery. The Annals of Thoracic Surgery. 2009;**88**(1):64-68

[106] Bohrer H, Gust R, Bottiger BW. Cardiopulmonary resuscitation after cardiac surgery. Journal of Cardiothoracic and Vascular Anesthesia. 1995;**9**:352

[107] Kempen PM, Allgood R. Right ventricular rupture during closed-chest cardiopulmonary resuscitation after pneumonectomy with pericardiotomy: A case report. Critical Care Medicine. 1999;**27**:1378-1379

[108] American Heart Association. Highlights of the 2015 American Heart Association Guidelines Update for CPR and ECC. Available from: www.heart.org/cpr [Accessed: 22 April 2016]

[109] Chan PS, Krumholz HM, Nichol G, Nallamothu BK, American Heart Association National Registry of Cardiopulmonary Resuscitation Investigators. Delayed time to defibrillation after in-hospital cardiac arrest. The New England Journal of Medicine. 2008;**358**(1):9-17

[110] Bradley SM, Liu W, Chan PS, et al. Defibrillation time intervals and outcomes of cardiac arrest in hospital: Retrospective cohort study from Get with the Guidelines-Resuscitation registry. BMJ. 2016;**353**:i1653

[111] Society of Thoracic Surgeons Task Force on Resuscitation After Cardiac Surgery. The Society of Thoracic Surgeons expert consensus for the resuscitation of patients who arrest after cardiac surgery. The Annals of Thoracic Surgery. 2017;**103**(3):1005-1020

[112] Sanders AB, Kern KB, Atlas M, et al. Importance of the duration of inadequate coronary perfusion pressure on resuscitation from cardiac arrest. Journal of the American College of Cardiology. 1985;**6**:113-118

[113] Twomey D, Das M, Subramanian H, et al. Is internal massage superior to external massage for patients suffering a cardiac arrest after cardiac surgery? Interactive Cardiovascular and Thoracic Surgery. 2008;7:151-156

[114] Paradis NA, Martin GB, Rivers EP, et al. Coronary perfusion pressure and the return of spontaneous circulation in human cardiopulmonary resuscitation. JAMA. 1990;**263**(8):1106-1113

[115] Pottle A, Bullock I, Thomas J, et al. Survival to discharge following open chest cardiac compression (OCCC). A 4-year retrospective audit in a Cardiothoracic Specialist Centre—Royal Brompton and Harefield NHS Trust, United Kingdom. Resuscitation. 2002;**52**(3):269-272

[116] Perkins GD, Ji C, Deakin CD, et al. A randomized trial of epinephrine in out-of-hospital cardiac arrest. The New England Journal of Medicine. 2018;**379**(8):711-721

[117] Dunning J, Fabbri A, Kolh PH, et al. Guideline for resuscitation in cardiac arrest after cardiac surgery. European Journal of Cardio-Thoracic Surgery. 2009;**36**:3-28

[118] Mhyre JM, Tsen LC, Einav S, Kuklina EV, Leffert LR, Bateman BT. Cardiac arrest during hospitalization for delivery in the United States, 1998-2011. Anesthesiology. 2014;**120**:810-818

[119] Lewis G. Saving mothers' lives: Reviewing maternal deaths to make motherhood safer 2003-2005. The Seventh Report on Confidential Enquiries into Maternal Deaths in the United Kingdom. London, UK: CEMACH; 2007

[120] Mhyre JM, Bateman BT. Tipping our CAPS to the UKOSS cardiac arrest in pregnancy study. BJOG. 2017;**124**:1382

[121] Rees GA, Willis BA. Resuscitation in late pregnancy. Anaesthesia. 1988;**43**:347-349

[122] Yun JG, Lee BK. Spatial relationship of the left ventricle in the supine position and the left lateral tilt position (implication for CPR in pregnant patients). Fire Science and Engineering. 2013;**27**:75-79

[123] Higuchi H, Takagi S, Zhang K, Furui I, Ozaki M. Effect of lateral tilt angle on the volume of the abdominal aorta and inferior vena cava in pregnant and nonpregnant women determined by magnetic resonance imaging. Anesthesiology. 2015;**122**:286-293

[124] Andersen LW, Granfeldt A, Callaway CW, et al. Association between tracheal intubation during adult in-hospital cardiac arrest and survival. JAMA. 2017;**317**:494-506

Chapter 2

Pediatric Cardiac Arrest

Priscilla Yu, Ivie D. Esangbedo, Lakshmi Raman and Cindy Darnell Bowens

Abstract

This chapter will focus on four important topics in pediatric cardiac arrest. We will highlight recent developments in pediatric CPR quality, medications used in cardiac arrest, ECPR, and post-cardiac arrest care (PCAC) and discuss the existing literature behind AHA guidelines and gaps in knowledge. Optimization of CPR quality is critical during cardiac arrest. We will summarize literature regarding current guidelines which target provider-centered goals and discuss evidence behind patient-centered goals. We will also discuss the evidence behind drugs used in the PALS guidelines. In cases of refractory cardiac arrest, ECMO can be lifesaving; however, there are still many gaps in our knowledge of this field. We will summarize the literature regarding determination of candidacy, cannulation strategies, resuscitation practices during ECPR, and outcomes. After a cardiac arrest, PCAC is crucial to minimize further injury from post-cardiac arrest syndrome (PCAS). The main goals of PCAC are to prevent further brain injury, treat myocardial dysfunction, and systemic ischemia/reperfusion injury. We will discuss AHA guidelines on oxygenation and ventilation goals, targeted temperature management, hemodynamic monitoring, and neuromonitoring.

Keywords: CPR quality, ECPR, extracorporeal cardiopulmonary resuscitation, pediatric cardiac arrest, post-cardiac arrest care

1. CPR quality

1.1 Introduction

There are distinct anatomic and physiologic differences between children and adults that influence not only the etiologies of cardiac arrest but also how we manage these two populations. Children are more at risk for the development of respiratory failure than adults. The discussion of the anatomic reasons behind this is outside the scope of this chapter. Given these anatomic differences between the respiratory systems of adults and children, it is not surprising that the etiology of cardiac arrest in children is usually hypoxia from respiratory failure. In contrast, in adults, the etiology of cardiac arrest is usually secondary to cardiac decompensation [1, 2].

The differences in chest wall compliance between children and adults can also affect their responses to closed chest compressions during CPR. Proposed mechanisms of blood flow during closed chest CPR include compression of the heart between the sternum and spine as well as chest compression (CC)-induced increases in intrathoracic pressure, resulting in pressure gradients from the right heart to the pulmonary vasculature to the left heart and into the systemic vasculature. Based on these mechanisms, it is thought that better chest wall compliance leads to better cardiac output during CPR. This may explain why infants have better outcomes from cardiac arrest after in-hospital cardiac arrest (IHCA) than older children [1]. There are also differences in their myocardial function. Younger children have a limited ability to increase their stroke volume in the face of demand compared to older children and adults and thus are more dependent on heart rate to maintain cardiac output. For these reasons, in the setting of bradycardia with poor perfusion in children, it is imperative to start CPR. In fact, Nadkarni et al. published a multicenter analysis of IHCA from the National Registry of Cardiopulmonary Resuscitation in 2006 and showed that the incidence of initial rhythm of bradycardia with poor perfusion was significantly higher in children than adults. Children receiving CPR for bradycardia who maintain pulses have much higher rates of survival to hospital discharge (SHD) than those who had pulseless cardiac arrest [2].

The AHA guidelines for CPR in children were last updated in 2015. This book chapter section will cover the most recent recommendations, the basis behind these recommendations, and the research that has accrued since the 2015 guidelines (as summarized in **Table 1**). Approximately 15,000 hospitalized children each year undergo CPR with outcomes improving over time [3]. An analysis of over 7000 pediatric pulseless IHCA events between 2000 and 2018 in the Get With the Guidelines-Resuscitation (GWTG-R) registry showed a 19% absolute increase in SHD over time [3]. Unfortunately, the etiology of these improved outcomes has yet to be elucidated. There are many factors that may have led to the increase in SHD in pediatric IHCA over time. One of the factors that may contribute to improved outcomes is improved CPR quality. The AHA guidelines focus on delivering five components of high- quality CPR, which are delivery of chest compressions of adequate rate and depth, ensuring full recoil between compressions, minimizing interruptions in chest compressions, and avoiding excessive ventilation [4]. Despite these guidelines, there have been multiple studies showing difficulty in achieving these targets during CPR. A single center prospective observational study sought to compare CPR quality before and after the institution of the 2010 AHA guidelines. The authors found that while there was an increase in CC depth, rate, and chest compression fraction (CCF) after the 2010 guidelines, it was difficult to achieve the target goals for rate and depth [5]. In 2018, the Pediatric Resuscitation Quality (pediRES-Q) Collaborative, a large multicenter international pediatric resuscitation quality improvement network, published a landscape study characterizing CPR metrics for children with IHCA. They analyzed 112 events and found that guideline compliance for rate and depth in children is poor, with the most difficulty achieving compliance in younger children [6].

There has been a shift from the "provider"-centric to a "patient"-centric approach to CPR. Instead of targeting a standard depth, rate, and ventilation rate (provider centric), the "patient"-centric approach involves incorporating physiologic monitoring and adjusting CPR to the patient's hemodynamic responses as assessed by more invasive monitors like arterial blood pressure and end tidal carbon dioxide ($ETCO_2$) level. This hemodynamic-directed CPR approach could explain the poor compliance with AHA guidelines (which are "provider" centric) that has been described in the literature.

1.1.1 Chest compression metrics

1.1.1.1 Chest compression rate

The 2015 update to the AHA guidelines continues to recommend a chest compression rate of 100–120/min. As stated in the 2015 evidence summary, there is

CPR quality marker	AHA pediatric recommendations	AHA adult recommendations	Most recent literature since AHA recommendations are released
Metric			
Rate	100–120 beats/min	100–120 beats/min	80–100 beats/min
Depth	1/3 AP diameter of the chest or about 4 cm in infants, >5 cm in children >1 year, and >5 cm but <6 cm in adolescents	>5 cm but <6 cm	No association between depth and outcomes
Pauses	No more than 10 s	No more than 10 s	No literature associated with outcomes
CCF	At least 60%	At least 60%	No literature associated with outcomes
Ventilation	No advanced airway: chest compression to ventilation ratio 15:2 Advanced airway: 10 breaths/min	No advanced airway: chest compression to ventilation ratio 30:2 Advanced airway: 10 breaths/min	Higher rates (≥30 breaths/min in children <1 year old and ≥25 breaths/min in older children) associated with improved outcomes compared to lower rates
Duty cycle	50%	50%	No association between duty cycle and outcomes
Chest recoil	Full	Full	
Physiologic markers			
$ETCO_2$	Reasonable to monitor, but no goals established	≥20 mm Hg	No association between $ETCO_2$ and outcomes
Arterial blood pressure	Reasonable to monitor, but no goals established	≥25 mm Hg	DBP ≥ 25 mm Hg in infants and DBP ≥ 30 mm Hg in children was associated with improved outcomes
Coronary perfusion pressure	Insufficient evidence to make a recommendation	≥20 mm Hg	No new evidence

Table 1.
AHA recommendations for various CPR quality markers in children vs. adults as well as the recent literature since guidelines are released.

insufficient data in children for a systematic review for CC rate, and therefore the recommendations are based on evidence for adults. Given simplicity in CPR training and insufficient pediatric evidence, the recommendation was that it is reasonable to use the adult basic life support (BLS) CC rate of 100–120 for children [4]. Since the 2015 update was published, there has been one pediatric study published on this subject. The Eunice Kennedy Shriver National Institute of Child Health and Human Development Collaborative Pediatric Critical Care Research Network (CPCCRN) is a network of seven pediatric ICUs that conducts investigations related to pediatric critical care practice. Between 2013 and 2016, the CPCCRN conducted the Pediatric Intensive Care Unit Quality of CPR (PICqCPR) study, a multicenter prospective observational study to evaluate the association between invasive arterial blood pressures during CPR and outcomes. Using the dataset, the primary aim of the study was to evaluate the association between CC rates and blood pressure and survival outcomes. The results of the study showed that when compared to

AHA guidelines of 100 to <120, higher rate categories were associated with lower systolic (SBP); however, there was no correlation to survival. Also when compared to the AHA guidelines of 100 to <120, a CC rate of 80 to <100 was associated with a higher rate of SHD and survival with favorable neurological outcome (FNO) compared to CC rates within guidelines [7].

1.1.1.2 Chest compression depth

The 2015 update to AHA guidelines recommend to compress at least 1/3 of the anterior–posterior (AP) diameter of the chest, which is about 4 cm in infants, 5 cm in children, and greater than 5 cm but no more than 6 cm in adolescents [4]. Two single-center pediatric studies were reviewed for the 2015 update to the AHA guidelines. The first study was a case series of six infants after cardiac surgery who had CPR. In those infants, aged 0–7 months, attempting to compress the chest to ½ the AP diameter increased the SBP significantly compared to attempts to compress the chest to 1/3 the AP diameter [8]. The second study looked at 87 chest compression events in children >1 year and showed that AHA compliant guideline CC depths >51 mm were associated with improved 24-h survival compared to more shallow CC depths [9]. Since the 2015 update, there has been only one study published. This was a multicenter prospective observational study that looked at out-of-hospital cardiac arrests (OHCA). They looked at 153 pediatric events (children 1–19 years of age) with CPR metric data and found that there was no association with CC depth and return of spontaneous circulation (ROSC) [10].

1.1.1.3 Minimizing interruptions in chest compressions

The 2015 AHA guidelines continue to emphasize minimizing interruptions in chest compressions, in particular to less than 10 s. Ideally, these pauses should be coordinated so that a pulse check, rhythm check, and compressor switch occur at the same time and should only occur every 2 min. There should be a person assigned to the role of the pulse check, positioned with his/her finger on the pulse before the pause to minimize the pause duration. Chest compression fraction is defined as the time spent doing chest compressions during CPR. The 2013 AHA consensus statement on CPR quality recommended a CCF of at least 80% [11]; however, the 2015 AHA BLS guidelines recommend a CCF of at least 60% [12]. Observational studies of cardiac arrests often show that pauses can be more prolonged and more frequent than expected. In a single-center observational study in a pediatric emergency room, 33 cardiac arrests were analyzed. While the majority of pauses were <10 s in duration, 33% of pauses were >10 s. The number of coordinated pauses were rare, only 7% of the time [13]. A more recent observational study of CPR quality in two pediatric emergency departments analyzed 81 cardiac arrests. While median CCF was 91% with a median pause duration of 4 s, 22% of pauses were prolonged (>10 s). Again, the number of coordinated pauses were rare (6%) and prolonged with a median of 19 s [14]. Although the AHA guidelines recommend to switch providers performing CC every 2 min to prevent rescuer fatigue and therefore inadequate CPR quality, they also acknowledge that when a CPR feedback device is used, some individuals can go longer than 2 min [15]. A single-center observational study that sought to characterize causes for interruptions found that provider switch accounted for the majority of pauses. Individuals performing CC for at least 120 s compared to those switching earlier had less leaning, increased CC depth, and better compliance for depth with AHA guidelines [16]. While there is limited evidence in adults to support these guidelines on duration of pauses and CCF, these recommendations have been applied to children. There are no pediatric studies to date evaluating the association between CC interruptions and outcomes. In 2019, a single-center observational study was published that sought to evaluate the hemodynamic consequences of interruptions in CC. Thirty-two IHCA events were analyzed. The median duration of pauses was brief at 2.4 s; however, BPs before and after the pauses did not differ significantly [17].

1.1.1.4 Ventilation

For patients without an invasive airway at the time of cardiac arrest, BLS guidelines recommend a compression to ventilation ratio of 15:2 in children if there are two providers (in contrast to 30:2 for adults). Although there is no data to support the optimal compression to ventilation ratio in children, the recommended ventilation rate takes into account a higher baseline respiratory rate in children. For children without advanced airways in place at the time of arrest, there is often an emphasis on tracheal intubation during an IHCA given the most common etiology of IHCA is respiratory failure. The 2019 focused update on PALS reaffirms the 2010 recommendation that during a pediatric OHCA, the use of bag mask ventilation (BMV) is reasonable compared to an advanced airway. The update also specifies that no recommendation for or against an advanced airway could be made. These recommendations were made based on the review of 14 studies of airway interventions in children who had cardiac arrests [18].

In contrast to the recommendation for a higher ventilation rate without an advanced airway, when an advanced airway is in place, AHA guidelines recommend that ventilation rates of 10 breaths/min be applied to all age groups during CPR in order to simplify training. During CPR, cardiac output is usually about 25% of normal, and thus lower ventilation rates are recommended to match the lower output state, given the detrimental effects of positive pressure ventilation on venous return and right heart afterload. However, the etiology of cardiac arrest in children is usually asphyxia in nature compared to the primary cardiac origin of most adult cardiac arrests, and thus the recommendations of equal ventilation rates in children as to adults have been questioned. In 2019, the CCPCRN published the only study to date that has analyzed the association of ventilation rates in pediatric cardiac arrests and survival outcomes. As part of the PICqCPR study, the authors analyzed 52 events in patients with an invasive airway in place at the time of the cardiac arrest. No events were within the guideline ventilation rate (defined as 10 ± 2 breaths/min), and more than half of the events were considered high ventilation rates (defined as > or equal to 30 breath/min in infants <1 year and > or equal to 25 in children >1 year). In fact, higher ventilation rates were associated with higher odds of SHD [19].

1.1.1.5 Duty cycle

The term "duty cycle" refers to the amount of time spent in the compression phase of CPR. AHA guidelines for adult cardiac arrest recommend a duty cycle of 50% [20]. There have been no pediatric recommendations since 2005 on duty cycle. The only pediatric study to date on duty cycle was published in 2016. It was a single-center observational study that analyzed 97 pediatric events and found no association with duty cycle and survival [21].

1.1.1.6 Chest recoil

AHA guidelines recommend full chest recoil in between compressions, to avoid leaning. In 2009, a single-center prospective observational study sought to evaluate the prevalence of leaning and the effect of real-time feedback devices on leaning. They evaluated 20 pediatric cardiac arrests and found that leaning was common during pediatric CPR; however, leaning occurred significantly less when a feedback device was used [22]. In 2013, the same pediatric center published another prospective observational study looking at the quality of CPR in children 1–8 years of age with a real-time feedback device. In eight events, they found the percentage of CPR epochs (defined as 30-s periods of resuscitation) achieving the target goal of leaning <20% of compressions was 79%. In particular, the percent epochs achieving target leaning goals was better in the feedback group than in the no feedback device [23]. There are no studies to date evaluating the association with leaning and outcomes in children.

1.1.2 Physiologic monitoring

1.1.2.1 End tidal CO_2

The 2015 PALS guidelines state that it is reasonable to use $ETCO_2$ to guide the quality of CPR in children, although specific values to guide therapy in children have not been established [24]. These recommendations were made on extrapolation of adult and animal data since no pediatric literature at the time of these guidelines had been shown that $ETCO_2$ monitoring improves outcomes. For adults, AHA recommendations are to titrate to an $ETCO_2 \geq 20$ mm Hg [11]. In 2018, using the PICqCPR data, the CCPCRN published the only pediatric study to date that evaluates the association of ETCO2 values and survival outcomes. Contrary to adult literature, the authors found that there was no association between $ETCO_2 \geq 20$ mm Hg and SHD [25].

1.1.2.2 Arterial blood pressure

Similar to the recommendation for $ETCO_2$ monitoring, the 2015 PALS guidelines state that it is reasonable to use BP to guide CPR quality if an invasive arterial line is already in place; however, no specific values to guide therapy have been established [24]. At the time, these recommendations were based on animal data without any pediatric human literature. Since then, the CCPCRN has published three studies using PICqCPR data, evaluating the association of intra-arrest diastolic blood pressure (DBP) and post-arrest outcomes. The first study evaluated 164 events and showed that maintaining a mean DBP ≥ 25 mm Hg in infants and DBP ≥ 30 mm Hg in children was associated with SHD and survival with FNO. There was no association between SBP and outcomes [26]. The second study evaluated 77 survivors of the first study and sought to assess the association between intra-arrest BP and functional outcomes. Unlike the parent study which showed an association between DBP and FNO, there was no association between DBP and functional outcomes. Again, there was no association with SBP and functional outcomes [27]. The third study evaluated the subgroup of patients with cardiac disease. The authors analyzed the hemodynamic waveforms of 113 patients with cardiac disease and found an association with the same DBP goals and SHD in surgical patients but not medical patients. They also noted the majority of patients with single ventricles and open chest were able to attain the DBP goals. In patients who went on to have ECPR, approximately half were able to attain the DBP goals; however, there was no association between DBP goals and SHD [28].

1.1.2.3 Coronary perfusion pressure

Coronary perfusion pressure (CoPP) can be estimated by subtracting the right atrial (RA) pressure from the aortic DBP. While the 2013 AHA Consensus

Statement on CPR quality recommends titrating CoPP to >20 mm Hg in adults if invasive arterial line and central venous catheter is in place, they state that there is insufficient evidence to make a CoPP goal for infants and children [11]. While no pediatric studies exist, one pediatric animal study showed improvement in a hemodynamic-directed approach to CPR. In a study with 4-week-old piglets, hemodynamic-directed CPR with compression depth titrated to SBP > 90 mm Hg and vasopressor administration to maintain CPP ≥ 20 mm Hg resulted in higher survival rate than standard care of CC depth 1/3 AP diameter [29].

1.1.3 CPR devices

The 2015 AHA guidelines state that it is reasonable to use audiovisual feedback devices during CPR to optimize CPR quality. As mentioned before, there have been studies showing improvement in pediatric CPR quality with the addition of a real-time CPR feedback device [22, 23]. However, a systematic review and meta-analysis of studies using real-time feedback devices has not shown improvement in patient outcomes [30].

While mechanical chest compression devices such as Autopulse and LUCAS have been used in adults, both devices are not intended for use in children [31, 32].

1.1.4 Debriefing

There have been multiple adult studies showing that the implementation of a debriefing program can lead to improved CPR quality and outcomes [33]. There are generally two approaches to debriefing, hot debriefs and cold debriefs. Hot debriefs occur usually within hours after a cardiac arrest with team members involved in the cardiac arrest and involve mainly the members' recall of the events and their immediate reactions. Cold debriefs occur at a later time, within weeks of an event with a larger audience that includes the immediate team members but also other ICU staff. The cold debrief involves a more comprehensive review of the cardiac arrest and can include more objective measures such as defibrillator CPR data and physiologic monitor data [34]. Pediatric studies on debriefings have been limited. A study of the content and process of hot debriefs from the pediRES-Q collaborative revealed approximately half of all cardiac arrests are followed by hot debriefs. The content of the hot debriefs are usually about cooperation/coordination, communication, and clinical standards [35]. The association between hot debriefs and outcomes still needs to be determined. A single-center prospective interventional study sought to evaluate the effectiveness of the implementation of a cold debriefing program on survival outcomes in children. They found that implementation of their program was associated with improved CPR quality and survival with FNO [36].

1.1.5 CPR duration

Despite excellent quality CPR, many clinicians question whether continuing resuscitation is futile for prolonged cardiac arrests. An analysis of the GWTG registry aimed to examine the effect of CPR duration for pediatric IHCA on outcomes. The authors concluded that CPR duration was independently associated with SHD and survival with FNO. However, among survivors, survival with FNO was 70% in those arrests occurring <15 min and 60% for those patients with arrests >35 min. Compared to medical patients, surgical cardiac patients had the highest adjusted OR for SHD and survival with FNO [37].

1.2 Summary

The 2015 AHA guidelines on pediatric CPR are based on extrapolation of evidence from adult and animal studies. Since then there has been a growing amount of literature that supports transitioning CPR from a "provider"-centric to "patient"-centric CPR. Recent literature has shown no change or worse outcomes when providers follow "provider"-centric guidelines that use standardized targets. Chest compression rates lower than recommended have been associated with improved outcomes. There has been no association shown between CC depth and outcomes. Ventilation rates higher than 2015 AHA guidelines are associated with improved outcomes. More recent evidence is emerging that demonstrates targeting a patient's physiologic response to CPR may be more beneficial. Evidence has shown that DBP greater than 25 mm Hg in infants and 30 mm Hg in older children are associated with improved outcomes. There are many CPR quality metrics to choose from to guide CPR. These metrics can help improve the quality of CPR from a system-wide standpoint.

2. Medications used in cardiac arrest

The 2015 PALS guidelines discussed three drugs used during resuscitation in children: epinephrine, amiodarone, and lidocaine [24]. **Table 2** highlights these medications, comparing recommendations from the 2015 PALS update and most recent literature that has been published since then. The 2015 PALS guidelines state that it is reasonable to use epinephrine during cardiac arrest. This guideline was based on two pediatric observational studies that were inconclusive and one adult study showing increased ROSC and survival to admission but no change in SHD [24]. Since the 2015 guidelines, an analysis of nonshockable pediatric cardiac arrests in the GWTG registry showed a delay in epinephrine administration was associated with decreased likelihood of survival to admission, ROSC, SHD, and survival with FNO [38]. Another GWTG analysis looked at the intervals between epinephrine administration. Guidelines currently state to give epinephrine every 3–5 min during CPR. This study showed that compared to intervals of 1–5 min as the reference, longer intervals were associated with improved SHD [39]. For shock refractory VF or pulseless VT, the 2015 guidelines changed to state that either amiodarone or lidocaine was acceptable. Previous guidelines had recommended amiodarone as the preferred drug over lidocaine. This is based on pediatric retrospective data that shows lidocaine is associated with improved ROSC and 24-h survival; however, there is no change in SHD [24]. The 2018 update to the PALS guidelines continued

Medication	2015 PALS guidelines	Most recent literature
Epinephrine	It is reasonable to give epinephrine at intervals every 3–5 min	1. Delay in epinephrine administration associated with worse outcomes 2. Longer intervals between epinephrine are associated with better outcomes
Amiodarone/ lidocaine	Either amiodarone or lidocaine is equally acceptable for shock refractory VF or pulseless VT	2018 PALS update: no change

Table 2.
Medications used during pediatric cardiac arrest: Current guidelines vs. most recent literature.

to reaffirm the 2015 guidelines. No new pediatric data was available for the updated review; however, the committee did not consider extrapolated adult data [40].

3. Pediatric ECPR

3.1 History and current use of extracorporeal cardiopulmonary resuscitation (ECPR) in pediatrics

Extracorporeal membrane oxygenation (ECMO) use for cardiopulmonary resuscitation (CPR) in children was first described in the literature by del Nido in 1992 [41]. Since then, utilization of extracorporeal cardiopulmonary resuscitation has expanded in all pediatric age groups. The current definition of ECPR according to the Extracorporeal Life Support Organization (ELSO) is "the application of rapid-deployment venoarterial ECMO, to provide circulatory support in patients in whom conventional CPR is unsuccessful in achieving sustained return of spontaneous circulation (ROSC). Sustained ROSC is deemed to have occurred when chest compressions are not required for 20 consecutive minutes and signs of circulation persist" [42]. This definition has been used since ELSO updated its data definitions in 2018. Pre-2018, the ELSO definition of ECPR was "ECMO used for initial resuscitation from cardiac arrest" and did not include patients who had achieved ROSC when they were being cannulated for ECMO [43]. Apart from the ELSO definitions, the definition of ECPR varies in clinical studies, and this presents challenges with medical communication and synthesis of research.

Based on ELSO registry data, there has been an increasing use of ECPR in pediatric patients over the years [44]. The overwhelming majority of pediatric ECPR use reported in the literature is for in-hospital cardiac arrest (IHCA) [44]. There are only few reports of ECPR deployed in pediatric patients for out-of-hospital cardiac arrest (OHCA); 2% of pediatric ECPR cases reported to ELSO were for OHCA according to the 2016 pediatric ELSO registry report [44, 45]. There is one case report of out-of-hospital ECMO deployment in a child ("pre-hospital ECPR") [46].

From reported literature, the incidence of ECPR use varies from 5 to 27% of all pediatric IHCA cases between 2000 and 2016 [37, 47–49]. Of pediatric IHCA cases reported to the American Heart Association (AHA) Get With the Guidelines®-Resuscitation registry between the years 2000 and 2008, the incidence of ECPR use was 5–7% overall and 19–21% in patients with a cardiac diagnosis [37, 47]. More recently, the incidence of ECPR use was 27.2% in cardiac arrest patients reported to the Pediatric Cardiac Critical Care Consortium (PC4) registry between 2014 and 2016 [49].

The AHA had not included ECPR in Pediatric Advanced Life Support (PALS) guidelines until 2005 when guidelines were updated to include a consideration of ECPR in patients with a reversible cause of arrest or whose underlying condition could be treated by heart transplantation and who were located at an institution that could rapidly deploy ECMO, where effective conventional CPR had been started promptly [50]. Subsequent PALS updates have included this cautious recommendation to consider ECPR, particularly for cardiac patients with IHCA [18, 24, 51].

3.2 Cannulation procedure during CPR

Determination of a patient's ECPR candidacy and feasibility of cannulation should preferably be done prior to cardiac arrest. Criteria for determination of candidacy may vary from center to center, and there are no universal guidelines for this. Though the AHA recommends considering ECMO for pediatric IHCA, there are no specific guidelines for the actual implementation of ECMO during CPR.

Site of cannulation varies in pediatrics and could be central or peripheral. Central (transthoracic) cannulation is more frequently performed in cardiac surgical patients, some of whom may already have an open sternum [52–54] . Peripheral cannulation could be via right neck vessels (internal jugular vein and carotid artery) or femoral vessels. Data is conflicting on the presence of a correlation between cannulation site and outcomes in pediatric ECPR [55–62].

Questions also remain surrounding (i) the appropriate timing of initiating a request for ECMO implementation during CPR, (ii) the use of timed cycled interruptions of chest compressions to allow for cannulation, and (iii) the ongoing administration of epinephrine (adrenaline) during ECPR cannulation. From a review of the literature, clinical practice varies in regard to how long after the initiation of chest compressions that ECMO is requested for pediatric IHCA [57, 60, 63–66]. A cross-sectional survey of pediatric cardiac intensive care practitioners published in 2018 showed that 38% of respondents reported activating ECMO after just one dose of epinephrine, while more than 80% called for ECMO after the second dose [67]. The timing of initiation of ECMO cannulation during CPR is important because it contributes to total CPR duration. Based on this, it would seem prudent to request ECMO early into the resuscitation effort. But caution must also be taken to avoid deployment prematurely, for example, if return of spontaneous circulation (ROSC) could have been achieved without ECMO. The effect of total CPR duration on survival and neurological outcomes after pediatric ECPR is unclear. In a recent large study using data from both ELSO and GWTG-R registries, a linear relationship was demonstrated between CPR duration and odds of death before hospital discharge [68]. Multiple single-center studies have also shown worse outcomes from pediatric ECPR if duration of CPR is longer [52, 60, 63, 64, 66, 69–72]. However, still other studies have shown no correlation between ECPR duration and outcomes [37, 53, 57, 73–79]. The patient population possibly dictates the effect of ECPR duration on outcome. Compared to other illness categories, pediatric cardiac surgical patients have been shown to have a higher probability of favorable neurologic outcomes despite ECPR of prolonged duration [37].

The use of timed cycled interruptions of chest compressions to facilitate cannulation during ECPR is practiced in some centers, but there is no literature to show how widespread this practice is or whether it has positive effects on outcomes. Without timed cycled interruptions, chest compressions are paused randomly, usually at the discretion of the cannulating surgeon, and they are paused for varying amounts of time. With timed cycled interruptions, pauses in chest compressions are on a cycle—compressions are not paused unless a minimum time has passed (e.g., 2 min), and they are only paused for a maximum amount of time (e.g., 30–45 s). With the cycled method, the cannulating surgeon is only able to work in short bursts of time, and it is possible that overall CPR duration is therefore longer. However, it is also likely that CPR "no-flow" time is less. This is an area that needs to be studied.

Epinephrine administration for CPR during ECMO cannulation is also an area of research interest. Proponents of the cessation of epinephrine administration during ECMO cannulation for CPR argue that ongoing administration would only increase systemic vascular resistance (which would impede ECMO flow subsequently and hamper myocardial recovery) and is futile for ROSC since the decision would have already been made to cannulate. However, the 2009 study of 199 pediatric ECPR recipients from GWTG-R registry demonstrated no statistically significant difference between survivors and non-survivors in cumulative dose of epinephrine received during ECPR [73]. Also, in the cross-sectional survey of pediatric cardiac critical care clinicians published in 2018, only 19% of respondents reported limiting epinephrine to 1–3 doses during CPR before ECMO cannulation [67].

3.3 Elements of an ECPR program

Deployment of ECPR requires that a well-coordinated, streamlined, and efficient sequence of activities takes place. For success of an ECPR program, it is essential that clinical teams are always ready since time is of the essence. Important elements to a successful ECPR program include (i) prior identification of patients that would be offered ECMO in the case of cardiac arrest, (ii) prior establishment of a system of emergently notifying all required parties in the event of cardiac arrest (e.g., through paging), (iii) ready availability of primed ECMO circuits and blood products, and (iv) effectively trained and prepared team members [80, 81].

Some ECPR programs have crystalloid-primed or non-blood colloid-primed circuits always on standby [57, 76, 81, 82]. Sixty-five percent of 1828 pediatric ECPR cases reported to ELSO from 2011 to 2015 had an ECMO circuit primed with blood products [44]. Different considerations go into the choice of prime solution for rapid deployment. Blood-primed circuits are dependent on the rapid availability of blood products and cannot be stored long-term. Some programs do not keep pre-primed circuits if blood can be obtained quickly [83]. Crystalloid-primed circuits may be stored for up to 30 days but may require adjustment of pH and addition of blood prior to use [57, 76, 81]. Cost must also be considered in the decision to have pre-primed circuits on standby. For example, as published in 2017 by Erek et al., their pediatric ECPR program in Turkey avoids pre-primed ECMO circuits due to cost. Instead they emergently deploy cardiopulmonary bypass circuits for ECPR then transition to ECMO circuits later in the course [52].

Teams must be effectively trained and prepared. Simulation has proven to be an effective method for ECPR team training and has been used in many programs around the world with good results [84–86].

3.4 Pediatric ECPR outcomes

Survival after ECPR in pediatrics is around 43% in all age groups, according to ELSO [44]. Only a few pediatric studies have compared conventional CPR (CCPR) with ECPR [48, 87, 88]. In an analysis published in 2016 of almost 600 pediatric IHCA patients from the GWTG-R registry, there were increased odds of survival to hospital discharge for patients who received ECPR compared to CCPR only (adjusted OR 2.76; 95% CI 2.08–3.65; $p < 0.0001$) [87]. An earlier study published in 2013 did not demonstrate an association between ECPR and improved survival to discharge compared to CCPR, but that study had a small ECPR subgroup and was unable to match controls [48].

Taeb et al. compared CPR quality between ECPR and CCPR in pediatric cardiac intensive care patients. They found that CPR duration was significantly longer for patients who received ECPR than those who received CCPR [30 min (9.5–33 min) vs. 5.5 min (4–12.5 min); $p = 0.016$]. Rate of ROSC, intensive care unit length of stay, and hospital length of stay were not different between the groups [88].

Neurological outcomes after ECPR are important metrics, but there is a general paucity of data on this topic. Multiple single-center and registry studies have reported on neurologic status at hospital discharge using the Pediatric Cerebral Performance Category (PCPC) scale [37, 57, 61, 64, 73, 81, 87, 89–91]. However, many of those studies have incomplete data, and designation of a patient's PCPC is also subjective. In addition, the definition of favorable neurologic outcome scores using PCPC varies. All these make interpretation of the data somewhat difficult. In the 2019 study of merged ELSO and GWTG-R data, discharge PCPC was only available in 48% of 241 pediatric ECPR survivors; 93% of those had a PCPC ≤ 2 which was considered favorable [68].

There is limited data on functional and neurobehavioral status in pediatric ECPR patients beyond hospital discharge [60, 63, 92–95]. Torres-Andres et al. assessed health-related quality of life after pediatric ECPR. Children with normal brain imaging at the time of ECMO decannulation had statistically higher quality of life scores compared to other children, and those with ischemic changes on brain imaging at decannulation had higher quality of life scores than those with hemorrhagic changes [96].

3.5 Transportation of pediatric cardiac arrest patients to ECMO centers

The decision to transport pediatric cardiac arrest patients with active chest compressions to a hospital that performs ECPR must be considered carefully. Literature on this subject is minimal. Prolonged CPR before ECMO cannulation has been shown in some studies to not result in worse mortality, especially in patients with cardiac diagnoses [77, 97, 98]. However, Eich et al. describe the outcomes of 12 pediatric patients who suffered near-drowning episodes between 1987 and 2005 and who were transported to a tertiary center in Germany for emergent cardiopulmonary bypass [45]. Only 5 of the 12 survived to hospital discharge, of which 3 were in a persistent vegetative state.

In deciding to transport pediatric patients receiving CPR, one must consider the following: etiology of cardiac arrest, origin of transport (i.e., out-of-hospital transport vs. interhospital transfer), the duration of "no-flow" time, the anticipated total duration of CPR, the physical distance to the ECMO center, effectiveness of CPR during transport, and safety of medical personnel performing compressions during transport. Safety and effectiveness of CPR during transport of children has not been studied [99].

3.6 Summary

In summary, ECPR use in pediatrics is on the rise. There is evidence of its positive impact, and it has been included in resuscitation guidelines for pediatric in-hospital cardiac arrest, in specific patients and where existing programs are available. It is important that hospitals establishing and running ECPR programs have detailed protocols and repeated training and rehearsing for ECPR.

4. Pediatric post-arrest care

4.1 Introduction

In 1966, the National Academy of Sciences published a consensus statement on CPR describing the ABCDs of resuscitation. In this document A denoted airway opened; B denoted breathing restored; C denoted circulation restored; and D denoted definitive therapy. Definitive therapy was described as therapy for the management of the cause(s) of the arrest and management of resulting pathology from the arrest [100]. Successful return of spontaneous circulation (ROSC) that is sustained often results in post-cardiac arrest syndrome (PCAS). PCAS is described in phases defined by time. The immediate post-arrest phase is described as the first 20 min after ROSC. This is followed by the early post-arrest phase which is described as between 20 min through 6–12 h after ROSC. The intermediate phase follows lasting up to 72 h following ROSC. Afterwards the recovery phase starts and lasts until disposition when the rehabilitation phase begins. These last two phases vary in duration [101].

Post-cardiac arrest syndrome encompasses (1) post-cardiac arrest brain injury, (2) post-cardiac arrest myocardial dysfunction, (3) systemic ischemia/reperfusion response, and (4) persistent precipitating pathology. The severity of illness from this pathology varies based on the extent of the ischemic insult, the cause of the cardiac arrest, and patient's prearrest state of health. The mechanism of post-cardiac arrest brain injury is complex and includes excitotoxicity, disrupted calcium homeostasis, free radical formation, protease cascades, and activation of cell death signaling pathways. Post-cardiac arrest brain injury is also influenced by what is often hyperemic reperfusion and frequent failure to achieve adequate cerebral reperfusion. Post-cardiac arrest myocardial dysfunction describes the transient global dysfunction that is seen immediately after ROSC. The systemic ischemia/reperfusion response describes the whole-body ischemia/reperfusion that occurs with hypoxia-induced activation of immunologic and coagulation pathways that is seen with cardiac arrest. Clinically this appears as intravascular volume depletion, impaired vasoregulation, impaired oxygen delivery, and increased susceptibility to infection. The persistence of the precipitating cause of the cardiac arrest often complicates the pathology of post-cardiac arrest syndrome. Specific treatment of the cause must be aligned with treatment of the PCAS [101]. In 2019, the AHA scientific statement estimated that more than 1800 children and infants were at risk for PCAS annually [102]. The individual components of PCAS are potentially treatable, and this has led to an emphasis on post-cardiac arrest care (PCAC).

PCAC varies depending on the phase of post-cardiac arrest syndrome and the setting in which care is being delivered. PCAC requires multisystem support and must begin promptly after ROSC. The goal of the treatment is to support end-organ function, treat PCAS, and correct the causal factor for the arrest. PCAC begins with the initiation of monitoring as soon after ROSC as feasible. This monitoring includes continuous cardiac telemetry, pulse oximetry, continuous capnography, continuous temperature monitoring, blood pressure measurement, and monitoring of urine output. Laboratory analysis is also important and includes blood gases, serum electrolytes, serum glucose, and calcium. Other monitoring to consider includes arterial lactate, central venous oxygen saturation, chest x-ray, renal function, hemoglobin concentration, coagulation function, and monitoring for signs of inflammation. Neurologic monitoring is useful in a comatose post-cardiac arrest patient. The goal of neurologic monitoring is to prevent secondary neurological injury and aid in prognostication. This monitoring could include serial exams and electroencephalogram [103]. Appendix **Figure A1** shows an example of a post-arrest care checklist.

4.2 Hemodynamics

There is no high-quality evidence to support a single strategy for providing optimal hemodynamic support in pediatric patients post-cardiac arrest. Post-cardiac arrest myocardial dysfunction treatment can be aided by monitoring arterial lactate and central venous oxygen saturation. Parenteral fluids, inotropes, and vasoactive medications are to be used as needed to provide hemodynamic support. Optimal use of parenteral fluids vs. vasopressors/inotropes has not yet been determined. At times hemodynamic stability will include management of arrhythmias. Medications to treat arrhythmias are dependent on the underlying cardiac pathology. Hemodynamic treatment should be adjusted to account for the patient's PCAS and prearrest characteristics. At times extracorporeal membrane oxygenation is initiated during CPR as described earlier in the chapter. The efficacy of ECMO for hemodynamic support after ROSC is unclear [104].

4.3 Oxygenation and ventilation

Optimizing oxygenation and ventilation after ROSC is essential and may be hindered by the cause of the arrest and the ongoing PCAS. Providing oxygen is a common therapy in critically ill children. There is no consistent data on the usefulness of hyperoxia after cardiac arrest in children. Treatment with a goal of providing normal paO2 using the lowest possible fraction of inspired oxygen to maintain an oxygen saturation of 94–99% is the current strategy [102]. It is important to manage ventilation as both hypercarbia and hypocarbia have deleterious effects on cerebral perfusion. Current data suggest that it is appropriate to target normocapnia or a PaCO2 specific for the patient's condition while minimizing hypercapnia and hypocapnia [24, 105]. While providing strategies to optimize oxygenation and ventilation, we must be mindful that therapeutic hypothermia can alter the arterial oxygen saturation and affect carbon dioxide production which will be reflected in the minute ventilation [106].

4.4 Targeted temperature management (TTM)

The 2019 American Heart Association update for Pediatric Advanced Life Support included endorsement of post-cardiac arrest continuous maintenance of patient temperature, also referred to as TTM. In 2019 ILCOR pediatric CoSTR summarized evidence supporting the use of TTM (32–34°C) in infants and children after cardiac arrest [107]. Referring to their work, the American Heart Association recommends continuous measurement of core temperature during TTM. Additionally, for infants and children between 24 h of age and 18 years of age who remain comatose after out of hospital cardiac arrest or IHCA, it is reasonable to use TTM at 32–34°C followed by TTM at 36–37.5°C. Initiating hypothermia can be achieve in many ways including cooling blankets, surface cooling with ice packets, or gastric lavage. Electrolyte derangements including hyperglycemia, hypokalemia, hypophosphatemia, hypomagnesaemia, and hypocalcemia can occur during induction of hypothermia. This electrolyte instability can lead to arrhythmias. While maintaining hypothermia, careful monitoring is required. The ideal strategy for rewarming has not yet been identified. In children, the rewarming is usually done at a rate no faster than 0.5°C every 2 h. This reduces the risk of cerebral hyperperfusion, vasogenic edema, and acute systemic hypotension [102]. During PCAC, a temperature >37.5°C should be avoided and aggressively treated [108].

There was data suggesting that earlier timing of hypothermia was associated with better outcomes. Moler and colleagues developed a trial to investigate if shorter time to goal temperature was associated with improved outcomes at 1 year. Using data from the Therapeutic Hypothermia After Pediatric Cardiac Arrest Out-of-Hosptial Trial (ThAPCA –OH), critically ill children from 38 pediatric intensive care units in the United States and Canada were randomized to therapeutic hypothermia or normothermia [109]. Median time to goal temperature in group 1 was 5.8 h and in group 2 was 8.8 h. However, outcomes between the groups did not differ. They concluded that earlier time to goal temperature was not associated with better outcomes [110].

4.5 Sedation

Similarly, to other critically ill children, children with PCAS will likely require treatment with sedatives, analgesics, and possibly neuromuscular blockade. There is insufficient data to describe optimal management of sedation and analgesia for pediatric patients with PCAS. With the use of TTM sedation, analgesia and neuromuscular blockade may be used to facilitate cooling and prevent shivering. Caution is advised when using neuromuscular blockade as this will hinder the clinical neurologic exam and will mask seizures.

4.6 Neurologic monitoring

Continuous EEG monitoring for pediatric patients who are encephalopathic following cardiac arrest and ROSC is recommended. This recommendation came forth from the recent consensus statement from the American Clinical Neurophysiology Society Critical Care Continuous EEG Guidelines Committee [111]. It is recommended that EEG monitoring be initiated as soon as possible and continue for 24–48 h. The recommendation also advises to continue monitoring for 24 h after patients treated with hypothermia are rewarmed to normothermia. There have not been studies to evaluate the effect of treatment of seizures in the post-cardiac arrest period on patient outcomes. Generally, most clinicians treat seizures as they can increase metabolic demand and contribute to secondary brain injury.

4.7 AKI and glucose control

The impact of the management of AKI and glucose control during PCAC is unclear. Data evaluating pediatric post-cardiac arrest AKI and glucose control management is scarce. AKI in critically ill children is associated with increased mortality and morbidity [112, 113]. It is important to monitor kidney function during PCAC as these patients are at risk to develop AKI. During PCAC, it is important to monitor for and treat hypoglycemia and hyperglycemia in post-cardiac arrest patients. Both hypoglycemia and hyperglycemia have been associated with poor outcomes in children [114]. There is no data that evaluates interventional studies of glucose control on PCAC pediatric patients.

4.8 Rehabilitation

Rehabilitation following cardiac arrest is vital. Children surviving cardiac arrest are at risk for alterations in their quality of life from physical, cognitive, and emotional disabilities. They are at risk for significant declines in neurobehavioral function across multiple functional domains [115]. There is also evidence that post-cardiac arrest patients are at risk for developing delirium [116]. There is little data on specific interventions during PCAC that will improve functional outcomes in children after cardiac arrest. More information is needed to identify specific rehabilitation interventions that can be used in PCAC that will improve outcomes for pediatric post-cardiac arrest patients [102].

4.9 Summary

To summarize, how we care for pediatric patients post successful ROSC after cardiac arrest critically influences their outcomes. Each component of post-cardiac arrest care requires focused management. This care is highly complex and time sensitive. Despite knowing how crucial this management is to the outcomes of patients post-cardiac arrest, significant gaps in knowledge remain. More work is needed to identify the most efficient approaches to provide this care for pediatric patients.

5. Conclusions

Many of the recommendations regarding CPR quality metrics in children are based on extrapolation of adult and animal data, given the scarcity of pediatric literature. Although current AHA guidelines focus on "provider"-centric CPR, the evidence for transitioning to a "patient"-centric guided CPR is growing. Along with

CPR quality, the choice of the right medications and dosing intervals is critical during a pediatric cardiac arrest and is also a field of pediatric resuscitation that is lacking evidence. Despite good-quality CPR, there are many times when ROSC does not occur. Although PALS guidelines state that ECPR can be considered in certain circumstances, there are still gaps in the literature regarding cannulation strategies and resuscitation practices during ECPR. After successful ROSC or return of circulation after ECPR, the medical management of a child is critical to ameliorate the effects of PCAS and prevent further injury to vital organs, in particular the brain.

Appendix

Post Arrest Care Checklist

1. **Optimize Ventilation and Oxygenation**
    - Maintain advanced airway
    - Maintain normoxia (SpO_2 94-98%)
    - Maintain normocapnia (maintain continuous $ETCO_2$)

2. **Circulation**
    - Maintain reliable IV access
    - Maintain invasive BP monitoring
    - Optimize hemodynamic status
        - Aim for age specific BP target
        - Monitor MAP, CVP, lactate, $ScvO_2$, urine output
    - Assess for and treat persistent shock
        - Identify and treat possible contributing factors
3. **Active temperature management**
    - Constant core temperature monitoring
    - Can choose either pathway
        - *Hypo*thermic: 32°C-34°C
        - *Normo*thermic: 35°C-37°C
    - Prevent and treat fever for 96 hours
4. **Monitor and Treat:**
    - Neurological status
        - Neuro checks q1 hour
        - Need for Sedation/Paralysis
            - Continuous EEG monitoring with paralysis
        - Seizures
            - Obtain EEG for clinical seizure
        - Hyperosmolar therapy to target Na >140
    - Glucose Control
    - Serial Laboratory Sampling:
        - Arterial blood gas
        - Venous blood gas
        - Lactate
        - Chemistry
        - Glucose
        - Liver Function
        - Coagulation Labs

Figure A1.
Post arrest care checklist.

Author details

Priscilla Yu, Ivie D. Esangbedo, Lakshmi Raman and Cindy Darnell Bowens*
University of Texas Southwestern Medical Center, Children's Health Medical Center, Critical Care Division, USA

*Address all correspondence to: cindy.bowens@utsouthwestern.edu

References

[1] Berg MD et al. In-hospital pediatric cardiac arrest. Pediatric Clinics of North America. 2008;**55**(3):589-604, x

[2] Nadkarni VM et al. First documented rhythm and clinical outcome from in-hospital cardiac arrest among children and adults. Journal of the American Medical Association. 2006;**295**(1):50-57

[3] Holmberg MJ et al. Trends in survival after pediatric In-hospital cardiac arrest in the United States. Circulation. 2019; **140**(17):1398-1408

[4] Atkins DL et al. Part 11: Pediatric basic life support and cardiopulmonary resuscitation quality: 2015 American Heart Association guidelines update for cardiopulmonary resuscitation and emergency cardiovascular care. Circulation. 2015;**132**(18 Suppl 2):S519-S525

[5] Sutton RM et al. Pushing harder, pushing faster, minimizing interruptions...but falling short of 2010 cardiopulmonary resuscitation targets during in-hospital pediatric and adolescent resuscitation. Resuscitation. 2013;**84**(12):1680-1684

[6] Niles DE et al. Characterization of pediatric In-hospital cardiopulmonary resuscitation quality metrics across an international resuscitation collaborative. Pediatric Critical Care Medicine. 2018; **19**(5):421-432

[7] Sutton RM et al. Chest compression rates and pediatric in-hospital cardiac arrest survival outcomes. Resuscitation. 2018;**130**:159-166

[8] Maher KO et al. Depth of sternal compression and intra-arterial blood pressure during CPR in infants following cardiac surgery. Resuscitation. 2009;**80**(6):662-664

[9] Sutton RM et al. 2010 American Heart Association recommended compression depths during pediatric in-hospital resuscitations are associated with survival. Resuscitation. 2014;**85**(9): 1179-1184

[10] Sutton RM et al. A quantitative analysis of out-of-hospital pediatric and adolescent resuscitation quality—A report from the ROC epistry-cardiac arrest. Resuscitation. 2015;**93**:150-157

[11] Meaney PA et al. Cardiopulmonary resuscitation quality: [Corrected] improving cardiac resuscitation outcomes both inside and outside the hospital: A consensus statement from the American Heart Association. Circulation. 2013;**128**(4):417-435

[12] Travers AH et al. Part 3: Adult basic life support and automated external defibrillation: 2015 international consensus on cardiopulmonary resuscitation and emergency cardiovascular care science with treatment recommendations. Circulation. 2015;**132**(16 Suppl 1):S51-S83

[13] Donoghue A et al. Videographic assessment of cardiopulmonary resuscitation quality in the pediatric emergency department. Resuscitation. 2015;**91**:19-25

[14] O'Connell KJ et al. Pauses in compressions during pediatric CPR: Opportunities for improving CPR quality. Resuscitation. 2019;**145**:158-165

[15] Berg MD et al. Part 13: Pediatric basic life support: 2010 American Heart Association guidelines for cardiopulmonary resuscitation and emergency cardiovascular care. Circulation. 2010;**122**(18 Suppl 3): S862-S875

[16] Sutton RM et al. Quantitative analysis of chest compression interruptions during in-hospital resuscitation of older children and

adolescents. Resuscitation. 2009;**80**(11): 1259-1263

[17] Morgan RW et al. Hemodynamic effects of chest compression interruptions during pediatric in-hospital cardiopulmonary resuscitation. Resuscitation. 2019;**139**:1-8

[18] Duff JP et al. 2019 American Heart Association focused update on pediatric advanced life support: An update to the American Heart Association guidelines for cardiopulmonary resuscitation and emergency cardiovascular care. Circulation. 2019;**140**(24):e904-e914

[19] Sutton RM et al. Ventilation rates and pediatric In-hospital cardiac arrest survival outcomes. Critical Care Medicine. 2019;**47**(11):1627-1636

[20] Berg MD et al. Pediatric basic life support: 2010 American Heart Association guidelines for cardiopulmonary resuscitation and emergency cardiovascular care. Pediatrics. 2010;**126**(5):e1345-e1360

[21] Wolfe H et al. Quantitative analysis of duty cycle in pediatric and adolescent in-hospital cardiac arrest. Resuscitation. 2016;**106**:65-69

[22] Niles D et al. Leaning is common during in-hospital pediatric CPR, and decreased with automated corrective feedback. Resuscitation. 2009;**80**(5): 553-557

[23] Sutton RM et al. First quantitative analysis of cardiopulmonary resuscitation quality during in-hospital cardiac arrests of young children. Resuscitation. 2014;**85**(1):70-74

[24] de Caen AR et al. Part 12: Pediatric advanced life support: 2015 American Heart Association guidelines update for cardiopulmonary resuscitation and emergency cardiovascular care. Circulation. 2015;**132**(18 Suppl 2):S526-S542

[25] Berg RA et al. End-tidal carbon dioxide during pediatric in-hospital cardiopulmonary resuscitation. Resuscitation. 2018;**133**:173-179

[26] Berg RA et al. Association between diastolic blood pressure during pediatric In-hospital cardiopulmonary resuscitation and survival. Circulation. 2018;**137**(17):1784-1795

[27] Wolfe HA et al. Functional outcomes among survivors of pediatric in-hospital cardiac arrest are associated with baseline neurologic and functional status, but not with diastolic blood pressure during CPR. Resuscitation. 2019;**143**:57-65

[28] Yates AR et al. Survival and cardiopulmonary resuscitation hemodynamics following cardiac arrest in children with surgical compared to medical heart disease. Pediatric Critical Care Medicine. 2019;**20**(12): 1126-1136

[29] Morgan RW et al. A hemodynamic-directed approach to pediatric cardiopulmonary resuscitation (HD-CPR) improves survival. Resuscitation. 2017;**111**:41-47

[30] Kirkbright S et al. Audiovisual feedback device use by health care professionals during CPR: A systematic review and meta-analysis of randomised and non-randomised trials. Resuscitation. 2014;**85**(4):460-471

[31] Lucas Chest Compression Systems. [Internet]. [cited: 11 May 2020]. Available from: https://www.lucas-cpr.com/files/7762374_101034-00%20Rev%20F%20LUCAS%203%20IFU%20US_lowres.pdf

[32] Zoll: AutoPulse Resuscitation System [Internet]. [cited: 11 May 2020]. Available from: https://api.zoll.com/-/media/public-site/products/autopulse/zoll-san-jose-upload/12555-001-rev-7-autopulse-system-user-guide.ashx

[33] Edelson DP et al. Improving in-hospital cardiac arrest process and outcomes with performance debriefing. Archives of Internal Medicine. 2008; **168**(10):1063-1069

[34] Couper K, Perkins GD. Debriefing after resuscitation. Current Opinion in Critical Care. 2013;**19**(3):188-194

[35] Sweberg T et al. Description of hot debriefings after in-hospital cardiac arrests in an international pediatric quality improvement collaborative. Resuscitation. 2018;**128**:181-187

[36] Wolfe H et al. Interdisciplinary ICU cardiac arrest debriefing improves survival outcomes. Critical Care Medicine. 2014;**42**(7):1688-1695

[37] Matos RI et al. Duration of cardiopulmonary resuscitation and illness category impact survival and neurologic outcomes for in-hospital pediatric cardiac arrests. Circulation. 2013;**127**(4):442-451

[38] Andersen LW et al. Time to epinephrine and survival after pediatric In-hospital cardiac arrest. Journal of the American Medical Association. 2015; **314**(8):802-810

[39] Hoyme DB et al. Epinephrine dosing interval and survival outcomes during pediatric in-hospital cardiac arrest. Resuscitation. 2017;**117**:18-23

[40] Duff JP et al. 2018 American Heart Association focused update on pediatric advanced life support: An update to the American Heart Association guidelines for cardiopulmonary resuscitation and emergency cardiovascular care. Circulation. 2018;**138**(23):e731-e739

[41] del Nido PJ et al. Extracorporeal membrane oxygenator rescue in children during cardiac arrest after cardiac surgery. Circulation. 1992;**86** (5 Suppl):II300-II304

[42] ELSO. ELSO Database Definitions 2018-2-1.pdf [Internet]. Available from: https://www.elso.org/Portals/0/Files/PDF/ELSO%20Database%20Definitions%202018-2-1.pdf [cited September 15, 2019]

[43] Extracorporeal Life Support Organization—ECMO and ECLS > Publications > Red Book. 5th ed. [Internet]. Available from: https://www.elso.org/Publications/RedBook5thEdition.aspx [cited 13 January 2020]

[44] Barbaro RP et al. Pediatric extracorporeal life support organization registry international report 2016. ASAIO Journal. 2017;**63**(4):456-463

[45] Eich C et al. Outcome of 12 drowned children with attempted resuscitation on cardiopulmonary bypass: An analysis of variables based on the "Utstein style for drowning". Resuscitation. 2007; **75**(1):42-52

[46] Arlt M et al. Out-of-hospital extracorporeal life support for cardiac arrest-a case report. Resuscitation. 2011; **82**(9):1243-1245

[47] Ortmann L et al. Outcomes after in-hospital cardiac arrest in children with cardiac disease: A report from get with the guidelines—Resuscitation. Circulation. 2011;**124**(21):2329-2337

[48] Lowry AW et al. Characterization of extracorporeal membrane oxygenation for pediatric cardiac arrest in the United States: Analysis of the kids' inpatient database. Pediatric Cardiology. 2013; **34**(6):1422-1430

[49] Alten JA et al. Epidemiology and outcomes of cardiac arrest in pediatric cardiac ICUs. Pediatric Critical Care Medicine. 2017;**18**(10):935-943

[50] American Heart Association. 2005 American Heart Association (AHA) guidelines for cardiopulmonary resuscitation (CPR) and emergency

cardiovascular care (ECC) of pediatric and neonatal patients: Pediatric advanced life support. Pediatrics. 2006; **117**(5):e1005-e1028

[51] Kleinman ME et al. Part 14: Pediatric advanced life support: 2010 American Heart Association guidelines for cardiopulmonary resuscitation and emergency cardiovascular care. Circulation. 2010;**122**(18 Suppl 3):S876-S908

[52] Erek E et al. Extracorporeal cardiopulmonary resuscitation for refractory cardiac arrest in children after cardiac surgery. Anatolian Journal of Cardiology. 2017;**17**(4):328-333

[53] Guo Z et al. Extracorporeal cardiopulmonary resuscitation in children after open heart surgery. Artificial Organs. 2019;**43**(7):633-640

[54] Zeybek C, Kemal Avsar M, Yildirim O, et al. Utilization of extracorporeal membrane oxygenation in pediatric cardiac surgery: A single center experience, 34 cases in 8 years. Iranian Journal of Pediatrics. 2017;**27**(6): e14402

[55] Barrett CS et al. Neurological injury after extracorporeal membrane oxygenation use to aid pediatric cardiopulmonary resuscitation. Pediatric Critical Care Medicine. 2009; **10**(4):445-451

[56] Chan T et al. Survival after extracorporeal cardiopulmonary resuscitation in infants and children with heart disease. The Journal of Thoracic and Cardiovascular Surgery. 2008;**136**(4):984-992

[57] Kane DA et al. Rapid-response extracorporeal membrane oxygenation to support cardiopulmonary resuscitation in children with cardiac disease. Circulation. 2010;**122**(11 Suppl):S241-S248

[58] Wolf MJ et al. Extracorporeal cardiopulmonary resuscitation for pediatric cardiac patients. The Annals of Thoracic Surgery. 2012;**94**(3):874-879; discussion 879-80

[59] Thiagarajan RR et al. Extracorporeal membrane oxygenation to aid cardiopulmonary resuscitation in infants and children. Circulation. 2007; **116**(15):1693-1700

[60] Torres-Andres F et al. Survival and long-term functional outcomes for children with cardiac arrest treated with extracorporeal cardiopulmonary resuscitation. Pediatric Critical Care Medicine. 2018;**19**(5):451-458

[61] Tsukahara K, Toida C, Muguruma T. Current experience and limitations of extracorporeal cardiopulmonary resuscitation for cardiac arrest in children: A single-center retrospective study. Journal of Intensive Care. 2014;**2**(1):68

[62] Shin HJ et al. Results of extracorporeal cardiopulmonary resuscitation in children. Korean Journal of Thoracic and Cardiovascular Surgery. 2016;**49**(3):151-156

[63] Garcia Guerra G et al. Survival and neurocognitive outcomes in pediatric extracorporeal-cardiopulmonary resuscitation. Resuscitation. 2015;**96**: 208-213

[64] Sivarajan VB et al. Duration of resuscitation prior to rescue extracorporeal membrane oxygenation impacts outcome in children with heart disease. Intensive Care Medicine. 2011; **37**(5):853-860

[65] Alsoufi B et al. Survival outcomes after rescue extracorporeal cardiopulmonary resuscitation in pediatric patients with refractory cardiac arrest. The Journal of Thoracic and Cardiovascular Surgery. 2007; **134**(4):952-959 e2

[66] Alsoufi B et al. Results of rapid-response extracorporeal cardiopulmonary resuscitation in children with refractory cardiac arrest following cardiac surgery. European Journal of Cardio-Thoracic Surgery. 2014;**45**(2):268-275

[67] Lasa JJ et al. Extracorporeal cardiopulmonary resuscitation in the pediatric cardiac population: In search of a standard of care. Pediatric Critical Care Medicine. 2018;**19**(2):125-130

[68] Bembea MM et al. Outcomes after extracorporeal cardiopulmonary resuscitation of pediatric In-hospital cardiac arrest: A report from the get with the guidelines-resuscitation and the extracorporeal life support organization registries. Critical Care Medicine. 2019;**47**(4):e278-e285

[69] Alsoufi B et al. Does single ventricle physiology affect survival of children requiring extracorporeal membrane oxygenation support following cardiac surgery? World Journal for Pediatric and Congenital Heart Surgery. 2014; **5**(1):7-15

[70] Delmo Walter EM et al. Rescue extracorporeal membrane oxygenation in children with refractory cardiac arrest. Interactive Cardiovascular and Thoracic Surgery. 2011;**12**(6):929-934

[71] Huang SC et al. Eleven years of experience with extracorporeal cardiopulmonary resuscitation for paediatric patients with in-hospital cardiac arrest. Resuscitation. 2012; **83**(6):710-714

[72] Aharon AS et al. Extracorporeal membrane oxygenation in children after repair of congenital cardiac lesions. The Annals of Thoracic Surgery. 2001;**72**(6): 2095-2101; discussion 2101-2

[73] Raymond TT et al. Outcomes among neonates, infants, and children after extracorporeal cardiopulmonary resuscitation for refractory inhospital pediatric cardiac arrest: A report from the National Registry of cardiopulmonary resuscitation. Pediatric Critical Care Medicine. 2010;**11**(3):362-371

[74] Allan CK et al. Emergent use of extracorporeal membrane oxygenation during pediatric cardiac catheterization. Pediatric Critical Care Medicine. 2006; **7**(3):212-219

[75] Beshish AG et al. Functional status change among children with extra-corporeal membrane oxygenation to support cardiopulmonary resuscitation in a pediatric cardiac ICU: A single institution report. Pediatric Critical Care Medicine. 2018;**19**(7):665-671

[76] Duncan BW et al. Use of rapid-deployment extracorporeal membrane oxygenation for the resuscitation of pediatric patients with heart disease after cardiac arrest. The Journal of Thoracic and Cardiovascular Surgery. 1998;**116**(2):305-311

[77] Kelly RB, Harrison RE. Outcome predictors of pediatric extracorporeal cardiopulmonary resuscitation. Pediatric Cardiology. 2010;**31**(5):626-633

[78] Polimenakos AC et al. Post-cardiotomy extracorporeal cardiopulmonary resuscitation in neonates with complex single ventricle: Analysis of outcomes. European Journal of Cardio-Thoracic Surgery. 2011;**40**(6): 1396-1405 discussion 1405

[79] Polimenakos AC et al. Post-cardiotomy rescue extracorporeal cardiopulmonary resuscitation in neonates with single ventricle after intractable cardiac arrest: Attrition after hospital discharge and predictors of outcome. Pediatric Cardiology. 2017; **38**(2):314-323

[80] Laussen PC, Guerguerian AM. Establishing and sustaining an ECPR program. Frontiers in Pediatrics. 2018;**6**:152

[81] Turek JW et al. Outcomes before and after implementation of a pediatric rapid-response extracorporeal membrane oxygenation program. The Annals of Thoracic Surgery. 2013;**95**(6): 2140-2146; discussion 2146-7

[82] Alsoufi B et al. Extra-corporeal life support following cardiac surgery in children: Analysis of risk factors and survival in a single institution. European Journal of Cardio-Thoracic Surgery. 2009;**35**(6):1004-1011; discussion 1011

[83] Ghez O et al. Absence of rapid deployment extracorporeal membrane oxygenation (ECMO) team does not preclude resuscitation ECMO in pediatric cardiac patients with good results. ASAIO Journal. 2007;**53**(6): 692-695

[84] Sawyer T et al. Impacts of a pediatric extracorporeal cardiopulmonary resuscitation (ECPR) simulation training program. Academic Pediatrics. 2019;**19**(5):566-571

[85] Puslecki M et al. BEST life-"bringing ECMO simulation to life"-how medical simulation improved a regional ECMO program. Artificial Organs. 2018;**42**(11): 1052-1061

[86] Su L et al. Implementation of an extracorporeal cardiopulmonary resuscitation simulation program reduces extracorporeal cardiopulmonary resuscitation times in real patients. Pediatric Critical Care Medicine. 2014;**15**(9):856-860

[87] Lasa JJ et al. Extracorporeal cardiopulmonary resuscitation (E-CPR) during pediatric In-hospital cardiopulmonary arrest is associated with improved survival to discharge: A report from the American Heart Association's get with the guidelines-resuscitation (GWTG-R) registry. Circulation. 2016;**133**(2):165-176

[88] Taeb M et al. Comparison of pediatric cardiopulmonary resuscitation quality in classic cardiopulmonary resuscitation and extracorporeal cardiopulmonary resuscitation events using video review. Pediatric Critical Care Medicine. 2018;**19**(9):831-838

[89] Burke CR et al. Pediatric extracorporeal cardiopulmonary resuscitation during nights and weekends. Resuscitation. 2017;**114**:47-52

[90] Huang SC et al. Extracorporeal membrane oxygenation rescue for cardiopulmonary resuscitation in pediatric patients. Critical Care Medicine. 2008;**36**(5):1607-1613

[91] Prodhan P et al. Outcomes after extracorporeal cardiopulmonary resuscitation (ECPR) following refractory pediatric cardiac arrest in the intensive care unit. Resuscitation. 2009; **80**(10):1124-1129

[92] Meert KL et al. Extracorporeal cardiopulmonary resuscitation: One-year survival and neurobehavioral outcome among infants and children with In-hospital cardiac arrest. Critical Care Medicine. 2019;**47**(3):393-402

[93] Meert KL et al. One-year survival and neurologic outcomes after pediatric open-chest cardiopulmonary resuscitation. The Annals of Thoracic Surgery. 2019;**107**(5):1441-1446

[94] Meert K et al. Paediatric in-hospital cardiac arrest: Factors associated with survival and neurobehavioural outcome one year later. Resuscitation. 2018;**124**: 96-105

[95] Meert K et al. One-year cognitive and neurologic outcomes in survivors of paediatric extracorporeal cardiopulmonary resuscitation. Resuscitation. 2019;**139**:299-307

[96] Ahmed OZ et al. Change in functional status among children treated in the intensive care unit after injury. Journal of Trauma and Acute Care Surgery. 2019;**86**(5):810-816

[97] Chrysostomou C et al. Short- and intermediate-term survival after extracorporeal membrane oxygenation in children with cardiac disease. The Journal of Thoracic and Cardiovascular Surgery. 2013;**146**(2):317-325

[98] Morris MC et al. Risk factors for mortality in 137 pediatric cardiac intensive care unit patients managed with extracorporeal membrane oxygenation. Critical Care Medicine. 2004;**32**(4):1061-1069

[99] Noje C et al. Interhospital transport of children undergoing cardiopulmonary resuscitation: A practical and ethical dilemma. Pediatric Critical Care Medicine. 2017;**18**(10): e477-e481

[100] Cardiopulmonary resuscitation. Statement by the Ad Hoc Committee on Cardiopulmonary Resuscitation of the Division of Medical Sciences, National Academy of Sciences—National Research Council. Journal of the American Medical Association. 1966;**198**(4):372-379

[101] Neumar RW et al. Post-cardiac arrest syndrome: Epidemiology, pathophysiology, treatment, and prognostication. A consensus statement from the International Liaison Committee on Resuscitation (American Heart Association, Australian and New Zealand Council on Resuscitation, European Resuscitation Council, Heart and Stroke Foundation of Canada, InterAmerican Heart Foundation, Resuscitation Council of Asia, and the Resuscitation Council of Southern Africa); the American Heart Association Emergency Cardiovascular Care Committee; the Council on Cardiovascular Surgery and Anesthesia; the Council on Cardiopulmonary, Perioperative, and Critical Care; the Council on Clinical Cardiology; and the Stroke Council. Circulation. 2008; **118**(23):2452-2483

[102] Topjian AA et al. Pediatric post-cardiac arrest care: A scientific statement from the American Heart Association. Circulation. 2019;**140**(6): e194-e233

[103] Bongiovanni F et al. Standardized EEG analysis to reduce the uncertainty of outcome prognostication after cardiac arrest. Intensive Care Medicine. 2020

[104] Holmberg MJ et al. Extracorporeal cardiopulmonary resuscitation for cardiac arrest: A systematic review. Resuscitation. 2018;**131**:91-100

[105] Gill C, Kissoon N. Pediatric life support update: 2015 American Heart Association highlights. Pediatric Emergency Care. 2017;**33**(8):585-593

[106] Karnatovskaia LV et al. Effect of therapeutic hypothermia on gas exchange and respiratory mechanics: A retrospective cohort study. Therapeutic Hypothermia and Temperature Management. 2014;**4**(2):88-95

[107] Soar J et al. 2019 International consensus on cardiopulmonary resuscitation and emergency cardiovascular care science with treatment recommendations: Summary from the basic life support; advanced life support; pediatric life support; neonatal life support; education, implementation, and teams; and first aid task forces. Circulation. 2019;**140**(24):e826-e880

[108] Duff JP et al. 2019 American Heart Association focused update on pediatric basic life support: An update to the American Heart Association guidelines for cardiopulmonary resuscitation and emergency cardiovascular care. Pediatrics. 2020;**145**(1):e20191361

[109] Moler FW et al. Therapeutic hypothermia after out-of-hospital cardiac arrest in children. The New England Journal of Medicine. 2015; **372**(20):1898-1908

[110] Moler FW et al. Pediatric out-of-hospital cardiac arrest: Time to goal target temperature and outcomes. Resuscitation. 2019;**135**:88-97

[111] Herman ST et al. Consensus statement on continuous EEG in critically ill adults and children, part I: Indications. Journal of Clinical Neurophysiology. 2015;**32**(2):87-95

[112] Soler YA et al. Pediatric risk, injury, failure, loss, end-stage renal disease score identifies acute kidney injury and predicts mortality in critically ill children: A prospective study. Pediatric Critical Care Medicine. 2013;**14**(4): e189-e195

[113] Alkandari O et al. Acute kidney injury is an independent risk factor for pediatric intensive care unit mortality, longer length of stay and prolonged mechanical ventilation in critically ill children: A two-center retrospective cohort study. Critical Care. 2011;**15**(3): R146

[114] Faustino EV, Apkon M. Persistent hyperglycemia in critically ill children. The Journal of Pediatrics. 2005;**146**(1): 30-34

[115] Slomine BS et al. Neurobehavioural outcomes in children after In-hospital cardiac arrest. Resuscitation. 2018;**124**: 80-89

[116] Boncyk CS et al. In the ICU - delirium post cardiac arrest. Current Opinion in Critical Care. 2019;**25**(3): 218-225

Chapter 3

Sudden Cardiac Death in Young Athletes

Leonid Makarov

Abstract

Sudden death (SD) is the most dangerous and irreversible outcome of diseases in clinical as well as in sports medicine. Between 1980 and 2011, the Sudden Death in Young Athletes Registry in the USA, which was developed based on mass media information, recorded 2406 cases of sudden death, which were observed in 29 diverse sports. In the USA 80% of all SD occurred in high school/middle school or collegiate student athletes, and 20% were engaged in organized youth, postgraduate. Statistical data vary greatly in different countries: SCD incidence rate in the USA is 7.47 and 1.33 per 1,000,000 exercising male and female school-age athletes, respectively, whereas in Italy, the rate is 2.6 cases in men and 1.1 in women per 100,000 individuals per year who are involved in active competitive sports. The European Heart Rhythm Association (EHRA) position paper concluded that as an overall estimate, 1–2 out of 100,000 athletes between of age of 12 and 35 years old die suddenly each year. It was shown that the risk of SCD is significantly higher in athletes than in nonathletes with the same heart condition in the general population, by more than five times for ARVC, 2.6 times for coronary artery disease, 1.5 times for myocarditis, and more than 2 times for cardiac conduction system diseases.

Keywords: sport, sudden cardiac death, young athletes

1. Introduction

Sudden death (SD) is the most dangerous and irreversible outcome of diseases in clinical [1] as well as in sports medicine [2–7]. SD in the sports definition includes cases of death that occurred immediately during exercise as well as within the first 1–24 hours from the onset of initial symptoms that have led to a change or cessation of physical activity. Most cases of SD in athletes are associated with sporting activity [6, 8]. In 2015 the European Guidelines for the Prevention of Sudden Death classified athletes into a separate group with a special risk of SD [9].

SD is traditionally considered to be associated primarily with heart diseases. But according to the data provided by the US National Collegiate Athletic Association (NCAA) athletes between 2003 and 2013, accidents are the leading cause of death in the SD structure of athletes (50%); however the leading position among somatic diseases undoubtedly belongs to sudden cardiac death (SCD) which constitutes 15% of all SD cases; the other causes of SD, both medical and nonmedical (suicide, homicide) do not exceed 10% [5].

IntechOpen

2. The epidemiology of SCD in sports

It is not easy to determine the accurate epidemiology of SCD in sports. Much depends on the selected inclusion criteria for the analysis, the age of the athletes, the level of athletic achievement, sporting experience, type of sports, and other factors. Therefore, studies carried out in different countries show an unequal SCD incidence rate in athletes. Between 1980 and 2011, the Sudden Death in Young Athletes Registry in the USA, which was developed based on mass media information, recorded 2406 cases of sudden death, which were observed in 29 divers sports [6]. In this paper 80% SD occurred in high school/middle school or collegiate student athletes, and 20% were engaged in organized youth, postgraduate.

SCD incidence rate determined in the USA was 7.47 and 1.33 per 1,000,000 exercising male and female school-age athletes, respectively [10]. The statistical data can however vary greatly in some areas. According to Corrado et al. [3], the SCD incidence rate in Italy was 2.6 cases in men and 1.1 in women per 100,000 individuals per year who are involved in active competitive sports. In recent years, with screening of athletes before active exercise, this figure decreased to 0.87 cases per 100,000 per year. In the USA, in children and adolescent athletes, SCD is registered in 0.66 cases per 100,000 exercising male school students and 1.45 per 100,000 male college students and 0.12 per 100,000 female school students and 0.28 per 100,000 female college students (Van Camp et al., [10]). In Ireland [11] the SCD incidence rate in sports was 1 case per 600,000, while in a French study [12], it was 0.26 per 100,000 per year. In a study conducted on Rhoda Island [13], the rate was 0.36 per 100,000 per year in individuals aged up to 30 years and 4.46 and 0.05 per 100,000 per year in men and women older than 30, respectively. The European Heart Rhythm Association (EHRA) position paper concluded that as an overall estimate, 1–2 out of 100,000 athletes between the ages of 12 and 35 years old die suddenly each year [8].

3. SCD and types of sports

The data on sports-associated SCD cases as well as those on epidemiology are quite varied, depending on national sporting traditions, age, gender, and group inclusion criteria (professional sports, school sports, general fitness activity). Most SCD causes in the USA [6], most SCD cases in young athletes in active competitive sports occurred in basketball and football, which accounted for 35 and 30%, respectively; soccer, cross-country/track, and baseball accounted for 8, 7, and 6% of the cases respectively; such sports as wrestling, boxing, swimming, ice hockey, and marathon running accounted for between 1 and 5%; and rugby, triathlon, martial arts, tennis, volleyball, gymnastics, figure skating, golf, and others accounted for less than 1%.

By another study from the USA (Harmon et al. [5]), the highest incidence rates of SCD per athletes were 1 in 8978 in men's basketball, 1 in 23,689 in men's soccer, and 1 in 35,951 in men's football. In women its rates were 1 in 57,611 in swimming and 1 in 77,061 in basketball.

SCDs not associated with commotio cordis (see below) were reported most frequently in children and adolescents involved in ice hockey, football, and basketball [14]. In Spain SCD was observed most often in cyclists (34.4%), soccer players (21.3% in the general group and 33.3% in athletes younger than 35 years), and gymnasts (8%). Fewer deaths occurred in basketball, rowing, marathon running, jogging, and mountain climbing [15]. In Italy [3] the highest number of SCD cases was registered in soccer (40%); 9% of the cases in swimming and rugby; 7% in cycle racing, running, and volleyball; and 3% of cases in judo, tennis, and gymnastics. It is clear that this rating of dangerous sports is based on a specific regional and temporal sample of published sports-related SCD cases and does not fully reflect all types of sports for which SCD were recorded. SCD cases associated with many other sports periodically come to public attention through the media. The studies by Quigley and Ragosta cited above most frequently recorded SCD when playing golf (31.3 and 23.4%, respectively), cricket (21.5%), and jogging and less often during basketball (10.2%), swimming (8%), and cycling races (6%). In a major study conducted in France [16], SCD was most frequently observed during cycling (30.6%), jogging (21.3%), and soccer (13.05%); in individuals of all ages playing sports and exercising regularly, SCD in other sports did not exceed 5% in this list.

4. Commotio cordis

The SCD cases associated with a blunt blow to the heart area and classified as death caused by heart contusion (contusion cordis) or concussion (commotio cordis) constitute a special group [14, 17–19]. Occurring in the vulnerable phase of the cardiac cycle (the beginning of T wave on ECG), this blow initiates fatal arrhythmias, ventricular fibrillation, or at once asystole. Under normal heart rate (60–80 bpm), this vulnerable period takes up approximately 2–3% of the time or up to 20% if the heart rate increases to 120 bpm or more. Therefore, athletes are more vulnerable to this grave complication during exercise. Young American athletes most frequently experience SCD in lacrosse, then hockey and basketball [14]. There have been reports of SCD occurring from a punch to the heart in martial arts, due to being struck with a hockey puck, or other circumstances. Commotio cordis is the cause of 2 [5] to 20% [6, 7, 14] of SCD cases in young athletes.

5. Gender and age of the victims

According to the US Registry, the age of inclusion in the analysis of SCD and cardiac arrest in athletes was limited to 39 years; 2153 deaths from all causes (89%) occurred in males and 253 deaths (11%) were in females (4). In mortality rate among the 842 athletes with autopsy-confirmed cardiovascular diagnoses, the incidence in males exceeded that in females by 6.5-fold, $P < .001$ ([6], 1172). An analysis of 61 cases of SCD that occurred during exercise in Spain in 1995–2001 revealed that the age of the athletes and those involved in sports reached 65 years (mean age 31.9 ± 14.2 years). In 59 cases vs. 2, the victims were male [15]. Among 60 squash players who died suddenly at the age of 22–66 years (46 ± 10.3), 59 individuals (98.3%) were also male [20]. However, women may dominate in some sports characterized by a relatively small number of SCDs or cardiac arrests, e.g., 90% in volleyball and 73% in softball [6]. The number of arrhythmias and SCD risk increases with age. However, this applies primarily to those who are not engaged in or who have retired from professional and competitive sports [6].

6. Circumstances of SCD and prodromal symptoms

When analyzing the circumstances of SCD in young athletes, it was observed that in 83% of cases, SCD occurred during or immediately after exercise, and only 17% was not associated with any physical activity [6]. In some cases, it was possible to obtain the medical histories of the victims or data on the presence of some specific diseases or conditions or potential symptoms preceding the fatal episode. In 60 squash players who died suddenly, Northcote et al. [20] were performed an analysis of prodromal symptoms before death. In a decreasing order of symptom frequency, athletes with sudden deaths complained of chest pain, increasing fatigue, non-specific gastrointestinal disorders, a burning sensation in the heart area, feeling short of breath, pain in the ears or neck, non-specific malaise, upper respiratory tract infections, dizziness and/or palpitations, and severe headache. Five of the victims (8.3%) had no significant symptoms before death. Prodromal symptoms were more frequent in athletes than in nonathletes of the same age who died suddenly, 32 vs. 23%, respectively, as observed by Corrado et al. [21]. This suggests that even minor, non-specific health complaints in regularly training athletes must be taken seriously by doctors, coaches, and the athletes themselves, as they may herald the onset of a life-threatening event. Some conditions in athletes, often considered to be undoubtedly life-threatening, such as syncope, to the contrary, are not always associated with a risk of sudden death, although that risk should always be ruled out first. For example, cardiac diseases with a high risk of SCD that required a withdrawal from the sports were revealed only in two (0.4%) of 474 young athletes with syncope [22]; these diseases were hypertrophic cardiomyopathy (HCM) in one case and arrhythmogenic right ventricular dysplasia/cardiomyopathy (ARVC) in the other. In our study [23], no diseases possessing a risk of SCD and requiring a withdrawal from sports have been identified in any of the 34 high-level athletes who had a history of syncope.

7. Causes of SCD

Elucidation of the etiological causes of SCD in athletes is one of the most controversial issues in this area. Meanwhile, it is one of the key issues for the development of scientifically based methods for SCD prevention, selection of individuals suitable for sports, and primary and secondary prevention of SCD. Due to new technologies in diagnostics and an increasing number of studies in this area, the opinions on the etiology of SCD have changed considerably. In the 1980s, among all SCD cases in young athletes in the USA, HCM was diagnosed in 36% of athletes who died suddenly, with the maximum left ventricular wall thickness from 15 to 40 mm (mean 23 ± 5 mm) and an average weight of the heart of 521 ± 113 g, followed by (in a descending order) coronary artery abnormalities and borderline left ventricular hypertrophy, interpreted as possible HCM [6]. However, we cannot exclude the possibility that it was exercise-induced cardiac hypertrophy (which is a component of the non-pathological athlete's heart), myocarditis, ARVC, and ion-channel cardiac disease or channelopathies (long or short QT syndrome, Brugada syndrome, idiopathic ventricular fibrillation, catecholaminergic ventricular tachycardia), i.e., diseases that can only be determined by an ECG prior to death. The long QT syndrome (LQTS) is the most dangerous ion-channel cardiac disease in young person and sports accordingly. Modern diagnostic of LQTS (in the absence of secondary causes for QT prolongation) is based on the ESC criteria [9]. At the present days, mutation in 16 various genes have been identified (LQTS1–LQTS16). The LQTS1 most dangerous during sports activity because 90% cardiac events (SCD, cardiac arrest, syncope) occur due adrenergic triggers and in water [24]. Other pathologies, such as mitral valve prolapse, aortic rupture, aortic stenosis, dilated cardiomyopathy, Wolff-Parkinson-White syndrome, rare non-specific myocardial damage (sarcoidosis), and other causes, were recorded in 1–2% of cases each.

A smaller (though with a more extended age range (11–65 years) analysis of sports-associated SCD cases in Spain [15] has demonstrated that in most cases the cause of SCD in all ages was ischemic heart disease (40.9%), arrhythmogenic cardiomyopathy (as in some cases there was not only right ventricular but biventricular dilatation, and this diagnosis was made) in 16.3% of cases, HCM (6.5%), left ventricular hypertrophy (4.9%), myocardial fibrosis (3.2%), nonatherosclerosis coronary artery abnormalities (3.2%), dilated cardiomyopathy (1.6%), etc. In 16.3% of cases, the cause of death remained unknown. When the observation group was divided into SCD cases occurring before and after 30 years of age, it was revealed that the majority of cases of ischemic heart disease were concentrated in the older age group (23 vs. 2 cases younger than 30 years) and that there was an equal number of cases of HCM, while ARVC, coronary artery abnormalities (so as spontaneous dissection), and all cases with uncertain autopsy results were more frequent among young individuals.

However, in the abovementioned French study [16] of SCD cases in athletes and persons regularly engaged in physical activity aged below 35 years, the percentage of HCM reached 10%, while cases classified as "unexplained death" accounted for 36%; according to the data from the US National Collegiate Athletic Association, published in 2015 [5], the structure of SCD included unexplained death (classified as sudden unexplained death - SUD) in 25% cases, confirmed HCM in 8%, and not otherwise specified HCM in 8%. The most up-to-date information on the subject is probably presented in the 2016 report by the British Registry of SCD in sports [4], where SUD in all age categories constituted 42% and HCM, 6%. Marked changes in the age dynamics of SCD etiology were also noted. In the age group of over 35 years, SUD constituted 28% (idiopathic left ventricular hypertrophy with fibrosis (ILVHF) accounted for the same percentage); at the age of 18–35 years, the proportion of SUD increased to 44% (ILVHF to 14%), and in the youngest group of <18 years, the frequency of SUD was the highest (56%), while ILVHF rates decreased to 10%. Rates of HCM and myocarditis confirmed by autopsy remained virtually unchanged with age at 6–8% for HCM and 1–2% for myocarditis. The frequency of identified ARVC moderately increased with age, from 6% in athletes under 18 years old to 14% at the age of 18–35 and 18% in athletes aged over 35 years.

8. Ethnic differences

There are some ethnic differences in SCD rates depending on its cause. In general, for over 27 years of observation in the USA, white males dominated in a large cohort of athletes who died suddenly (46%), followed by African Americans and other minority (43%), and white and black and other minority females (8 and 3%) [6]. However, an analysis of specifically cardiovascular SCD in those who died from HCM and coronary artery abnormalities revealed significantly higher (more than twofold) rates in African Americans, while Caucasians were still at the top of the list for ARVC and primary electrical diseases (channelopathy). In the European study [21], the range of diseases identified in athletes suddenly dying was almost the same, yet there were significant differences in the frequency of the main variants of myocardial damage; ARVC was detected in 24% of cases, HCM in 2%, and myocarditis in 10%. If the proportion of the three major variants of myocardial damage (ARVC, HCM, and myocarditis), detected in suddenly dying young American and Italian athletes, is compared, similar aggregate values are obtained, namely, 38% in Italy and 46% in the USA. Taking into account all potential ethnic differences or autopsy reports, there may be a different interpretation of similar pathomorphological changes.

Nevertheless, it is obvious that the main risk group for SCD in athletes includes those with life-threatening cardiac arrhythmias and myocardial changes. However, the risk of SCD is significantly higher in athletes than in nonathletes with the same heart condition in the general population—by more than 5 times for ARVC, 2.6 times for coronary artery disease, 1.5 times for myocarditis, and more than 2 times for cardiac conduction system diseases [6].

9. SCD prevention in athletes

Solutions to this problem vary from country to country. In the USA, a group of American Heart Association (AHA) experts has proposed 12 steps that can help in the prevention of SCD in athletes at the initial screening stage [25]. These include the following conditions and medical history features:

Medical history:

1. Chest pain/discomfort on exertion

2. Sudden fainting/presyncope

3. Vertigo (dizziness) on exertion

4. Heart murmurs

5. High blood pressure (> 140/90 or more on the first measurement)

Family history:

1. Sudden death of the first-degree relatives aged under 50 years (first of all parents, brothers, sisters, and grandparents)

2. Cardiovascular disease in close relatives under 50 years

3. Cardiomyopathy, LQTS, Marfan syndrome, ARVC, or other conditions with a risk of life-threatening arrhythmias or coronary artery disease in relatives

Physical examination:

1. Femoral pulse

2. Marfan syndrome manifestations

3. Sitting BP measurements

It is noteworthy that an ECG is not included in this screening list. Supporting this approach, the guideline authors note that the rates of SCD in athletes in the USA and Italy (where an ECG is a compulsory component of the medical checkup in athletes before training) are about the same. A prospective cohort study in individuals aged below 36 years engaged in competitive sports was conducted in the Italian region of Veneto between 1979 and 1999. The most frequent cause of SCD in the study was ARVC (24%), followed by ischemic heart disease of atherosclerotic etiology (20%), abnormal outlet of coronary arteries (14%), and mitral valve prolapse (12%) [2]. Among older athletes (> 35–40 years), more than half of the cases of SCD were associated with ischemic heart disease, as in the general population.

Some other American studies support the use of an ECG as part of a medical checkup of athletes at the early stages. A large study of 5615 young athletes conducted in Nevada (USA) demonstrated that the sensitivity of an ECG in the identification of serious cardiovascular pathology was 70% compared to 3% in the group of athletes where only a medical history and physical examination were used [26]. The specificity of ECG was 97.4%. Only 0.4% (22 of 5615) were withdrawn from sporting competitions. The estimated "cost" of a life saved by using only clinical and medical history data in this study was USD 84,000, while by adding an ECG, it may be reduced almost twofold (USD 44,000).

In the Japanese study [27], the researchers evaluated ECG screening results in 68,503 school students, and the SCD incidence in adolescents involved in competitive sports was on average 1.32 per 100,000 per year. Three deaths occurred in children without preceding syncope or SCD cases in the family history. In one 14-year-old boy, HCM had been identified earlier, at the pre-screening stage, and he was withdrawn from the sport, but he still died suddenly while jogging. In two other cases (13- and 16-year-old boys), SCD occurred while playing handball and basketball, and both had a normal ECG, and no pathological changes were identified during autopsy. The estimated "cost" of a life saved by using ECG screening in this study was USD 8000 (26).

Together with history and physical examination, the mandatory instrumental part of the cardiac examination in members of Russian junior national teams (less 18 years old) consists of a 12-lead resting ECG (with using original normal ECG criteria, which were elaborated at 500 young elite athletes) [28], EchoCG, and bicycle ergometry or treadmill test. A more thorough examination (Holter monitoring, analysis of heart rate turbulence, ventricular late potentials, magnetic resonance therapy, tilt test, etc.) depends on the changes detected at the preliminary stage, as well as medical history features, such as syncope, sudden death in the family, ECG changes, etc.

Despite a rather sizable document, it seems to us that for so-called elite athletes in high-level sports, it would be beneficial to include Holter monitoring, for special indication in athletes with syncope, arrhythmias, palpitation, and pathological changes of ECG—long or short QT and others [29, 30].

The European experience, which formed the basis for the International Olympic Committee recommendations, includes gathering a detailed medical history with an emphasis placed on the identification of complaints of potentially arrhythmogenic origin (palpitations, heart pain, etc.), syncope, cardiovascular disease, and cases of SCD in the family, especially at a young (under 50 years) age, and physical and ECG examinations, especially focusing on abnormal heart murmurs, alterations in blood pressure, ECG criteria of heart chamber hypertrophy, signs of myocardial ischemia, shortening or lengthening of the QT and PR intervals, and ventricular and supraventricular tachyarrhythmias [2]. The use of such screening, including an ECG in assessing the risk of SCD for 25 years in Italy, has shown that the incidence of SCD in young athletes aged 12–35 years engaged in competitive sports declined from 3.6 SCD cases per 100,000 per year (one death per 27,777 athletes) in 1979–1981 to 0.4 deaths per 100,000 per year (one death per 250,000 athletes) in 2003–2004. In general, SCD in athletes included in the screening decreased by 89%, whereas the incidence of SCD in the population not covered by the screening has not changed during the period [2]. This was due primarily to an increase in early detection and withdrawal from competitive sports of young people suffering from HCM, ARVC, and dilated cardiomyopathy (from 4.4% in 1979 to 9.4% in 2004). ECG changes may be the only early marker of a risk of life-threatening arrhythmias and SCD in athletes. However, the interpretation of ECG in athletes has its own peculiarities; any potentially life-threatening changes may be affected by conditions specific only to sports. For instance, the QT interval is longer in athletes [31]; its shortening was revealed when using some anabolic agents in athleticism [32]. The emergence of new, noninvasive methods of electrocardiological diagnostics seems to be promising for risk group stratification in sports. Certain features of the QT interval frequency adaptation [33] and microvolt T-wave alternans [34, 35] may aid in the stratification of athletes with electrical instability of the heart and an increased risk of life-threatening arrhythmias and SCD, and they may differentiate pathological and non-pathological transformations of the athlete's heart. The 2015 European Society of Cardiology Guidelines for the prevention of SCD proposes the following algorithm of SCD prevention in athletes [9]:

Prevention of sudden cardiac death in athletes (ESC).

Recommendations	Class	Level	Reference
Careful history taking to uncover underlying cardiovascular disease, rhythm disorder, and syncopal episodes or family history of SCD is recommended in athletes	I	C	This panel of experts
Upon identification of ECG abnormalities suggestive of structural heart disease, echocardiography and/or CMR imaging is recommended	I	C	This panel of experts
Upon identification of ECG abnormalities suggestive of structural heart disease, echocardiography and/or CMR imaging is recommended	IIa	C	This panel of experts
Physical examination and resting 12-lead ECG should be considered for pre-participation screening in younger athletes	IIa	C	This panel of experts
Middle-aged individuals engaging in high-intensity exercise should be screened with history, physical examination, SCORE, and resting ECG	IIa	C	[36]
Staff at sporting facilities should be trained in cardiopulmonary resuscitation and on the appropriate use of automatic external defibrillators	IIa	C	[37, 38]

ESC = European Society of Cardiology, CMR = cardiac magnetic resonance, ECG = electrocardiogram, SCD = sudden cardiac death, SCORE = systematic coronary risk evaluation, Class = class of recommendation (I, IIa, IIb, III), Level = level of evidence (A, B, C), Reference = reference(s) supporting recommendations.

The main fatal arrhythmia leading to death is ventricular fibrillation. If this develops, the most effective method for treatment is electric defibrillation. As was shown above, the majority of SCD cases in athletes occur during engagement in sports [2, 6], in contrast to similar data from nonathletes where up to 80% of SCD cases are registered at home [29, 30]. This enables the creation of a system of more effective medical aid in the first few minutes after cardiac arrest during physical activity. According to the US National Registry of Sudden Death, in cases of sudden death associated with exercise in young people over the period from 2000 and 2006, the percentage of survival in the latter 3 years of the study almost doubled compared to the first 3 years, reaching 14–17% [39]. And only in 2006, similar rates of successful recovery after cardiac arrest were achieved by using automatic external defibrillators (AED), which are publicly available, and electrical defibrillation performed by specialized emergency teams [39]. There were many reports of successful defibrillation in cardiac arrest in athletes during physical activity or competition [19].

Labor costs, effectiveness, and economic costs of comprehensive preventive screening in 785 athletes aged 5–65 years who are engaged in high-intensity sports [38] were also evaluated. As a result of this screening, newly diagnosed cardiovascular diseases were identified in 2.8% of athletes; economic costs were USD 199 per athlete. The researchers consider such a screening to be warranted and affordable. The guidelines also highlight the importance of training coaches and staff in sports centers on the actions needed in case of emergency, performing cardiopulmonary resuscitation and the use of AED, both in athletes and spectators during major competitions [37].

Regular physical activity in the young is the most effective prophylactic for all cardiac diseases, but SCD in young athletes remains rare but a very tragic event for the family, friends, and society, which can arise deep negative resonance media about sports. Prevention of SCD in the young athletes is based on careful pre-participation screening of young athletes for identifying diseases with risk of SCD during sports activity and to elaborate a detailed plan of the first aid during and after cardiac events in sports competition and any sports activity, it is necessary to perform careful pre-participation screening of young athletes for identifying diseases with high risk of SCD during sports activity and to elaborate a detailed plan of the first aid after cardiac events during sports competition and any sports activity.

Author details

Leonid Makarov
Center for Syncope and Cardiac Arrhythmias in Children and Adolescents, Central Children Clinical Hospital Russian Federal Medico Biology Agency (FMBA of Russia), Academy of Postgraduated Education FMBA of Russia, Moscow, Russia

*Address all correspondence to: dr.leonidmakarov@mail.ru

References

[1] Myerburg RJ, Castellanos A. Cardiac arrest and sudden cardiac death. In: Braunwald E, editor. Heart Disease: A Textbook of Cardiovascular Medicine. New York: WB Saunders Publishing Co; 1997. pp. 742-779

[2] Corrado D, Basso C, Pavei A, Michieli P, Schiavon M, Thiene G. Trends in sudden cardiovascular death in young competitive athletes after implementation of a preparticipation screening program. Journal of the American Medical Association. 2006;**296**:1593-1601

[3] Corrado D, Antonio P, Hans HB, Luc V, Alessandro B, Mats B, et al. Cardiovascular preparticipation screening of young competitive athletes for prevention of sudden death: Proposal for a common European protocol. European Heart Journal. 2005;**26**:516-524

[4] Finocchiaro G, Papadakis M, Robertus J-L, Dhutia H, Alexandros KS, Maite T, et al. Etiology of sudden death in sports: Insights from a United Kingdom regional registry. Journal of the American College of Cardiology. 2016;**67**(18):2108-2115

[5] Harmon KG, Asif IM, Maleszewski JJ, Owens DS, Prutkin JM, Salerno JC, et al. Incidence, cause, and comparative frequency of sudden cardiac death in National Collegiate Athletic Association athletes a decade in review. Circulation. 2015;**132**:10-19

[6] Maron BJ, Haas TS, Ahluwalia A, Murphy CJ, Garberich RF. Demographics and epidemiology of sudden deaths in young competitive athletes: From the United States National Registry. The American Journal of Medicine. 2016;**129**:1170-1177

[7] Maron BJ, Pelliccia A. The heart of trained athletes: Cardiac remodeling and the risks of sports, including sudden death. Circulation. 2006;**114**:1633-1644

[8] Mont L, Pelliccia A, Sharma S, Biffi A, Borjesson M, Terradellas JB, et al. Pre-participation cardiovascular evaluation for athletic participants to prevent sudden death: Position paper from the EHRA and the EACPR, branches of the ESC. Endorsed by APHRS, HRS, and SOLAECE. European Journal of Preventive Cardiology. 2017;**24**(1):41-69

[9] Priori SG, Blomstrom-Lundqvist C, Mazzanti A, Blom N, Borggrefe M, John C, et al. ESC guidelines for the management of patients with ventricular arrhythmias and the prevention of sudden cardiac death. European Heart Journal. 2015;**36**(41):2793-2867

[10] Van Camp SP, Bloor CM, Mueller FO, Cantu RC, Olson HG. Nontraumatic sports death in high school and college athletes. Medicine & Science in Sports & Exercise. 1995;**27**(5):641-647

[11] Quigley F. A survey of the causes of sudden death in sport in the Republic of Ireland. British Journal of Sports Medicine. 2000;**34**:258-261

[12] Tabib A, Miras A, Taniere P, Loire R. Undetected cardiac lesions cause unexpected sudden cardiac death during occasional sport activity. A report on 80 cases. European Heart Journal. 1999;**20**:900-903

[13] Ragosta M, Jeannie C, Sturner WQ, Thompson PD. Death during recreational exercise in the state of Rhode Island. Medicine and Science in Sports and Exercise. 1984;**16**:339-342

[14] Maron BJ, Doerer JJ, Haas TS, Estes NA, Hodges James S, Link MS. Commotio cordis

and epidemiologe of sudden death in competitive lacrosse. Pediatrics. 2009;**124**(3):966-971. DOI: 10.1542/peds.2009-0167

[15] Paz S-MM, Aguilera B. Causes of sudden death during sports activities in Spain. Revista Española de Cardiología. 2002;**55**(4):347-358

[16] Marijon E, Tafflet M, Celermajer DS, Dumas F, Perier M-C, Mustafic H, et al. Sports-related sudden death in the general population. Circulation. 2011;**124**:672-681

[17] Bode F, Franz M, Wilke I, Bonnemeier H, Schunkert Y, Wiegand UKH. Ventricular fibrillation induced by stretch pulse: Implications for sudden death due to commotio cordis. Journal of Cardiovascular Electrophysiology. 2006;***17***:1011, 2006-1017

[18] Link MS, Maron BJ, Wang PJ, Vander Brink BA, Zhu W, Estes MNA. Upper and lower limits of vulnerability to sudden arrhythmic death with chest-wall impact (commotio cordis). Journal of the American College of Cardiology. 2003;**41**:99-104

[19] Strasburger J, Maron BJ. Commotio Cordis. New England Journal Medicine. 2002;**347**(16):17

[20] Northcote R, Flannigan C, Ballantyne D. Sudden death and vigorous exercise–A study of 60 deaths associated with squash. British Heart Journal. 1986;**55**(2):198-203

[21] Corrado D, Cristina B, Giulio R, Maurizio S, Gaetano T. Does sports activity enhance the risk of sudden death in adolescents and young adults? Journal of the American College of Cardiology. 2003;**42**(11):1959-1963

[22] Colivicchi F, Ammirati F, Santini M. Epidemiology and prognostic implications of syncope in young competing athletes. European Heart Journal. 2004;**25**(19):1749-1753

[23] Makarov L, Komoliatova V. Syncope in the young elite athletes. European Heart Journal. 2013;**34**(Suppl 1):1363

[24] Panhuyzen-Godkoops N, Arthur W. Channelopathy in athletes. In: Pellicia A, Heinbuchel H, Corrado D, Sharma S, editors. The ESC Textbook of Sport Cardiology. UK: Oxford University Press; 2019. pp. 253-264

[25] Maron BJ, Thompson PD, Ackerman MJ, Gary B, Stuart B, David C, et al. American Heart Association Council on nutrition, physical activity, and metabolism recommendations and considerations related to preparticipation screening for cardiovascular abnormalities in competitive athletes: 2007 update: A scientific statement from the American Heart Association Council on nutrition, physical activity, and metabolism: Endorsed by the American College of Cardiology Foundation. Circulation. 2007;**115**(12):1643-1455

[26] Fuller CM, McNulty CV, Spring DA, Arger RM, Bruce SS, Chryssos BE, et al. Prospective screening of 5,615 high school athletes for risk of sudden cardiac death. Medicine & Science in Sports & Exercise. 1997;**29**:1131-1138

[27] Tanaka Y, Yoshinaga M, Anan R, Tanaka Y, Nomura Y, Oku S, et al. Usefulness and cost effectiveness of cardiovascular screening of young adolescents. Medicine & Science in Sports & Exercise. 2006;**38**:2-6

[28] Makarov L, Vera K, Vlad K, Natalia F, Irina K. The peculiarity of the rest electrocardiograms in young elite athletes. The European Journal of Preventive Cardiology. 2013;**20**(1)

[29] Makarov L, Komoliatova V, Kiseleva I, Fedina N, Besportochny D. The role of Holter monitoring in the

examination of young elite athletes. The European Journal of Preventive Cardiology. 2015a;**22**:S126

[30] Makarov L, Komoliatova V, Fedina N, Solokhin Y. Prevalence of out-of-hospital sudden cardiac death in Moscow in 2005-2009. Advances in Epidemiology. 2015b. 6 p. Article ID: 310878

[31] Moss AJ. What duration of the QTc interval athletes from competitive sports? European Heart Journal. 2007;**28**:2825-2826

[32] Ali Babaee Bigi M, Amir A, Arsalan A. Short QT interval: A novel predictor of androgen abuse in strength trained athletes. Annals of Noninvasive Electrocardiology. 2009;**4**(1):35-39

[33] Genovesi S, Daniele Z, Emanuela R, Maria GV, Andrea S, Marco S-B. Effects of exercise training on heart rate and QT interval in healthy young individuals: Are there gender differences? Europace. 2007;**9**:55-60

[34] Inama G, Claudio P, Ornella D, Massimiiano N, Giorgio D, Rita P, et al. Microvolt T-wave alternans for risk stratification in athletes with ventricular arrhythmias: Correlation with programmed ventricular stimulation. Annals of Noninvasive Electrocardiology. 2008;**13**:14-21

[35] Madias JE. Athletes, ventricular arrhythmias, electrophysiological testing, microvolt T-wave alternans, and a follow-up of 30 ± 21 months: A need for follow-up updates. Annals of Noninvasive Electrocardiology. 2008;**13**:319-320

[36] Nolan JP, Soar J, Zideman DA, Biarent D, Bossaert LL, Deakin C, et al. Group ERCGW. European resuscitation council guidelines for resuscitation 2010 section 1. Executive summary. Resuscitation. 2010;**81**:1219-1276

[37] Borjesson M, Serratosa L, Francois C, Corrado D, Drezner D, Dugmore DL, et al. Consensus document regarding cardiovascular safety at sports arenas: Position stand from the European Association of Cardiovascular Prevention and Rehabilitation (EACPR), section of sports cardiology. European Heart Journal. 2011;**32**:2119-2124

[38] Menafoglio A, Di Valentino M, Porretta AP, Foglia P, Segatto J-M, Siragusa P, et al. Cardiovascular evaluation of middle-aged individuals engaged in high-intensity sport activities: Implications for workload, yield and economic costs. British Journal of Sports Medicine. 2014;**49**:757-761

[39] Drezner JA, SDY CJ, Harmon Kimberly G, Linette D. Survival trends in the United States following exercise-related sudden cardiac arrest in the youth: 2000—2006. Heart Rhythm. 2008;**5**:794-799

Chapter 4

The Wearable Cardioverter-Defibrillator

Peter Magnusson, Joseph V. Pergolizzi and Jo Ann LeQuang

Abstract

The wearable cardioverter-defibrillator (WCD) is a rechargeable external device that can be worn under the clothing all day long and protects the wearer from potentially life-threatening ventricular tachyarrhythmias. When a dangerous arrhythmia is detected, the WCD can deliver high-energy shocks. The WCD has been shown to be effective in accurately detecting and appropriately treating ventricular tachycardia (VT) and ventricular fibrillation (VF). It is intended for temporary use as a bridge to an implantable cardioverter-defibrillator (ICD), heart transplantation, or left ventricular assist device; patients with heart failure with reduced ejection fraction may benefit from the WCD while their condition improves. It can be used temporarily after explant of an ICD until reimplantation is deemed possible. In select patients with myocardial infarction, a WCD may be useful during the immediate period after infarction. It is indicated for use when a permanently implanted ICD must be explanted because of infection; the patient can use the WCD until the infection resolves, and a new ICD can be implanted. The role of the WCD is emerging as an important therapeutic option to protect patients at elevated risk of sudden cardiac death (SCD).

Keywords: arrhythmia, cardiomyopathy, heart failure, heart transplantation, implantable cardioverter-defibrillator, sudden cardiac death, wearable cardioverter-defibrillator (WCD)

1. Introduction

Sudden cardiac death (SCD) is mainly due to ventricular tachyarrhythmias even though bradycardia may occur. The population at risk for SCD is heterogeneous and includes those whose risk is based on a transient arrhythmia-provoking electrical event, structural heart disease, a channelopathy, heart failure, cardiomyopathy, or other underlying conditions [1]. For patients at elevated risk for potentially life-threatening ventricular tachyarrhythmias but with a transient contraindication for an implantable cardioverter-defibrillator (ICD) therapy, the wearable cardioverter-defibrillator (WCD) is an important therapeutic option (LifeVest 4000®, Zoll, Pittsburgh, Pennsylvania, USA). The external vest delivers high-energy rescue therapy in the event a ventricular tachyarrhythmia is detected along with electrogram storage and remote monitoring [2]. First introduced to market in 2001, the WCD is intended for short-term use, typically for a few months [3].

IntechOpen

2. The WCD and its function

Currently, there is only one WCD, the LifeVest 4000®, and no other similar products are on the market. The WCD weighs 800 g and is available in a range of sizes with adjustable straps and an elasticized belt to fit snugly next to the skin under clothing (**Figure 1**). The WCD has three pad-style electrodes for defibrillation and four more electrodes for arrhythmia detection (sensing). It is equipped with a battery-powered defibrillation unit capable of generating several high-energy shocks. When the WCD prepares to deliver a shock, it delivers a small amount of gel to the skin at each electrode, and a biphasic waveform of 75 or 150 J is delivered [4].

The WCD detects arrhythmias using an algorithm of heart rate (including rate stability and onset of arrhythmia) and waveform morphology. In the presence of noise or when a waveform template is not available, the detection function can work using rate alone. Once an arrhythmia is detected, the device signals the patient for about 30 s, allowing the wearer to abort the shock by manually depressing two response buttons. If the rate drops below the detection threshold during this 30-s waiting period, the detection is delayed or the shock prevented, depending on whether the slower rate was brief and temporary or persisted [5]. The WCD offers programmable parameters in that the ventricular fibrillation (VF) zone can be set between 120 and 250 beats per minute (bpm) and the ventricular tachycardia (VT) zone can be programmed from 120 bpm to the lower bound of the VF zone [6]. The clinician may also program the time from arrhythmia detection to therapy delivery from 60 to 180 s for the VT zone and 25 to 40 s for the VF zone [5].

The WCD is rechargeable and comes with two lithium-ion batteries. One battery is used at all times in the device, while the other may be charged in about 3.5 h using a proprietary charging station. Battery life is approximately 2 days, but even if the battery signals the patient that it is getting low, there is usually sufficient charge retained for 10 shocks of 150 J each. During an arrhythmic episode, the WCD will deliver up to five shocks. If the arrhythmia persists, the device detects again and repeats the cycle until the rhythm is converted or the battery is exhausted [5]. Once the WCD delivers therapy, it should be replaced.

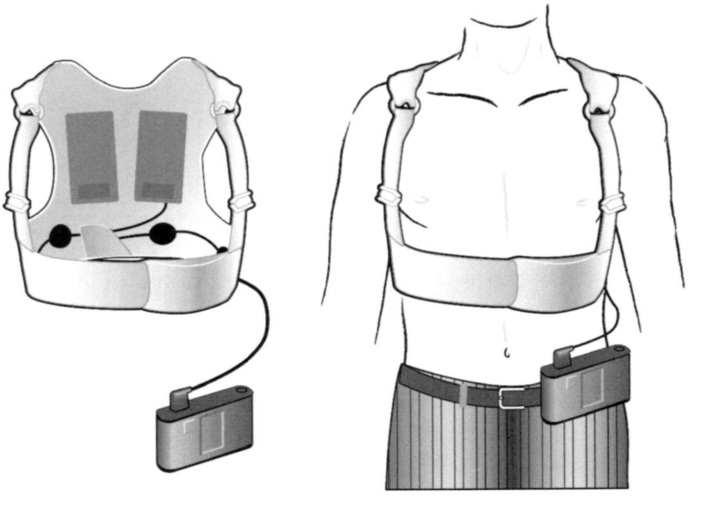

Figure 1.
The WCD (LifeVest 4000® from Zoll) is worn like a vest and is powered by a rechargeable battery, capable of delivering high-energy shocks to convert a potentially life-threatening ventricular tachyarrhythmia. Art by Todd Cooper.

DOI: http://dx.doi.org/10.5772/intechopen.90663

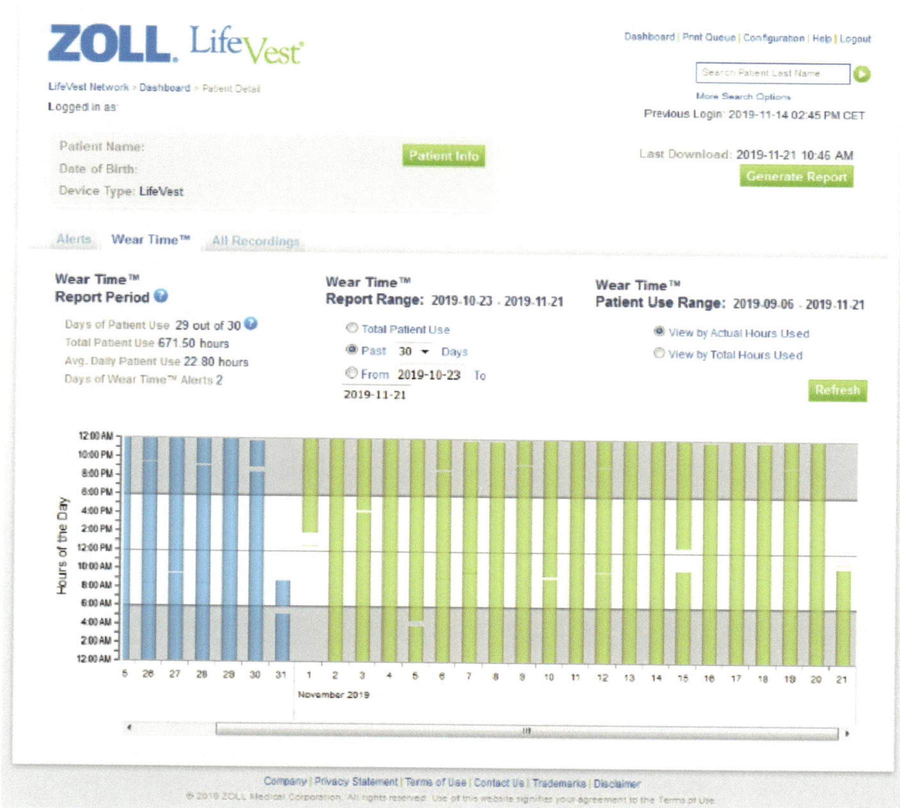

Figure 2.
The wear time: report on the WCD.

Patients are given a transmitter which can transmit data from the WCD directly to the clinic via a secure server. Remote transmissions do not require any patient intervention. Like cardiac implantable electronic devices, the WCD can be programmed to send out alerts when specific triggering events occur. The remote monitoring system records the number of hours per day that the patient wears the WCD, and the patient can activate the device to record an electrogram in the event of symptoms. While the WCD will attempt to make a daily remote transmission, if this is not possible, data transmission should occur at least once a week, and monthly in-clinic visits are recommended for WCD patients [5]. Reports from the WCD are shown in **Figures 2** and **3**.

3. Guidelines for the WCD

The American College of Cardiology, American Heart Association, and European Society of Cardiology (ACC/AHA/ESC) 2006 guidelines for the management of patients with ventricular arrhythmias and the prevention of sudden cardiac death was the first society-based recommendation for the use of WCD in patients at transient high risk for VF, such as patients waiting for heart transplant; patients at high risk following an acute myocardial infarction or invasive cardiac procedure; and patients whose ICD had to be temporarily explanted, for example, because of an infection [7]. The International Society for Heart and Lung Transplantation

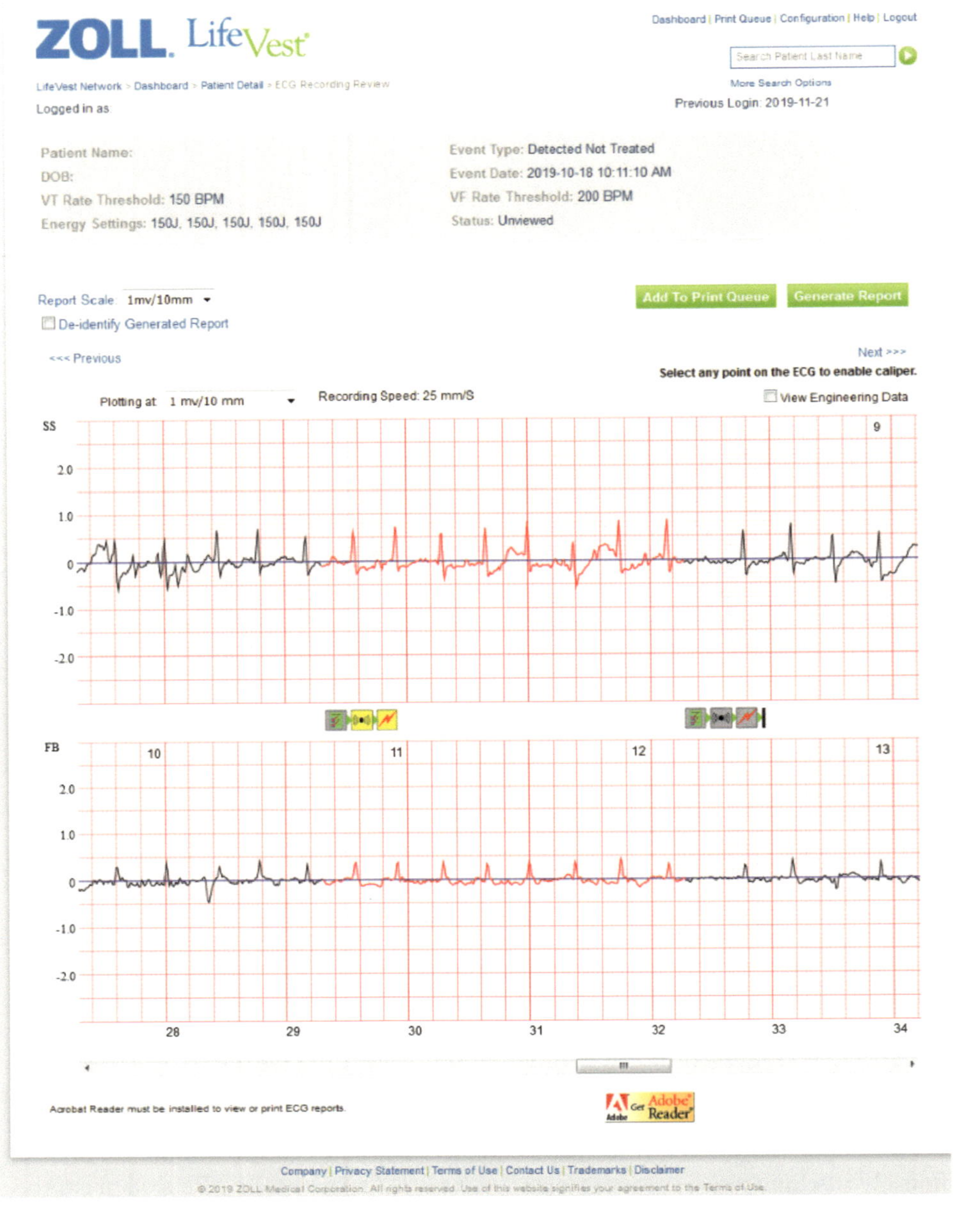

Figure 3.
Report from the WCD about a tachycardia that was detected but did not require therapy delivery.

guidance made the WCD a Class I indication for Status 1B patients awaiting transplant at home [8]. In 2009, the Heart Rhythm Society expert consensus recommended that the WCD be considered as an alternative treatment for patients who needed early ICD revision following device explant in the setting of suspected continuing infection [9]. In 2013, the ACC/AHA guideline stated that the utility of the WCD in high-risk patients in the first 4 to 6 weeks after myocardial infarction was being investigated [10]. The European Heart Rhythm Association, Heart Rhythm Society, and Asia Pacific Heart Rhythm Society (EHRA/HRS/APHRS) Expert Consensus on Ventricular Arrhythmias stated that patients with heart failure with reduced ejection fraction after a myocardial infarction (with or without revascularization) may benefit from WCD use in weeks to months until recovery [11]. Many patients who might be potential WCD candidates are not routinely included in clinical trials, and the HRS/ACC/AHA Expert Consensus Statement of 2014 suggested that the WCD may be considered as a "bridge to ICD" in certain patients [12]. The following year, in 2015, ESC guidelines suggested that the WCD might be used in patients with transiently impaired LV function, naming certain specific conditions such as myocardial infarction, peripartum cardiomyopathy, and myocarditis, and in patients awaiting heart transplantation or a left ventricular assist device [13].

In 2016, the AHA issued a science advisory about the WCD which was endorsed by the HRS [14]. Among their key concepts: they viewed the WCD as a temporary means for preventing arrhythmic death without the need of bystander response; despite limited evidence from randomized controlled trials, observational data support the notion that the WCD can detect and terminate ventricular tachyarrhythmias; and the use of a WCD is reasonable when there is a clear ICD indication and a current, transient contraindication to ICD implantation. According to this advisory, the role of a WCD is less clear when the risk of arrhythmias is transient, but a WCD still may be appropriate. The most controversial use of the WCD is in patients in the early recovery phase after myocardial infarction or with a newly diagnosed form of nonischemic cardiomyopathy. Many of these patients will not need a permanent ICD but will experience a period of time when they are at increased risk of SCD. Evidence for use of the WCD was C-level (expert opinion) and may be summarized as:

- The use of WCD is reasonable when there is an indication for an ICD, but a transient contraindication or interruption in ICD care (such as infection) temporarily prevents implantation (Class IIa).

- The use of WCD is reasonable as a bridge to more definitive therapy, such as heart transplant (Class IIa).

- The use of WCD may be reasonable if there is concern about an elevated SCD risk that is expected to resolve over time or with treatment, for example, ischemic heart disease following revascularization or nonischemic cardiomyopathy being initiated on guideline-directed medical therapy (Class IIb).

- The WCD may be appropriate as a bridge therapy when patients are at elevated risk for SCD in cases where an ICD would reduce the risk of SCD but not improve overall survival, such as within 40 days following acute myocardial infarction (Class IIb).

- WCDs should not be used when the risk for potentially life-threatening nonarrhythmic causes is expected to exceed the risk of ventricular arrhythmias, especially in those situations where longevity is not expected to exceed 6 months (Class III).

4. Clinical trials and other evidence

There are many observational studies about the use of the WCD, but to date only one large randomized clinical trial has been published, the Vest Prevention of Early

Study description	Appropriate therapy	Inappropriate therapy	Wear time	Comments
Acute myocardial infarction				
Barraud et al. 24 consecutive patients with LVEF <30% and recent myocardial revascularization	Two VT occurred (8.3%); one terminated spontaneously, and one was successfully treated	None	Mean 3.0 ± 1.3 months duration Daily wear time 21.5 hours/day	The WCD offered life-saving intervention for one patient
Kondo et al. 24 patients with myocardial infarction	Two patients (8.3%) received appropriate shock; both first shocks were successful	None	Median duration of WCD therapy was 33 days (range 20–67 days) Median daily wear time 23.1 h/day One patient excluded because of irregular use of WCD	In total, 58% went on to get ICD. Ejection fraction improved over baseline ($p < 0.01$) with 50% having an ejection fraction >35% Two patients (8.3%) died of fatal but non-arrhythmic events within 3 months
Controlled studies				
Olgin et al. VEST 2302 patients with myocardial infarction with ejection fraction ≤35% 1524 in WCD arm 778 controls	20 patients (1.3% of WCD group)	Nine patients (0.6% of WCD group)	Mean follow-up was 84.3 ± 15.6 days Wear time for WCD patients was median 18.0 h/d (3.8–22.7) with decreasing wear time over course of study	Arrhythmic death occurred in 1.6% and 2.4% of WCD and controls, respectively (not significant) All-cause mortality rates were 3.1% and 4.9% for WCD and controls, respectively ($p = 0.04$) Of the 48 WCD patients who died, only 12 were wearing the WCD at time of death
Heart failure				
Barsheshet et al. 75 heart failure patients prescribed a WCD in an observational study at 2 centers, SWIFT	Eight arrhythmic events occurred in 6.6% of patients (n = 5), all successful	None	Median wearing duration was 59 days, 80% of patients wore the WCD more than 50% of the day	At the end of study, 28% received an ICD
Duncker et al. PROLONG study 156 patients with ejection fraction ≤35% prescribed WCD for 3 months and then re-evaluated	Eleven patients received a total of 12 appropriate shocks	None	Cumulative 42.7 patient-years of wear time; mean time per patient was 101 ± 89 days Wear time 21.7 ± 4.0 h/day	48/156 discontinued therapy before 3 months (noncompliance, early improvement of ejection fraction, ICD implanted, etc.)

Study description	Appropriate therapy	Inappropriate therapy	Wear time	Comments
				33% of patients improved within 3 months to ejection fraction >35%
Heart transplantation				
Opreanu et al. 121 patients awaiting heart transplantation National registry based on convenience sample 55% NICM, 17% ICM, 27% mixed 32% were NYHA Class III and 34% Class IV	Seven patients (6%)	Two patients (1.7%)	Median wear time 39 days Median daily use 20 h/day	Eleven patients (9%) died in the study
Hemodialysis				
Wan et al. 75 hemodialysis patients with a history of SCA	75 patients (100%) experienced at least 1 SCA event while wearing the WCD 84 total events 136 total shocks delivered	Not reported	Mean duration of wear 62.9 ± 73.1 day (2–308 days) Mean daily wear 18.9 ± 4.6 h/day	Among patients with shockable rhythms, 30-day survival rate was 63.0%
Infected device				
Ellenbogen et al. 8058 patients who had an ICD removed for infection and used WCD as bridge to reimplant	334 patients (4%) experienced 406 VT/VF events, of which 348/406 (86%) were treated by WCD, all successfully 54 patients aborted shocks for arrhythmias that resolved spontaneously 12-month cumulative event rate 10%	159 patients (2%), no associated deaths	Median wear duration 53 days (25–94) Daily wear time not reported	Risk of VT/VF was highest in initial weeks after ICD removal at 0.9%, 0.7%, and 0.7% for first, second, and third weeks, respectively 30-day post-event survival rate was 81% overall 80% of patients in this study got an ICD
Observational studies from a single center				
Bhaskaran et al. Eight WCD patients	None	None	Median duration 77 days Mean daily wear 23.4 ± 0.6 h/day	1/8 patients in the study were noncompliant with WCD

Study description	Appropriate therapy	Inappropriate therapy	Wear time	Comments
Erath et al. 102 WCD patients	Four patients (3.9%)	Two patients (2.0%), both due to SVT	Median duration 54 days Median daily wear 23 h/day	55% received an ICD
Naniwadekar et al. 140 WCD patients 32% ICM, 46% NICM 85.9% African-Americans	Two patients (1.4%) received a total of two appropriate shocks	Two patients (1.4%) received a total of four inappropriate shocks (two SVT, two artifacts)	Median duration 43 days (7–83 days) Mean daily wear time 17.3 ± 7.5 h/day	Seven patients died 32% received an ICD
Roger et al. 105 consecutive patients with newly diagnosed ICM or NICM and ejection fraction ≤35%	Five patients (4.8%)	None	Mean duration of wear 68.8 ± 50.4 days Mean wear time 21.5 ± 3.5 h/day	At the end of WCD wear, 54.8% of ICM and 48.8% of NICM patients indicated for primary prevention ICD
Sasaki et al. Nine patients at risk for SCD	One patient (11.1%)	None	Median duration of use 21 days [7–31] Median wear time 23.7 h/day (23.6–23.9)	One patient died of worsening heart failure 67% received an ICD
Pediatric				
Spar et al. 455 patients (age 3–17 years)	Six patients (1.3%) received a total of 13 shocks	Two patients (0.4%)	Median duration of use 33 days (1–999) Median wear time 20.6 h/day (0.3–23.8)	Seven patients died, none of whom were wearing the WCD at time of death
Psychological aspects				
Weiss et al. 123 WCD patients from a multicenter registry administered several surveys	NA	NA	NA (study followed patients for 6 weeks)	Depressive symptoms decreased from 21% at baseline to 7% after 6 weeks of using the WCD Anxiety decreased from 52% at baseline to 25% at week 6
Registries				
Chung et al. National postmarket registry Retrospective analysis	First shock success was 100% (75/75) for unconscious VA and	Inappropriate shocks occurred in 1.9% of patients in 4788 months of use, or 1.4% per month	Mean duration of wear 52.6 ± 69.9 days (range 1–1590 days)	14.2% of patients discontinued WCD Overall survival rate was 99.2% but

Study description	Appropriate therapy	Inappropriate therapy	Wear time	Comments
3569 WCD patients Compared against Social Security Death Index	99% (79/80) for all VA 89.5% survival of VA events	Multiple reasons for inappropriate shock. Some of these shocks could have been aborted by patients, but patients did respond	Median daily wear time was 21.7 h/day 52% of patients wore WCD >90% of day	no significant difference compared to first ICD implant patients
Daimee et al. 1732 grouped as older (≥65, n = 722) and younger (<65 years, n = 1010)	Older patients had higher event rates per 100 patient-years for sustained VT and VF (32.0 vs. 9.8, (p = 0.027) Older patients, especially those with ICM were more likely to have VT/VF treated with shock (6.9 vs. 2.4, p = 0.034)	Not reported except as being "rare"	Older patients had significantly longer wear times (median 22.8 h/day vs. 22.3 h/day $p < 0.001$)	Younger patients with NICM had higher event rates per 100 patient-years for atrial arrhythmias (150.0 vs. 74.9, p = 0.055) Older patients were more likely to get an ICD after WCD (41.8% vs. 36.5%, p = 0.034)
Kutyifa et al. 3195 (805 with ICM, 927 with NICM, 268 with congenital heart disease) WEARIT-II Registry	41 patients had 120 episodes of sustained VT, of whom 54% received an appropriate shock	0.5% of patients got an inappropriate shock	Median duration of wear was 90 days Median wear time 22.5 h/day	At the end of WCD use, 42% got an ICD; most frequent reason not to get an ICD was improved ejection fraction
Lamichhane et al. 220 WCD patients in manufacturer's postmarket registry of individuals who wore the WCD > 1 year 33.2% of the patients were African-Americans	4.1% A total of 13 sustained VT episodes with 92.3% success rate (12/13 shocks)	3.6%	Mean duration was 451 ± 290 days Median wear time 20.4 h/day (15.5–22.9)	Two patients died (one refractory VT and one bradycardia transitioning to asystole), and 59% of patients stopped using the WCD before the study ended, either because they got an ICD, their condition improved, they had another intervention (transplant), or other reasons
Retrospective analyses				
Bossory et al. 201 patients from 1 center prescribed a WCD with 1 year follow-up	Five patients (2.5%), nine shocks	One patient (0.5%), SVT	Mean duration was 63 ± 53.7 days Mean wear time 23.0 ± 0.62 h/day	79% of WCDs were prescribed by clinicians who were not EPs

Study description	Appropriate therapy	Inappropriate therapy	Wear time	Comments
Dillon et al. 2105 WCD patients in a retrospective analysis of arrhythmia detection	1.58 appropriate shocks per 100 patient-months 54 total appropriate shocks	0.99 inappropriate shocks per 100 patient-months 34 total inappropriate shocks, most due to interference (47.1%)	Data for 1 year were analyzed Median duration of use was 36 days (3–365) Median wear time 21.3 h/day (0–23.9)	Most frequent reason for wearing the WCD was myocardial infarction, but study included several indications
Ellenbogen et al. population came from 234 consecutive in-hospital episodes of VT/VF in 173 in-hospital patients who had a WCD for primary prevention, history of VA, or other reasons, including device explant; 40% had a history of myocardial infarction	100% had an appropriate shock 68% occurred during weekdays, and 55% of events happened in the daytime	Not reported	Median follow-up 6 days while patients were in the hospital	Most VA occurred in unmonitored units, the ICU, and the ED 24-h survival following therapy delivery was >90%
Quast et al. 79 WCD patients	Two patients (2.6%) for annual rate of 13.6%	One patient (1.3%) for annual rate of 6.7%	Median duration 73 days (50.0–109.8) Median daily wear time 23.3 h/day (22.6–23.7)	In 52.2% ejection fraction improved enough that ICD implant was not necessary
Salehi et al. 127 patients with CM and self-reported excessive alcohol use	Seven patients (5.5%) had nine sustained VT episodes, 100% successful conversion	Not reported	Median duration 51 days Median wear time 18.0 h/day	11 patients (8.6%) died during the 100 days of follow-up, but no deaths were caused by WCD shock failure or undersense
Singh et al. 639 WCD patients ICM and NICM	None for NICM patients Six ICM patients (2.2%), of whom five survived the shock and four survived to hospital discharge	Three NICM patients (1.2%) 0.7% of ICM	Mean duration 61 days (25–102) Mean daily wear 22 h/day	
Uncontrolled studies				
Beiert et al. 114 patients ICM (31.6%) NICM (45.6%) Congenital heart disease (5.3%)	6.1% (no NICM patients were shocked) One patient had an appropriate but ineffective shock and was externally defibrillated	64 patients (56.6%) were signaled inappropriately for a shock, almost all due to artifacts. All shocks were aborted by the	Median duration 52.0 days (range 25–90) Daily wear time 23.1 h/day (19.0–23.8)	One patient in this study died of asystole

DOI: http://dx.doi.org/10.5772/intechopen.90663

Study description	Appropriate therapy	Inappropriate therapy	Wear time	Comments
Infected device removal (11.4%) and others		patients, no inappropriate shocks delivered		
Feldman et al. WEARIT (n = 177) and BIROAD (n = 112) studies WEARIT patients had symptomatic heart failure and ejection fraction < 30% BIROAD patients had acute myocardial infarction and were in waiting period of 30–40 days before an ICD could be implanted	Eight appropriate shocks of which 75% were successful The two unsuccessful shocks were deemed related to improperly placed electrodes	Six inappropriate shocks (0.67% unnecessary shocks/month)	Mean duration of use was 3.1 months (2.6 for BIROAD and 3.4 for WEARIT groups, respectively) Daily wear time not reported	12 patients died (5 of whom were not wearing WCD, and 1 wore it improperly) 68 patients dropped out of study for adverse events or discomfort wearing the WCD
Wassnig et al. 6043 WCD patients	94 patients (1.6%) were shocked Incidence rate 8.5% (95% CI, 6.7–10.7) per 100 patient-years for men and 7.9% (95% CI, 4.8–12.3) for women 94% success rate	26 patients (0.4%), incidence 2.3 (95% CI, 1.5–3.4) per 100 patient-years In 10 cases, the reason was SVT	Median duration varied from 49 to 66 days Median daily wear varied from 22.7 to 23.5 h/day	Patients with explanted ICDs had higher average rates of shock (19.3 per 100 patient-years, 95% CI, 12.2–29.0)
Zylla et al. 106 real-life cases taken from 2010 to 2016	One patient (0.94%) shocked for VF, successful	Two patients (1.9%) 12.3% had an average of >1 inappropriate shock alarms per day (shocks aborted)	Median duration of wear 58.5 days Mean wear time 22.7 h/day Younger patients (≤ 50 years) less compliant	17% discontinued therapy for various reasons: discomfort, frequent alarms, reimbursement problems, technical issues

AMI, acute myocardial infarction; CI, confidence interval; CM, cardiomyopathy; EP, electrophysiologist; ICD, implantable cardioverter-defibrillator; ICM, ischemic cardiomyopathy; NICM, nonischemic cardiomyopathy; NYHA, New York Heart Association; SCA, sudden cardiac arrest; SCD, sudden cardiac death; SVT, supraventricular tachycardia; VA, ventricular arrhythmia; VF, ventricular fibrillation; VT, ventricular tachycardia; WCD, wearable cardioverter-defibrillator.

Table 1.
An overview of the main uses of the WCD, therapy deliveries, and key findings [15, 17–44].

Sudden Death (VEST) study (n = 2302) [15]. All patients had had a recent myocardial infarction and a left ventricular ejection fraction ≤35%; some but not all patients had undergone revascularization. Patients were randomized into two arms: guideline-directed medical treatment (control) or a WCD. In the first 90 days after myocardial infarction, the WCD did not result in a lower rate of arrhythmic death, but total mortality was lower in the WCD group (3.1% vs. 4.9%, $p = 0.04$, uncorrected) [15]. Despite the fact that the VEST study did not result in a lower rate of arrhythmic death for WCD patients, there are important aspects of this study that deserve deeper scrutiny. Unwitnessed arrhythmic death is difficult to ascertain, and five of the nine VEST subjects deemed to have died due to an arrhythmia were wearing the WCD at the time, and the WCD showed no evidence of a tachyarrhythmia. Since arrhythmic death is rare, even a small number of misinterpretations in a study like this may skew results. Moreover, the study was designed assuming patients would wear the WCD at least 70% of the time, and compliance dropped as the study progressed. Since fewer patients wearing the WCD died, it has been argued that there was not a single active treatment group in the study (WCD group) but rather two: patients randomized to the WCD group broken down into those who wore the WCD and those who did not [16]. Of the patients in the WCD arm of the study who died, 75% were not wearing the WCD at the time [15].

Early after the WCD was first cleared to market, an observational study called the Wearable Defibrillator Investigative Trial (WEARIT) enrolled 177 ambulatory patients who had New York Heart Association (NYHA) functional Class III or IV heart failure and an ejection fraction <30%. It was subsequently combined with a similar observational study, the Bridge to ICD in patients at risk of sudden arrhythmic death (BIROAD), which enrolled patients who had an AMI and needed bridge therapy for up to 3 months (n = 112). In 901 patient-months, the mean duration of wear was 3.1 months. Among the WEARIT patients, there were two appropriate and successful therapy deliveries in the same patient several days apart, and there were four appropriate, successful therapies delivered in two of the BIROAD patients. Two unsuccessful therapy deliveries occurred, both of which involved the improper wear of the WCD. Altogether, 12 patients died over the course of the study, none of whom were wearing the WCD at the time. Over the 901 patient-months, there were 6 inappropriate therapy deliveries in 6 patients (0.7% per month) [17].

The WEARIT-II Registry enrolled 2000 patients, of whom 805 were diagnosed with ischemic cardiomyopathy, 927 with nonischemic cardiomyopathy, and 268 with congenital heart disease [18]. During the study, 41 patients experienced a total of 120 episodes of VT, of whom 54% received an appropriate shock. Inappropriate shocks occurred in 0.5% of patients. Many of the patients in WEARIT-II had improved their ejection fraction over the course of time they wore the WCD, and at the end of WCD treatment, only 42% got an ICD.

The Study of Wearable Cardioverter Defibrillator in Advanced Heart-Failure Patients (SWIFT) was a nonrandomized prospective study at two centers evaluating the use of the WCD in 75 patients hospitalized with advanced heart failure symptoms and LV dysfunction. Patients wore the WCD for 3 months after hospital discharge. Two-thirds of the patients (66%) had nonischemic cardiomyopathy. Eight arrhythmic events occurred in five patients, all successfully terminated by the WCD. No inappropriate therapies were delivered, and no patients died in the course of the study. When the study concluded, 28% were implanted with an ICD [19].

A summary of these trials appears in **Table 1**.

5. Patient populations

5.1 Transient contraindication for an ICD

One of the main reasons for WCD use is ICD system infection, which poses a clinical challenge in that the best course of action is to extract the device and lead(s), submit the patient to a course of antibiotic therapy, and then replace the ICD system with a new device [7, 9, 45]. The rate of infections associated with cardiac implantable electronic systems continues to increase, even at high-volume centers [46]. Antimicrobial therapy may last 10–14 days or longer, depending on the nature of the infection and the patient's response. During this time, the patient is without an ICD. Leaving the ICD in place while treating an infection is associated with a high mortality rate (31–66%) [47, 48], but removing the device also increases the patient's mortality rate, albeit from 8–27% [49–51]. Thus, the clinician faces three challenges: if the device is replaced too early, the patient risks re-infection; if the patient is deprived of the device too long, there is a risk for potentially life-threatening arrhythmias; and placing the patient under close monitoring in the hospital or a long-term care facility is cost prohibitive and deleterious to the patient's quality of life. In such cases, the use of a WCD can be a valuable interim solution for arrhythmic rescue.

In a study of 97 ICD patients whose devices had to be explanted for infection, patients were prescribed a WCD for the mean antimicrobial treatment course of 21 days. As they recovered from infection, two patients experienced a total of four VT episodes, all of which could be successfully treated [52]. In a retrospective analysis of 8058 patients who received a WCD from 2002 to 2014 when an infected ICD was removed, 4% experienced ventricular tachyarrhythmias, and the rate of arrhythmic episodes was greatest in the first 3 weeks after device explantation (0.9, 0.7, and 0.7%, respectively), and the risk for ventricular tachyarrhythmias after device removal was 4% during the first 2 months and 10% at 1 year [25].

5.2 Bridge to cardiac transplantation/left ventricular assist device

Heart transplantation or the use of a left ventricular assist device is the only potentially long-term therapeutic option for some patients, but during the waiting period, patients are at high risk for dangerous arrhythmias and may have other comorbid conditions as well. In a study of 121 patients prescribed with the WCD while waiting to receive a donor heart (mean 127 days), 7 patients (5.8%) were shocked appropriately, and all survived [23]. Two inappropriate therapy deliveries occurred deemed to be caused by rapid ventricular response to atrial fibrillation. In this study, two patients died of asystole during the waiting period; asystole is not treated by the WCD because it lacks a pacing capability [23].

5.3 Low ejection fraction in reimbursement-mandated waiting period

In the USA and other parts of the world, patients with an ejection fraction ≤35% may be required by reimbursement authorities and guidelines to wait out a specific period of time before an ICD may be implanted; these time periods range from 30 to 90 days. This includes patients with cardiomyopathy.

5.4 NYHA Class IV heart failure

This group of patients meets the requirements for Class IV heart failure but is not otherwise indicated or qualified to receive an ICD. Some of these patients may be waiting for cardiac transplantation, while others may be contraindicated for ICD implant for other reasons (frailty, comorbidities, patient refusal, and so on). The Study of Wearable Cardioverter Defibrillator in Advanced Heart-Failure Patients (SWIFT) was a prospective study of 75 advanced heart failure patients at 2 centers. All patients had low ejection fraction (21.5 ± 10.4% at baseline), were prescribed a WCD, and were followed up for 3 months. In the SWIFT study, 66% of patients had nonischemic cardiomyopathy. Over the course of the study, eight arrhythmic events occurred in five patients, including three episodes of nonsustained VT and one episode of polymorphic VT; all episodes were appropriately treated. No patient in the study received inappropriate therapy delivery. At the end of the study, 28% of patients went on to permanent device implantation, and the cumulative mortality rate at 3 years in this population was 21% for patients with nonischemic cardiomyopathy compared to 21% for those with ischemic cardiomyopathy [19].

5.5 Ischemic and nonischemic cardiomyopathy

Patients with ischemic cardiomyopathy may be indicated for a primary prevention ICD if they have an ejection fraction ≤35% and NYHA functional Class II or III or if they have an ejection fraction ≤30% with NYHA Class I [53]. Nonischemic cardiomyopathy covers a range of conditions that may include inflammatory, toxic, metabolic, genetic, or autoimmunological processes, and arrhythmic activity, including SCD, may be one of the first symptoms of nonischemic cardiomyopathy [5, 13]. Such patients typically fall into the reimbursement-mandated waiting period before a primary prevention ICD can be implanted, and many patients with recent-onset cardiomyopathy recover left ventricular ejection fraction and even experience reverse remodeling to the point that ICD implantation is unwarranted [5]. In cardiomyopathy patients, it is not clear if and how long patients should wait before ICD implantation is either deemed reasonable or unnecessary [5]. Ischemic cardiomyopathy patients may have higher rates of events than nonischemic cardiomyopathy patients [42]. Pharmacological therapy for cardiomyopathy may also improve the ejection fraction, and the WCD may be helpful as medical therapy is optimized [53].

In a retrospective single-center study of patients from June 2004 to May 2015, focus was placed on patients with newly diagnosed cardiomyopathy (254 nonischemic and 271 ischemic) [41]. Patients wore the WCD for a median of 61 days (interquartile range 25–102 days) and for a median of 22 h/day (17–23 h). The study produced 56.7 patient-years of data for nonischemic cardiomyopathy patients, during which no patients got appropriate shocks, but 1.2% (n = 3) were shocked inappropriately. There were 46.7 patient-years of data for ischemic cardiomyopathy, where 2.2% (n = 6) were shocked appropriately and two inappropriately (0.7%) [41].

5.6 Acute myocardial infarction

The role of defibrillation has been controversial in acute myocardial infarction (AMI) patients since the defibrillator in acute myocardial infarction trial (DINAMIT) reported that early ICD implantation failed to confer a mortality benefit in this arrhythmia-rich population [54]. Current guidelines recommend that following myocardial infarction, patients with compromised left ventricular function do not receive an ICD for a 3-month to 40-day waiting period, whether or not they have been revascularized [53]. In the weeks immediately following a myocardial infarction, patients are vulnerable to a number of potentially lethal conditions, many unrelated to ventricular tachyarrhythmias, so that the mortality rate for myocardial infarction patients with or without an ICD is roughly the same (7.2% for both, assuming linear mortality rates in the first 3 months, based on DINAMIT study data) [54]. This imposes a "waiting period" on myocardial infarction patients before a device may be implanted and during which time they may be especially vulnerable to SCD. For many patients and clinicians, this creates a tension between abiding by evidence-based guidelines and meeting reimbursement requirements yet still providing reasonable means to rescue post-AMI patients from SCD [6]. The WCD has been proposed as an interim device for this population during this waiting period before a permanent ICD may be implanted. Further complicating this picture is the fact that some myocardial infarction patients will recover left ventricular function in the weeks following their heart attack to the point that they do not require an ICD at all. Thus, it may be argued that for these patients, the use of the WCD may be to provide possible rescue during recovery from the myocardial infarction and to avoid unnecessary ICD implantation [6].

It has been observed that myocardial infarction patients prescribed a WCD and shocked appropriately and successfully to convert a ventricular tachyarrhythmia nevertheless have high mortality rates. While this remains to be elucidated, it suggests that either ventricular tachyarrhythmias in the immediate aftermath of a heart attack are indicative of poor outcomes or the arrhythmia and/or the rescue shock has a destabilizing effect on the patient [55]. The Valsartan in acute myocardial infarction trial (VALIANT) evaluated 14,609 myocardial infarction patients with low ejection fraction for SCD. VALIANT reported myocardial infarction patients with an ejection fraction ≤30% had a mortality of 2.3% per month in the first 30 days after the myocardial infarction (and that 83% of all patients who died of sudden unexpected death died within the first 30 days of hospital discharge). Every decrease of 5% in the ejection fraction was associated with a 21% increase in SCD risk in the first 30 days after myocardial infarction [56].

The Vest Prevention of Early Sudden Death (VEST) trial found that in myocardial infarction patients with low ejection fractions (≤35%), the WCD did not significantly reduce arrhythmia-associated deaths compared to the control group who did not have a WCD [15]. The rates of arrhythmic death were 1.6% in the WCD and 2.4% in the control group (relative risk 0.67, 95% confidence interval, 0.37–1.21, $p = 0.18$) [15]. It must be noted in this connection that arrhythmic death can be challenging to adjudicate when the patient dies without a witness. However, even comparing all-cause mortality data did not provide a significant benefit for WCD patients over those who did not have a WCD [15].

5.7 Renal failure

Compared to one SCD death per 1000 patient-years in the general population, hemodialysis patients face a 50-fold greater risk of arrhythmic death at 43 deaths per 1000 patient-years [57, 58]. Patients on hemodialysis present clinical challenges in that they are often comorbid and frequently geriatric, may be frail, and are prone to infections. End-stage renal disease and hemodialysis expose these patients to a very considerable risk of arrhythmic death, but many hemodialysis patients are not appropriate candidates for ICD therapy. Compared to historical data, the WCD has been associated with improved survival in renal failure patients [24].

5.8 Other conditions

5.8.1 Takotsubo cardiomyopathy

Takotsubo cardiomyopathy, sometimes called "broken-heart syndrome," is a form of cardiomyopathy where the myocardium weakens and remodels. This condition is potentially reversible, but while patients experience the cardiomyopathy, they are at risk for potentially life-threatening ventricular tachyarrhythmias, and some develop concomitant QT interval prolongation, further increasing their risk for arrhythmia [5]. In a study based on all data from the USA involving WCD wear from 2007 through 2012, a total of 102 takotsubo patients were identified by the ICD-9 code 429.83. This population was overwhelmingly female (89%) with an initial ejection fraction of 27 ± 6% who wore the WCD for a mean duration of 44 ± 31 days with a mean follow-up of 440 ± 374 days. During the WCD wear time, 2% of patients (n = 2) received an appropriate shock, 1% (n = 1) received two inappropriate shocks, and 2% (n = 2) suffered bradyarrhythmias that required pacing. Two patients in the study died (one asystole and one from an arrhythmia while not wearing the WCD) [59].

5.8.2 Peripartum cardiomyopathy

Peripartum cardiomyopathy results in left ventricular dysfunction that can predispose the patient to SCD. About half of these patients will recover significantly or entirely over the course of about 6 months even without intervention; however, some will not, and all are at high risk for arrhythmias during the course of the condition [5]. In a study of 12 consecutive women with peripartum cardiomyopathy observed at a single center (of whom seven wore the WCD), four episodes of VF occurred in three of the patients wearing the WCD, all of which were successfully terminated. One patient experienced numerous alarms for inappropriate shocks but was able to abort them so that no inappropriate shocks occurred. No deaths occurred. During therapy for heart failure, over the course of the 12-month follow-up, ejection fractions improved significantly from 24.0 ± 11.8% at baseline to 46.6 ± 7.6%. Patients with a lower ejection fraction at baseline improved more than those with a higher ejection fraction at baseline [60].

5.8.3 Long QT syndrome

Long QT syndrome (LQTS) is a heritable and potentially fatal cardiac channelopathy that exposes patients to the risk of SCD. LQTS patients are typically treated with beta blockade, left cardiac sympathetic denervation, and, in some cases, a permanent ICD. It is unclear what, if any, role the WCD might play for treating LQTS. A retrospective review of 1027 LQTS patients who were prescribed a WCD as a bridge to possible ICD implantation or other treatments found no inappropriate shocks that were administered by the WCD and only 1 patient received an appropriate shock to terminate VF [61]. Since LQTS is a lifelong condition, the WCD is not an optimal permanent solution in this population, but it may be helpful as newly diagnosed patients consider their therapeutic options or for LQTS patients on medical therapy who are entering high-risk periods of life, such as having to take a medication that might prolong their QT interval further or in postpartum women [61].

6. Special populations

The WCD is available in different sizes and has an elasticized waistband and adjustable straps, making it suitable for use in a variety of patients, including children. The role of the WCD in certain special populations is being addressed, but there is limited evidence about these groups.

6.1 Pediatric patients

Guidance is available to schools and teachers for children prescribed the WCD. In particular, it is important that educators realize that unlike the automatic external defibrillator systems available in many schools, the WCD will detect arrhythmias and treat them without any bystander intervention [62, 63]. Children seem to adjust well to the WCD. In a study of 231 pediatric WCD patients between the ages of 8 and 17 years monitored a median of 39 days with daily wear time around 21 h/day, a step-counter accelerometer device reported that activity levels for these children increased significantly over baseline in the first 3 weeks after getting the WCD ($p < 0.001$) [64]. This suggests that the WCD does not inhibit or curtail the children's activities and may help them achieve recommended levels of daily exercise.

6.2 Cancer patients

Some patients with cancer may be at elevated risk for dangerous arrhythmias because of chemotherapy-induced cardiomyopathy or long QT syndrome caused by drugs but may be contraindicated for device implant because of their malignancy or other reasons [65].

6.3 Geriatric patients

The prevalence of cardiovascular disease is high in the geriatric population, but there may be reluctance to consider an older patient for WCD therapy, in particular because it may be uncomfortable or feel restricting to them. In a large study of 1732 patients with ischemic and nonischemic cardiomyopathy, patients were grouped by age into younger (<65 years) and older groups (≥65 years). The older group ($n = 722$) wore the WCD more hours per day (median 22.8 vs. 22.3, $p < 0.001$) and had higher rates of events (31.95 vs. 9.82, $p = 0.027$). Younger patients with nonischemic cardiomyopathy had a higher rate of atrial arrhythmias (150.1 vs. 74.9, $p = 0.055$), and more following WCD therapy, a greater number of older than younger patients got a permanent ICD (41.8% vs. 36.5%, $p = 0.034$). Patients in both age groups tolerated WCD therapy well [34].

7. Appropriate and inappropriate therapy

The WCD has been shown to deliver appropriate high-energy therapy to convert dangerous ventricular tachyarrhythmias. In a postmarket registry of 3569 WCD patients (mean duration wear was 52.6 ± 69.9 days), first shock success occurred in 99% of cases (79/80) for all episodes of conscious VT/VF and in 100% of cases ($n = 76$) of unconscious VT/VF [33]. Because the WCD is an external device, it is far more exposed to sources of electromagnetic interference (noise) than implanted devices, which may result in oversensing, inappropriate arrhythmia detection, and inappropriate therapy delivery. Patients are signaled about 30 s prior to therapy delivery and may abort the shock by pressing two buttons [39, 40]. For this reason, the rate of inappropriate therapy delivery with the WCD is relatively low, occurring in approximately 0.4–3.0% of patients [6, 18, 33, 43]. See **Table 1**.

The WCD delivers rescue shock therapy only and has no pacing capability. Asystole, a recognized risk factor for dangerous ventricular tachyarrhythmias, may occur in patients with compromised cardiovascular function, such as low ejection fraction. While an ICD can detect and offer pacing support during an asystole episode, the WCD cannot pace such patients, and there is a risk that an untreated asystole may be fatal [66].

8. Patient factors

There are specific patient factors that warrant consideration when prescribing this novel therapeutic option. Many patients will have no concept of what a WCD is or how it works.

8.1 Patient education

Manufacturer's representatives may be available to help train patients in the proper function of the WCD, and, if they are not available, the clinical team should make sure the patient knows how to wear the vest, how to adjust it for proper fit, how to replace the battery, how to charge the battery, and how to transfer data from the WCD to the network. For this reason, the WCD requires the patient be able to understand and manage these tasks and be willing to do them. An initial training session should make sure the patient can put on the vest and insert batteries that may last an hour or more. It may be helpful for a second follow-up contact with the trainer over the course of the next few days to help with any questions or problems the patient may still have. The manufacturer has a 24-h technical support hotline for urgent questions [5].

8.2 Compliance

Compliance is an issue in all areas of medicine but particularly in the case of the WCD which patients may find restrictive or uncomfortable. A postmarket registry study ($n = 3569$) found that patients who used the WCD for a longer duration of time (days of wear) were significantly more likely to wear in more hours per day ($p < 0.001$) [33]. Over time, the WCD has been redesigned to make it lighter in weight and more comfortable for extended wear. Remote monitoring can alert the clinic as to actual wear time for an individual patient [67]. Compliance may be encouraged by educating the patient as to the nature of ventricular tachyarrhythmias and how the device protects them.

8.3 Psychological factors

It has been speculated that patients prescribed a WCD may experience emotional distress and view the device as a constant worrisome reminder of their own mortality. Patients may also feel isolated if they do not know anyone else who has ever worn such a device. Patients have sometimes reported that they find the device symbolic of their own vulnerability [33]. Of course, such adverse emotions may occur in all patients facing the sudden news that they have a serious cardiovascular condition regardless of whether they are prescribed a WCD or some other therapy. Psychological distress is an important clinical consideration because it is potentially modifiable. There may be ways to reduce depressive or anxious symptoms in clinically meaningful ways. Depression worsens outcomes and actually serves as a predictor for both mortality and shock therapy [68, 69]. Depression has been associated with a nearly doubled risk for all-cause mortality in ICD patients [69]. Furthermore, depression and anxiety may adversely affect patient compliance, adherence to pharmacological therapy, and lifestyle.

In another study of 123 patients considered WCD candidates, at baseline 21% showed signs of clinically depressive symptoms, and 52% had anxiety. Six weeks after WCD therapy commenced, rates of depression and anxiety dropped to 7 and 25%, respectively [32]. It is not clear if patients recovered their emotional equilibrium as a result of WCD therapy or as a matter of course as they got used to their new identities as cardiac patients.

8.4 Device-device compatibility

When a patient has more than one electronic cardiac device, the potential of device-device interaction exists. The literature reports one case of a fatal device-device interaction between a permanent pacemaker and a WCD [70]. In this case, the patient received unipolar dual-chamber pacing, but when he developed VF, no therapy was delivered as the device inappropriately detected the large unipolar pacing spikes as cardiac signals [70].

A study sponsored by Zoll examined pacing in 60 patients testing the AAI, VVI, and DDD modes in both unipolar and bipolar device configurations to determine if the WCD would detect the pacing spikes; patients were signaled before shock delivery and could use the patient response buttons to avert the therapy delivery. Only unipolar DDD pacing was detected by the WCD's algorithm and only in 10% of patients (6/60). This study suggests that pacing may occur concomitantly with WCD use if unipolar configurations are avoided [2]. If unipolar pacing must be used in a particular patient, then the WCD is contraindicated. Another study of the concomitant use of the WCD and a pacemaker showed that double-counting and waveform alterations might also occur in certain bipolar pacing modes and in single-chamber as well as dual-chamber pacing [44]. Caution is urged in using the WCD in patients with pacing support from an implanted pacemaker system.

9. Costs

The WCD is "rented" to patients for a monthly fee, and reimbursement provisions vary by country. Since costs can be substantial, there is a need to better stratify patients into those who truly need a WCD for arrhythmic rescue and those who might be unlikely to benefit from it [41]. Cost-effectiveness models show that the number needed to treat to save 1 life with a WCD falls in the range of 70–110 patients over a median of 53–57 days [26]. There are situations in which the WCD poses a decided cost advantage. For example, cardiomyopathy patients who might otherwise be considered a candidate for permanent primary prevention ICD implantation may benefit from using the WCD during a recovery period; data shows that ~60% of such patients will recover to the point that an ICD implantation is not necessary [18, 33, 41]. Thus, the costs for the temporary use of the WCD may be offset by the decision not to implant an ICD. In patients whose ICD must be removed for infection, it is sometimes necessary to keep the patient in the hospital or discharge him or her to a skilled nursing facility for weeks during antimicrobial therapy and recovery. The patient is at risk for SCD throughout this time. A cost-effectiveness analysis found that the WCD was cost-effective in this situation in that it allowed the patient to be discharged home; the analysis is based on the assumption that there was a 2-week 5.6% risk of SCD in the population and the patient had to wait at least 2 weeks before ICD replacement [71].

10. Future directions

The WCD technology effectively treats VT/VF, but bradycardia pacing support would likely prevent SCD to an even greater extent. Adding pacing capability to the WCD would be an important and life-saving step forward.

A major obstacle in WCD therapy remains patient adherence. Unfortunately, not all patients are motivated to comply with the prescription to use the WCD, and unnecessary deaths occur because of poor compliance. Therefore, motivating the patient to adhere to therapy is of utmost importance. A combined approach with technology reminders (e.g., text messages via smartphones) and close follow-up by device professionals is crucial.

Much has been accomplished in the past 30 years to better treat the risk of SCD, and the WCD is definitely an important milestone in our advancing knowledge. Nevertheless, much more needs to be done to reduce the rates of arrhythmic death even more.

A Class II recall of the WCD occurred in January 2018, covering 33,000 devices. This problem, in which certain vests displayed a warning message to the effect that they could not charge sufficiently to deliver therapy, has been addressed.

11. Conclusions

The WCD is an important advancement in the armamentarium for cardiovascular disease and demonstrates safe, effective therapy, but patient compliance remains a concern. The WCD is an interim therapeutic alternative to the ICD. In some cases, the WCD may help patients recover significant systolic function to the point that an ICD is no longer necessary. Patients who need the WCD should receive individual one-on-one instruction in how to use the device, and clinicians should be prepared that there may be a degree of psychological distress. Nevertheless, these devices are important advancement in cardiac care for people at risk of dangerous arrhythmias.

Acknowledgements

The authors gratefully acknowledge Todd Cooper of Coyote Studios in Green Valley, California, for the artwork in **Figure 1**.

Conflict of interest

Peter Magnusson has received speaker fees or grants from Abbott, Alnylam, Bayer, AstraZeneca, BMS, Boehringer Ingelheim, Lilly, Novo Nordisk, Internetmedicin, Octopus Medical, Pfizer, and Zoll.

Joseph Pergolizzi is a principal at Native Cardio, Inc.

Jo Ann LeQuang has no relevant disclosures.

Author details

Peter Magnusson[1,2], Joseph V. Pergolizzi[3] and Jo Ann LeQuang[3]*

1 Centre for Research and Development, Uppsala, Sweden

2 Department of Medicine, Cardiology Research Unit, Karolinska Institutet, Sweden

3 NEMA Research, Inc., Naples, Florida, USA

*Address all correspondence to: joannlequang@gmail.com

References

[1] Lloyd-Jones D, Adams RJ, Brown TM, Carnethon M, Dai S, De Simone G, et al. Executive summary: Heart disease and stroke statistics—2010 update: A report from the American Heart Association. Circulation. 2010;**121**(7):948-954

[2] Schmitt J, Abaci G, Johnson V, Erkapic D, Gemein C, Chasan R, et al. Safety of the wearable cardioverter defibrillator (WCD) in patients with implanted pacemakers. Pacing and Clinical Electrophysiology. 2017;**40**(3): 271-277

[3] Kovacs B, Reek S, Krasniqi N, Eriksson U, Duru F. Extended use of the wearable cardioverter-defibrillator: Which patients are most likely to benefit? Cardiology Research & Practice. 2018:1-8

[4] Agarwal M, Narcisse D, Khouzam N, Khouzam RN. Wearable cardioverter defibrillator "the Lifevest": Device design, limitations, and areas of improvement. Current Problems in Cardiology. 2018;**43**(2):45-55

[5] Reek S, Burri H, Roberts PR, Perings C, Epstein AE, Klein HU, et al. The wearable cardioverter-defibrillator: Current technology and evolving indications. Europace. 2017;**19**(3): 335-345

[6] Epstein AE, Abraham WT, Bianco NR, Kern KB, Mirro M, Rao SV, et al. Wearable cardioverter-defibrillator use in patients perceived to be at high risk early post-myocardial infarction. Journal of the American College of Cardiology. 2013;**62**(21): 2000-2007

[7] Zipes DP, Camm AJ, Borggrefe M, Buxton AE, Chaitman B, Fromer M, et al. ACC/AHA/ESC 2006 guidelines for management of patients with ventricular arrhythmias and the prevention of sudden cardiac death: A report of the American College of Cardiology/American Heart Association task force and the European Society of Cardiology Committee for practice guidelines (writing committee to develop guidelines for Management of Patients with Ventricular Arrhythmias and the prevention of sudden cardiac death). Journal of the American College of Cardiology. 2006;**48**(5):e247-e346

[8] Gronda E, Bourge RC, Costanzo MR, Deng M, Mancini D, Martinelli L, et al. Heart rhythm considerations in heart transplant candidates and considerations for ventricular assist devices: International Society for Heart and Lung Transplantation guidelines for the care of cardiac transplant candidates—2006. The Journal of Heart and Lung Transplantation. 2006;**25**(9):1043-1056

[9] Wilkoff BL, Love CJ, Byrd CL, Bongiorni MG, Carrillo RG, Crossley GH 3rd, et al. Transvenous lead extraction: Heart Rhythm Society expert consensus on facilities, training, indications, and patient management: This document was endorsed by the American Heart Association (AHA). Heart Rhythm. 2009;**6**(7):1085-1104

[10] O'Gara PT, Kushner FG, Ascheim DD, Casey DE Jr, Chung MK, de Lemos JA, et al. ACCF/AHA guideline for the management of ST-elevation myocardial infarction: Executive summary: A report of the American College of Cardiology Foundation/American Heart Association Task Force on Practice Guidelines: Developed in collaboration with the American College of Emergency Physicians and Society for Cardiovascular Angiography and Interventions. Catheterization and Cardiovascular Interventions. 2013, 2013;**82**(1):E1-E27

[11] Pedersen CT, Kay GN, Kalman J, Borggrefe M, Della-Bella P, Dickfeld T, et al. EHRA/HRS/APHRS expert consensus on ventricular arrhythmias. Heart Rhythm. 2014;**11**(10):e166-e196

[12] Kusumoto FM, Calkins H, Boehmer J, Buxton AE, Chung MK, Gold MR, et al. HRS/ACC/AHA expert consensus statement on the use of implantable cardioverter-defibrillator therapy in patients who are not included or not well represented in clinical trials. Circulation. 2014;**130**(1):94-125

[13] Priori SG, Blomstrom-Lundqvist C, Mazzanti A, Blom N, Borggrefe M, Camm J, et al. ESC Guidelines for the management of patients with ventricular arrhythmias and the prevention of sudden cardiac death: The Task Force for the Management of Patients with Ventricular Arrhythmias and the Prevention of Sudden Cardiac Death of the European Society of Cardiology (ESC) Endorsed by: Association for European Paediatric and Congenital Cardiology (AEPC). Europace. 2015;**17**(11):1601-1687

[14] Piccini PJ, Allen AL, Kudenchuk JP, Page LR, Patel RM, Turakhia PM. Wearable cardioverter-defibrillator therapy for the prevention of sudden cardiac death: A science advisory from the American Heart Association. Circulation. 2016;**133**(17):1715-1727

[15] Olgin JE, Pletcher MJ, Vittinghoff E, Wranicz J, Malik R, Morin DP, et al. Wearable cardioverter–defibrillator after myocardial infarction. New England Journal of Medicine. 2018; **379**(13):1205-1215

[16] Mirro MJ, Keltner EE, Roebuck AE, Sears SF. Playing it close to the VEST and the clinical guidelines: Clinical guideline compliance in HFrEF patients—Role of WCD. Pacing and Clinical Electrophysiology. 2018;**41**(10): 1314-1320

[17] Feldman AM, Klein H, Tchou P, Murali S, Hall WJ, Mancini D, et al. Use of a wearable defibrillator in terminating tachyarrhythmias in patients at high risk for sudden death: Results of the WEARIT/BIROAD. Pacing and Clinical Electrophysiology. 2004;**27**(1):4-9

[18] Kutyifa V, Moss AJ, Klein H, Biton Y, McNitt S, MacKecknie B, et al. Use of the wearable cardioverter defibrillator in high-risk cardiac patients: Data from the prospective registry of patients using the wearable cardioverter defibrillator (WEARIT-II registry). Circulation. 2015;**132**(17): 1613-1619

[19] Barsheshet A, Kutyifa V, Vamvouris T, Moss AJ, Biton Y, Chen L, et al. Study of the wearable cardioverter defibrillator in advanced heart-failure patients (SWIFT). Journal of Cardiovascular Electrophysiology. 2017; **28**(7):778-784

[20] Barraud J, Pinon P, Laine M, Cautela J, Orabona M, Koutbi L, et al. Ventricular arrhythmia occurrence and compliance in patients treated with the wearable cardioverter defibrillator following percutaneous coronary intervention. Heart, Lung and Circulation. 2018;**27**(8):984-988

[21] Kondo Y, Linhart M, Andrié RP, Schwab JO. Usefulness of the wearable cardioverter defibrillator in patients in the early post-myocardial infarction phase with high risk of sudden cardiac death: A single-center European experience. Journal of Arrhythmia. 2015;**31**(5):293-295

[22] Duncker D, König T, Hohmann S, Bauersachs J, Veltmann C. Avoiding untimely implantable cardioverter/defibrillator implantation by intensified heart failure therapy optimization supported by the wearable cardioverter/defibrillator—The PROLONG study.

Journal of the American Heart Association. 2017;**6**(1)

[23] Opreanu M, Wan C, Singh V, Salehi N, Ahmad J, Szymkiewicz SJ, et al. Wearable cardioverter-defibrillator as a bridge to cardiac transplantation: A national database analysis. The Journal of Heart and Lung Transplantation. 2015;**34**(10):1305-1309

[24] Wan C, Herzog CA, Zareba W, Szymkiewicz SJ. Sudden cardiac arrest in hemodialysis patients with wearable cardioverter defibrillator. Annals of Noninvasive Electrocardiology. 2014; **19**(3):247-257

[25] Ellenbogen KA, Koneru JN, Sharma PS, Deshpande S, Wan C, Szymkiewicz SJ. Benefit of the wearable cardioverter-defibrillator in protecting patients after implantable-cardioverter defibrillator explant: Results from the National Registry. Clinical Electrophysiology. 2017;**3**(3):243-250

[26] Bhaskaran A, Bartlett M, Kovoor P, Davis LM. The wearable cardioverter defibrillator: An early single Centre Australian experience. Some pitfalls and caveats for use. Heart, Lung & Circulation. 2016;**25**(2):155-159

[27] Erath JW, Vamos MS, Sirat AH, Hohnloser SH. The wearable cardioverter-defibrillator in a real-world clinical setting: Experience in 102 consecutive patients. Clinical Research in Cardiology. 2017;**106**(4):300-306

[28] Naniwadekar A, Alnabelsi T, Joshi K, Obasare E, Greenspan A, Mainigi S. Real world utilization and impact of the wearable cardioverter-defibrillator in a community setting. Indian Pacing and Electrophysiology Journal. 2017;**17**(3):65-69

[29] Roger S, Susanne R, Stefanie LR, Anna H, Siegfried L, Ibrahim E-B, et al. Therapy optimization in patients with heart failure: The role of the wearable cardioverter-defibrillator in a real-world setting. BMC Cardiovascular Disorders. 2018;**18**(1)

[30] Sasaki S, Tomita H, Shibutani S, Izumiyama K, Higuma T, Itoh T, et al. Usefulness of the wearable cardioverter-defibrillator in patients at high risk for sudden cardiac death. Circulation Journal: Official Journal of the Japanese Circulation Society. 2014;**78**(12): 2987-2989

[31] Spar SD, Bianco RN, Knilans KT, Czosek JR, Anderson BJ. The US experience of the wearable cardioverter-defibrillator in pediatric patients. Circulation: Arrhythmia and Electrophysiology. 2018;**11**(7): e006163

[32] Weiss M, Michels G, Eberhardt F, Fehske W, Winter S, Baer F, et al. Anxiety, depression and quality of life in acute high risk cardiac disease patients eligible for wearable cardioverter defibrillator: Results from the prospective multicenter CRED-registry. PLoS One. 2019;**14**(3): e0213261

[33] Chung M, Szymkiewicz S, M S, Zishiri E, Niebauer M, Lindsay B, et al. Aggregate national experience with the wearable cardioverter-defibrillator. Journal of the American College of Cardiology. 2010;**56**(3):194-203

[34] Daimee UA, Vermilye K, Moss AJ, Goldenberg I, Klein HU, McNitt S, et al. Experience with the wearable cardioverter-defibrillator in older patients: Results from the Prospective Registry of patients using the wearable cardioverter-defibrillator. Heart Rhythm. 2018;**15**(9):1379-1386

[35] Lamichhane MC, Gardiner JR, Bianco NJ, Szymkiewicz SK, Thakur RK. National experience with long-term use of the wearable cardioverter defibrillator in patients with cardiomyopathy. Journal of

Interventional Cardiac Electrophysiology. 2017;**48**(1):11-19

[36] Bossory L, Schubert S, Afzal MR, Weiss R, Tyler J, Kalbfleisch S, et al. Clinical experience with wearable cardioverter defibrillators at a tertiary electrophysiology program. Pacing and Clinical Electrophysiology. 2018;**41**(11): 1491-1494

[37] Dillon KA, Szymkiewicz SJ, Kaib TE. Evaluation of the effectiveness of a wearable cardioverter defibrillator detection algorithm. Journal of Electrocardiology. 2010;**43**(1):63-67

[38] Ellenbogen KA, Wan C, Shavelle DM. Outcome of patients with in-hospital ventricular tachycardia and ventricular fibrillation arrest while using a wearable cardioverter defibrillator. The American Journal of Cardiology. 2018;**121**(2):205-209

[39] Quast AF, van Dijk VF, Wilde AA, Knops RE, Boersma LV. Outpatient treatment with the wearable cardioverter defibrillator: Clinical experience in two Dutch centres. Netherlands Heart Journal. 2017;**25**(5): 312-317

[40] Salehi N, Nasiri M, Bianco NR, Opreanu M, Singh V, Satija V, et al. The wearable cardioverter defibrillator in nonischemic cardiomyopathy: A US national database analysis. Canadian Journal of Cardiology. 2016;**32**(10):1247. e1-e6

[41] Singh M, Wang NC, Jain S, Voigt AH, Saba S, EC A. Utility of the wearable cardioverter-defibrillator in patients with newly diagnosed cardiomyopathy: A decade-long single-center experience. Journal of the American College of Cardiology. 2015; **66**:2607-2613

[42] Beiert T, Malotki R, Kraemer N, Stöckigt F, Linhart M, Nickenig G, et al. A real world wearable cardioverter defibrillator experience—Very high appropriate shock rate in ischemic cardiomyopathy patients at a European single-center. Journal of Electrocardiology. 2017, 2017;**50**(5): 603-609

[43] Wassnig NK, Gunther M, Quick S, Pfluecke C, Rottstadt F, Szymkiewicz SJ, et al. Experience with the wearable cardioverter-defibrillator in patients at high risk for sudden cardiac death. Circulation. 2016;**134**(9): 635-643

[44] Zylla MM, Hillmann HA, Proctor TA, Kieser MA, Scholz EA, Zitron EA, et al. Use of the wearable cardioverter-defibrillator (WCD) and WCD-based remote rhythm monitoring in a real-life patient cohort. Heart and Vessels. 2018;**33**(11):1390-1402

[45] Margey R, McCann H, Blake G, Keelan E, Galvin J, Lynch M, et al. Contemporary management of and outcomes from cardiac device related infections. Europace. 2010;**12**(1):64-70

[46] Greenspon A, Patel J, Lau E, Ochoa J, Frisch D, Ho R, et al. 16-year trends in infection burden for pacemakers and implantable cardioverter-defibrillators in the United States 1993 to 2008. Journal of the American College of Cardiology. 2011; **10**:1001-1006

[47] Sohail MR, Uslan DZ, Khan AH, Friedman PA, Hayes DL, Wilson WR, et al. Infective endocarditis complicating permanent pacemaker and implantable cardioverter-defibrillator infection. Mayo Clinic Proceedings. 2008;**83**(1):46-53

[48] Klug D, Lacroix D, Savoye C, Goullard L, Grandmougin D, Hennequin JL, et al. Systemic infection related to endocarditis on pacemaker leads: Clinical presentation and management. Circulation. 1997;**95**(8): 2098-2107

[49] Baddour LM, Epstein AE, Erickson CC, Knight BP, Levison ME, Lockhart PB, et al. Update on cardiovascular implantable electronic device infections and their management: A scientific statement from the American Heart Association. Circulation. 2010;**121**(3):458-477

[50] Klug D, Balde M, Pavin D, Hidden-Lucet F, Clementy J, Sadoul N, et al. Risk factors related to infections of implanted pacemakers and cardioverter-defibrillators: Results of a large prospective study. Circulation. 2007;**116**(12):1349-1355

[51] Chua JD, Wilkoff BL, Lee I, Juratli N, Longworth DL, Gordon SM. Diagnosis and management of infections involving implantable electrophysiologic cardiac devices. Annals of Internal Medicine. 2000; **133**(8):604-608

[52] Tanawuttiwat T, Garisto JD, Salow A, Glad JM, Szymkiewicz S, Saltzman HE, et al. Protection from outpatient sudden cardiac death following ICD removal using a wearable cardioverter defibrillator. Pacing and Clinical Electrophysiology. 2014;**37**(5): 562-568

[53] Epstein A, DiMarco J, Ellenbogen K, Estes N, Freedman R, Gettes L, et al. ACC/AHA/HRS 2008 guidelines for device-based therapy of cardiac rhythm abnormalities: Executive summary. Journal of the American College of Cardiology. 2008;**51**(21):2085-2105

[54] Hohnloser SH, Kuck KH, Dorian P, Roberts RS, Hampton JR, Hatala R, et al. Prophylactic use of an implantable cardioverter-defibrillator after acute myocardial infarction. The New England Journal of Medicine. 2004; **351**(24):2481-2488

[55] Zei PC. Is the wearable cardioverter-defibrillator the answer for early post-myocardial infarction patients at risk for sudden death?: Mind the gap. Journal of the American College of Cardiology. 2013;**62**(21):2008-2009

[56] Solomon SD, Zelenkofske S, McMurray JJ, Finn PV, Velazquez E, Ertl G, et al. Sudden death in patients with myocardial infarction and left ventricular dysfunction, heart failure, or both. The New England Journal of Medicine. 2005;**352**(25):2581-2588

[57] Chugh SS, Jui J, Gunson K, Stecker EC, John BT, Thompson B, et al. Current burden of sudden cardiac death: Multiple source surveillance versus retrospective death certificate-based review in a large U.S. community. Journal of the American College of Cardiology. 2004;**44**(6):1268-1275

[58] Priori SG, Aliot E, Blomstrom-Lundqvist C, Bossaert L, Breithardt G, Brugada P, et al. Task force on sudden cardiac death of the European Society of Cardiology. European Heart Journal. 2001;**22**(16):1374-1450

[59] Deeprasertkul P, Opreanu M, Bianco N, Thakur R. National experience with wearable cardioverter-defibrillator use in Takotsubo Cardiomyopathy. Journal of the American College of Cardiology. 2013; **61**(10):E361

[60] Duncker D, Haghikia A, König T, Hohmann S, Gutleben KJ, Westenfeld R, et al. Risk for ventricular fibrillation in peripartum cardiomyopathy with severely reduced left ventricular function—Value of the wearable cardioverter/defibrillator. European Journal of Heart Failure. 2014; **16**(12):1331-1336

[61] Owen HJ, Bos JM, Ackerman MJ. Wearable cardioverter defibrillators for patients with long QT syndrome. International Journal of Cardiology. 2018;**268**:132-136

[62] Everitt MD, Saarel EV. Use of the wearable external cardiac defibrillator in children. Pacing and Clinical Electrophysiology. 2010;**33**(6):742-746

[63] Burch AE, Spar DS, Sears SF. Wearable cardioverter defibrillators in schools: A guide for parents and educators. Pacing & Clinical Electrophysiology. 2017;**40**(12): 1479-1482

[64] Huber NL, Burch AE, Bianco NR, Spar DS, Sears SF. Children with wearable cardioverter defibrillators: Examining activity levels via accelerometer. Progress in Pediatric Cardiology. 2019

[65] Everitt M, Verma A, Saarel E. The wearable external cardiac defibrillator for cancer patients at risk for sudden cardiac death. Community Oncology. 2011;**8**(9):400-403

[66] Gang UJ, Jons C, Jorgensen RM, Abildstrom SZ, Haarbo J, Messier MD, et al. Heart rhythm at the time of death documented by an implantable loop recorder. Europace. 2010;**12**(2):254-260

[67] Barraud J, Cautela J, Orabona M, Pinto J, Missenard O, Laine M, et al. Wearable cardioverter defibrillator: Bridge or alternative to implantation? World Journal of Cardiology. 2017;**9**(6): 531-538

[68] Whang W, Albert CM, Sears SF Jr, Lampert R, Conti JB, Wang PJ, et al. Depression as a predictor for appropriate shocks among patients with implantable cardioverter-defibrillators: results from the Triggers of Ventricular Arrhythmias (TOVA) study. Journal of the American College of Cardiology. 2005;**45**(7):1090-1095

[69] Mastenbroek MH, Versteeg H, Jordaens L, Theuns DA, Pedersen SS. Ventricular tachyarrhythmias and mortality in patients with an implantable cardioverter defibrillator: Impact of depression in the MIDAS cohort. Psychosomatic Medicine. 2014; **76**(1):58-65

[70] LaPage MJ, Canter CE, Rhee EK. A fatal device-device interaction between a wearable automated defibrillator and a unipolar ventricular pacemaker. Pacing and Clinical Electrophysiology. 2008; **31**(7):912-915

[71] Healy CA, Carrillo RG. Wearable cardioverter-defibrillator for prevention of sudden cardiac death after infected implantable cardioverter-defibrillator removal: A cost-effectiveness evaluation. Heart Rhythm. 2015;**12**(7): 1565-1573

Chapter 5

Inherited Ventricular Arrhythmias, the Channelopathies and SCD; Current Knowledge and Future Speculation – Epidemiology and Basic Electrophysiology

Abdullah Abdulrhman Al Abdulgader

Abstract

This chapter represents advanced scientific exploration in the different disciplines of SCD and channelopathy. Epidemiology of SCD and channelopathy is given special attention. The essence of detailed electrophysiological bases of the different diseases of channelopathies and the diverse cellular pathways mandated detailed discussion that can open the closed doors that we faced to the next generation(s). Special sections have been devoted to spatial as well as temporal heterogeneity of the cardiac action potential. Genetic heterogeneity and allelic heterogeneity are two prominent findings of channelopathies that confirm the fact of the major overlap in the field. The way we present the clinical findings is a true call for the next generation(s) of clinicians and researchers to revolutionize the field in the near future. Detailed management plans based on the up to date basic sciences findings for the different channelopathies give better therapeutic options for the clinicians in the field. Unique to this chapter is the new directions to look for channelopathies beyond the human body. The new understanding of the psychophysiological well-being of HRV and the sympathovagal balance extending to cosmic resonances and its possible effect on cardiac ion channels carries new era of promising preventive, diagnostic and therapeutic options.

Keywords: arrhythmia, Brugada syndrome (BrS), cardiac coherence (CC), catecholaminergic polymorphic ventricular tachycardia, ERS early repolarization syndrome, heart rate variability, long QT syndrome (LQTS), progressive cardiac conduction disease, sudden cardiac death, Schumann resonance, solar geomagnetic activity, SNP, SQTS

1. Introduction

One of the most devastating life moments that may impact the whole life of a person, family and society is sudden death experience of close relative or beloved. The whole medical provision is dedicated to prevent or delay death while

IntechOpen

maintaining good quality of life (QOL). For this reason, sudden loss of human life is creating the most serious challenge for medical professionals and decision-makers.

Sudden cardiac death (SCD) is defined as death occurring unexpectedly in the first hour after symptoms commence [1]. In the United States, around 300,000 deaths are occurring every year because of SCD [2]. It is conspicuous that this huge loss in the world communities is creating a major social impact. This impact is undoubtedly more destructive with the loss of young member of the family [3]. Ion channels in the myocardial cellular membrane are responsible for creating the basic unit of the electromagnetic foundation in humans known as cardiac action potential (AP). This is the result of an elegant interplay of ions at the cellular level. Genetic mutations in these channels can predispose to wide spectrum of clinical presentations and syndromes referred collectively to channelopathies (ionopathies). The basic pathology is genetic mutations creating disturbance in the process of critical ions traffic (Na^+, Ca^{2+}, K^+) across the cell membrane. The delicate miraculous balance in this ion traffic is the basic unit of the normal action potential. Disturbance of this balance in terms of loss or gain of function is the source of the fatal heart rhythm. Sadly, life-threatening arrhythmias and sudden cardiac death can be the first presenting symptom. Scientists and clinicians are racing in the last two decades in a unique complementary scientific effort to reconcile the rapidly growing body of knowledge of the molecular mechanisms and clinical correlates of SCD. In this chapter, we will review the epidemiology of the sudden cardiac death (SCD), then we will discuss the basic science of cellular action potential and its anomalies. We will navigate in detail in the genetic characterization of arrhythmic phenotypes, which started in 1995 with discovery of LQTS mutations, and the subsequent characterization of the diversity of genetic and molecular derangements, which can lead to channelopathies and the fatal rhythms.

2. Epidemiology of sudden cardiac death

Incidence and prevalence calculation in any disease in medicine is inevitably underestimation of the actual figures. This is due to the fact that underdiagnosis is the role. The most common cause of sudden death (SD) is SCD. Sudden cardiac death (SCD) is defined as sudden death within 1 h of the appearance of witnessed symptom or within 24 h of unwitnessed symptom in an individual without potentially lethal diagnosis [1].

Many cases of SCD have identifiable abnormalities such as hypertrophic cardiomyopathy, arrhythmogenic right ventricular cardiomyopathy, coronary artery anomalies or myocarditis [4]. However, a significant proportion of SD (3–53%) has no identifiable cause on autopsy examination, and these are labelled sudden unexpected death (SUD). Cardiac channelopathies (used interchangeably with ionopathy) account for approximately one-third of SUD cases. Worldwide records demonstrated that around 3,700,000 death per annum are due to SCD. In the western world (the United States and Europe), 1–2 death per 2000 of the general population are lost due to SCD. SCD in male gender is 3 times higher than female [2]. Channelopathies such as long QT syndrome (LQTS), Brugada syndrome (BrS), catecholaminergic polymorphic ventricular tachycardia (CPVT), short QT syndrome (SQTS), early repolarization syndrome (ERS) and idiopathic VF are estimated to be responsible for 10% of SCDs [5]. It is believed that about one-third of SUD cases are due to channelopathies.

2.1 Epidemiology of channelopathies

2.1.1 Long QT syndrome

Long QT syndrome (LQTS) is an inherited genetically heterogeneous group of arrhythmias characterized by a prolonged QTc interval in the 12-lead ECGs (with QTc values >470 ms for males and >480 ms for females, representing approximate 99th percentile values). The prevalence of LQTS in what seems to be healthy live births in Italy is 1:2500 [6]. In New Zealand, the reported prevalence is 1:4500 [7]. In Korean males, they reported QT prolongation (equal or more than 460 ms) as 1:5000 [8]. In Japanese males with high likelihood of LQTS score >3.5, the prevalence was similar to Italy (approximately 1:2500) [9].

In conclusion, the Asian reported prevalence is comparable to the west (1:5000–1:2500). At least 17 genes were identified contributing to LQTS. Mutations have been found in more than half of them (40–70%) [10]. In spite of the complexity of the subject, clinicians need to know for their practice more than 75% of mutations in congenital LQTS are located in the KCNQ1 (LQT1), KCNH2 (LQT2) or SCN5A (LQT3) genes [10]. The prevalence of the different gene mutations for LQT1, LQT2, LQT3 and others is 52%, 33%, 7% and 1.2%, respectively. A Japanese survey of 41 individuals reported genotypes in 71% constituting LQT1 38%, LQT2 38%, LQT3 21% and LQT8 3% [11]. The International LQTS Registry documented cardiac events (syncope, cardiac arrest and SCD) in LQTS individuals to be 63% for LQT1, 46% for LQT2 and 18% for LQT3 [12]. Cardiac events in LQT3, although being the less frequent, were shown to be more lethal than the other two types [12]. The triggers of the different LQTS are of special diagnostic indication. LQT1 is known to be triggered by exercise (typically swimming), while LQT2 has been linked to emotional events, like startle (typically alarm clocks) and delivery [13]. LQT3 is the 'inevitable' as it occurs during periods of rest or sleep. During childhood, boys with LQTS tends to develop more fatal attacks, compared to girls. After childhood, the incidence is comparable [14].

2.1.2 Short QT syndrome (SQTS)

SQTS was described in 2000, and it is a clinical entity characterized by short QT intervals on ECG (generally, QTc < 350 ms), high incidence of VT/VF, absence of structural heart disease, familial history of SCD and resuscitated cardiac arrest [15]. It is the severest form of the major channelopathies, with cardiac arrest/SCD being the most common presentation. Events occur during rest, sleep or exertion [4]. For this reason, high index of suspicion should be practiced in order to be able to diagnose this type of malignant channelopathies. Among 10,984 Japanese with approximately equal sex distribution, 1:3400 individuals showed QTc less than 300 ms [16]. Parts of idiopathic VF cases are likely to be borderline or latent SQTS individuals. SQTS was diagnosed in 12% of idiopathic VF survivors [17]. The course of SQTS individuals is more malignant with higher risk of recurrence of life-threatening arrhythmias and SCDs [18].

2.1.3 Brugada syndrome (BrS)

There is general impression that BrS incidence is underestimated. In one publication, BrS accounts for 4–12% of SCD [4]. It appears to be related to mutations affecting Na^+ channels. There are currently more than 300 mutations described, mostly autosomal dominant, affecting the SCN5A gene, leading to loss of Na^+ channel function in a variety of ways (interestingly, mutations in other parts of this gene lead to LQTS3). Other genes affecting the Na^+ channel are also implicated in BrS. BrS is characterized electrocardiographically by classical finding of coved ST-segment elevation in anterior precordial leads. Cardiac events secondary to ventricular tachycardia typically occur in young adults but have been described in children and infants [4]. Individuals with BrS develop a monomorphic ventricular tachycardia; often precipitated during sleep or rest, and during febrile illnesses [19].

It is thought that some SCN5A mutations alter the Na^+ channel in a temperature-dependent manner. Males have arrhythmic events more frequently, and there is thought to be a gender effect on ion channel expression [20]. The estimated prevalence of BrS ranges from 0.02 to 0.1% in Europe and from 0.1 to 0.25% in Asia [5]. Lai Tai means the southern pattern (referring to the mode of death during sleep) is a famous horror term in Thailand and 'Pokkuri'. The death secret has been diagnosed as Brugada syndrome, which is thought to be endemic heart electrical disease in this part of the world [21]. Later on, Europeans were shown to have similar prevalence [5]. About one-third of cases have been attributed to SCN5A mutations [22]. Mutations attributed to CACNA1C and CACNB2 are seen in around 12% of cases. Minor percentages are due to other gene mutations like GPD1L, SCN1B, KCNE3 and SCN3B [23–27]. In 50–80% of patients with BrS, VF or VT can be induced by ventricular extra stimuli in an EPS. There is dispersion of opinions in the ionopathy literature regarding the prognostic value of VT/VF inducibility in EPS. Nobuyuki Murakoshi and colleague consider inducibility as a poor prognostic factor, while many other authors do not believe of any significant correlation [5].

2.1.4 Early repolarization syndrome (ERS)

ERS is characterized by elevation of the QRS-ST junction (J point) and QRS notching or slurring (J wave) in multiple leads, especially the inferior and/or left precordial leads [28]. The slurred J point elevation which was interpreted by cardiology communities as normal electrocardiographic variant distracted Haissaguerre et al. who reported very important observation in this regard. Among 207 victims of idiopathic VF, 30% were found to have the slurred J point pattern (ER pattern) compared to 5% of controls [29].

In the Framingham Heart Study, the ER pattern was found in 6.1% of American and European persons and 5.8% in Finnish population [30, 31]. In Asia, the story seems to be more impressive. J wave elevation of at least 0.05 mV was detected in 7.26% of Chinese subjects [32]. In Japan, the incidence rate was 715 per 100,000 person-years [33].

In general, reviewing todays medical literature will reveal ERS prevalence figures which range from approximately 6 to 13% in the general population [34]. Male sex, younger age, lower systolic blood pressure, higher Sokolow-Lyon index for LVH calculation (S in V_1 + R in V_5 or V_6 (whichever is larger) $\geq$ 35 mm ($\geq$7 large squares) or R in aVL $\geq$ 11 mm) and lower Cornell voltage (S in V_3 + R in aVL > 28 mm (men) or S in V_3 + R in aVL > 20 mm (women)) are independently associated with the presence of the ER pattern [30]. An important observation in that regard points to the proportionality of ER amplitude to the risk of arrhythmic death.

ER of 0.2 mV or more in ECG inferior leads was shown to have much increased risk than those without. This was concluded after long mean follow-up of 29–41 years [35]. Notching of the J point was found to be associated with worse prognosis [5]. The rapid rise of ST segment and dominance of ST pattern in athletes was found to be benign variant of ERS. Looking with eye of scrutiny will show the similarities of clinical, electrocardiographic and genetic aspects between BrS and ERS. Future research could prove both syndromes to be a spectrum of one pathology.

2.1.5 Catecholaminergic polymorphic ventricular tachycardia (CPVT)

Catecholaminergic polymorphic ventricular tachycardia (CPVT) is an inherited arrhythmogenic disorder characterized by polymorphic VT induced by physical or emotional stress without any detectable morphological abnormalities in the heart [36]. Two important gene mutations has been described: mutations in genes encoding cardiac ryanodine type 2 receptor (RYR2) [autosomal dominant] and calsequestrin 2 (CASQ2) [autosomal recessive] [37, 38]. A subunit for inward-rectifier potassium channels called Kir2.1. Mutation in this subunit (KCNJ2) is responsible of a third variant of CPVT [39]. A Japanese report of 50 cases ranks the CPVT mutations frequency as follows: RYR2 (56%), CASQ (22%) and KCNJ2 (22%) [40]. CPVT is gaining more attention although being a rare disease compared to other channelopathies (1:10,000) because of its tendency to affect children and young adults [41]. In fact, CPVT is considered as highly malignant heart rhythm if neglected. In those situations, by the age of 20–30 years, the mortality is 30–50% [42].

2.1.6 Heart channelopathies and systemic involvement

Action potential is the basic unit of human body electricity. It is conceivable that ionopathic involvement of other systems is a fact. This will result in symptoms and syndromes that deserve attention for proper risk stratification of ionopathic subjects. Behere and Weindling elaborated on this in their unique review [43].

Jervell and Lange-Nielsen syndrome (JLNS) has been associated with about 4% of patients with the bilateral sensorineural loss [44]. However, Chang et al. challenged this concept. They thought that this association may have been overestimated in the era before genetic testing, and newer studies seem to reflect the similar rate of LQTS causing mutations in deaf children, as in the general population [45]. There is overlap between seizure disorders and cardiac channelopathies. Sudden unexpected death in epilepsy (SUDEP) has an incidence of 6–9/1000 person-years in epilepsy surgery programs. Channelopathy-associated mutations have been identified in 13% of patients with SUDEP [46]. Seizures triggered by exercise, emotion, sudden stimuli, seizures unresponsive to anti-seizure medications and seizures in the setting of family history of SD, syncope or obvious electrocardiographic abnormalities should all be viewed with high index of suspicion for underlying channelopathy [47]. In patients with BrS, fever is a well-known arrhythmogenic trigger because SCN5A mutations alter the temperature sensitivity of fast inactivation of the Na^+ channel. This may cause 'apparent life-threatening events (ALTEs)' and even SUD or sudden infant death syndrome (SIDS) in susceptible infants in the setting of febrile illnesses [48]. As many as 30% of victims of drowning-related deaths have been found to have cardiac channelopathies [49, 50]. Patients with SCN5A mutations have been found to have irritable bowel syndrome (IBS). In a recent study, 2% of patients with IBS were found to have SCN5A mutations, and in one case, mexiletine administration even caused normalization of bowel habits. It is hypothesized that channelopathies are involved in the pathogenesis of some forms of IBS [51]. There is also a co-existence of iron-deficiency anaemia, hypergastrinemia and gastric hyperplasia associated with LQT1. This suggests not only a role for the gene KCNQ1 in gastric secretion but also a role for gastrin as a marker of arrhythmia severity [52, 53]. Interestingly, in a study from the United States, 36% of patients with drug-induced LQTS possessed known arrhythmia-associated mutations [54].

2.1.7 Cardiac channelopathies and sudden infant death syndrome (SIDS)

SIDS is defined as SD of seemingly healthy children of age <1 year. The incidence of SIDS varies across the world [54]. About 10–20% of SIDS cases are attributed to genetic mutations associated with channelopathies [19, 54, 55]. Mutations associated with LQTS1 and LQTS3 have been related to SIDS [54]. Mutations in the genes encoding the beta sub-units of Na channels have also been implicated [56]. Interestingly, a loss of function mutation in the K^+ channel encoding gene KCNJ8 has also been associated with SIDS. It is hypothesized that this mutation causes maladaptation to stress such as endotoxemia [55]. A Japanese study looking more broadly at the characteristics of all infantile LQTS found that 84% of all cases were diagnosed in the foetal or neonatal period. LQTS1 was associated with most risk of a first cardiac event, but LQTS2 and LQTS3 more exclusively caused VT or TdP [11]. QT intervals were found to be longest around 2 months of age [57]. Foetal magnetocardiography and echocardiography have been used to assess foetal LQTS. Sinus bradycardia is a common finding. Trans-placental magnesium and lidocaine, and prenatal beta-blocker therapies have been used for management [58]. While less commonly studied or identified, mutations associated with CPVT, SQTS, and BS have been linked to SIDS [54].

3. The basic electrophysiology of the myocyte and myocardium in ion channel disease

Basic understanding of the electrophysiology of cardiac cells action potential (AP) and its anomalies constitutes the corner stone to dive and disclose the secrets of ionopathies and the resultant fatal cardiac rhythm. Basic research uses molecular techniques, as well as animal models. Phases of the ventricular action potential with description of major events (**Figure 1**) proved extremely useful in improving the arrhythmia communities' knowledge of inherited arrhythmogenic syndromes. The discussion of the myocyte action potential is invariably the discussion of the ion channels of the cellular membrane since the delicate trans-membrane traffic of ions is the source of cardiac action potential during normal electrophysiological function of the heart. It is critical to perceive that abnormal heart rhythms including the fatal ventricular arrhythmias are primarily due to abnormal formation or mutations of those trans-membrane pores or its regulatory subunits. Mutations in any of the genes involved in regulation of cardiac ion channels may potentially result in arrhythmias and may be classified as arising from either abnormal AP formation or abnormal AP propagation. Martin CA et al. authored unique review in this regard [59].

3.1 Abnormal AP formation and propagation

Aberrancy of AP formation can be interpreted through three main mechanisms: reentry, triggered activity or automaticity. Acceleration of depolarization of pacemaker tissue will end up with autonomous formation of AP called enhanced automaticity. This can be precipitated by underlying sympathovagal imbalance in favour of excessive sympathetic tone, hypokalaemia or drugs such as digitalis. Triggered activity referred to extra systole generated outside the primary pacemaker tissue [59]. The underlying mechanism is called afterdepolarization, which is oscillations of cardiac cell membrane potential generated before the previous AP, ending up with premature new AP. If this premature AP magnitude is reaching threshold, it will produce triggered beat. According to the timing of this triggered activity, it can be early or late. Triggered activity during repolarization of the original AP is called early afterdepolarization (EAD). It occurs when AP duration is prolonged until a degree where L-type Ca^{2+} channels are recovered from inactivation during the time of membrane depolarization. Inward ICa-L current will initiate the new premature depolarization of the membrane and will initiate the afterdepolarization [60]. Triggered activity after completion of repolarization or near completion is called delayed afterdepolarization (DAD). It occurs due to enhanced Ca^{2+} release from the cellular calcium store organelle called sarcoplasmic

DOI: http://dx.doi.org/10.5772/intechopen.92073

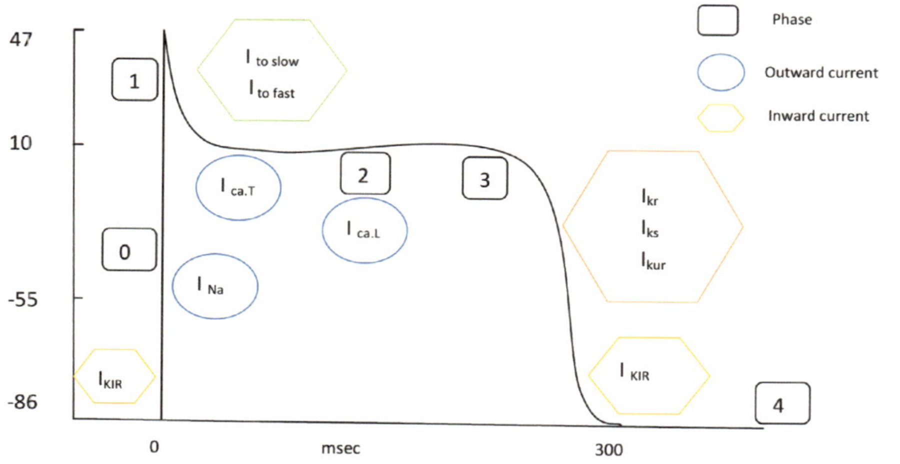

Phase 0 Rapid depolarization	Phase 1 Early repolarization	Phase 2 Action potential plateau	Phase 3 Final rapid repolarization	Phase 4 Resting membrane depolarization and diastolic depolarization
Excitatory stimulus or pacemaker potential depolarizes cell membrane beyond −70 mV At −70 mV, Na^+ channels are activated and allow inward current I_{Na} (channel NaV1.5). This current is brief but enormous, peaking the membrane potential at +47 mV.	The increase in potential from phase 0 results in opening of outward K^+channels and inward Ca^{2+} channels. There is repolarization from +47 mV to +10 mV due to rapid closure of $I_{Nav1.5}$ and activation of transient outward K^+current I_{Kto}, slow (channel KV1.4) and I_{Kto}, fast (channel KV4.2/4.3)	The membrane potential remains depolarized near 0 mV. Plateau phase is maintained by two inward Ca^{2+} currents – $I_{Ca.T}$ (channel CaVT.2) and $I_{Ca.L}$ (channel CaV1.2) and four outward K^+ currents	As the time dependent inward currents above inactivate, the outward K^+ currents dominate and cause rapid repolarization. These are rapid I_{Kr} (channel KHERG), ultrarapid I_{Kur} (channel KV1.5) and slow I_{KS} (channel KLVQT1)	The outward K^+ channels in phase 3 deactivate, the membrane is repolarized to -40 mV. The inward rectifier current I_{Kir} (channel Kir2.1) continues to drive the membrane potential to -70 mV, and the voltage dependent Na^+ channel which causes phase 0 remains inactivated till this happens

Figure 1.
Phases of the ventricular action potential with description of major events [59].

reticulum (SR) due to either activation of the Na^+/Ca^{2+} exchanger or Ca^{2+}-activated Cl-current. Classical examples of this Ca^{2+} overload environment is during digitalis toxicity or Catecholaminergic Polymorphic VT [61] (**Figure 2A**). The reentrant mechanism is unique. It requires an electrical obstacle around which AP is able to go around, disproportionately conducting exit pathways, one conducting fast and the other conducting slow and finally unidirectional conduction block. It is the most important mechanism as it is widely spread in much pathologies and most importantly the only type that is amenable for study and ablation in electrophysiology laboratory. The most common arrhythmias in clinical electrophysiology like atrioventricular nodal reentry tachycardia (AVNRT) and atrioventricular reentrant tachycardia (AVRT) are both reentrant and amenable for ablation. It is the underlying mechanism in patients with ventricular scarring, usually from old myocardial infarction, cardiomyopathy and infiltrative disease (**Figure 2B**).

3.2 Spatial electrophysiological heterogeneity

The human heart has been created in miraculous way where the structure supports and complements the function. After initiation of the normal impulse in the

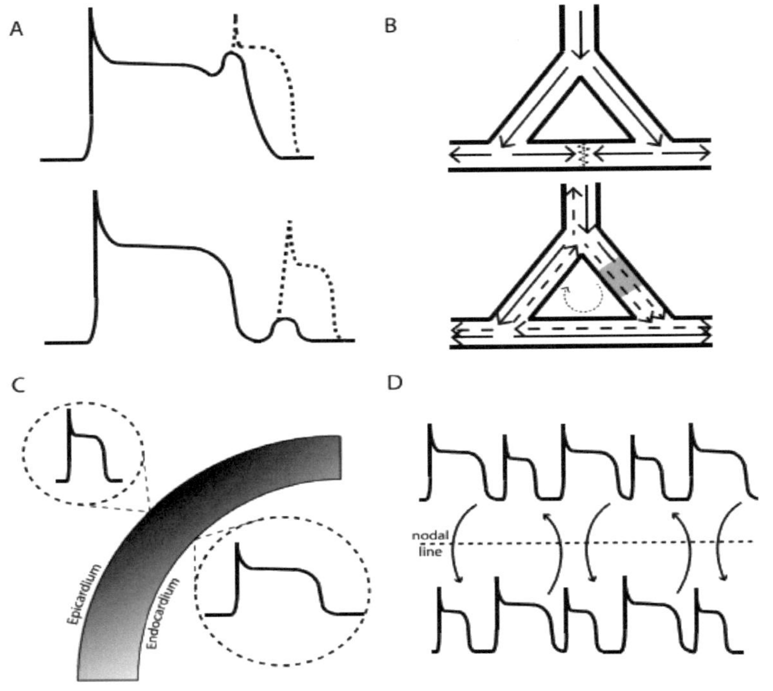

Figure 2.
Different mechanisms of arrhythmias [59]: (A) triggered activity: early after depolarization (EAD) (upper trace) and delayed after depolarization (DAD) (lower trace). Dotted lines represent formation of new AP. (B) Reentrant circuit: normal impulse propagation in two equal conduction velocities with collision in the middle and termination of the impulse (upper diagram). Presence of slow limb in the circuit (solid line) will end up with the normal impulse pass through and circulates around the other limb which is the fast limb at a time where its refractoriness is over (dotted). This will end up with excitation of the myocardium and initiation of tachycardia (lower diagram). (C) Transmural gradients due to heterogeneity of AP in different locations: shorter AP in epicardium compared to endocardium will end up with reexcitation. (D) Heterogenity of AP timing: creating duration alternans with the result of nodal line when the alternans time out creating block predisposing to reentry in the presence of triggered impulse.

sinus node, the wave of action potentials is characterized by highly sophisticated levels of gradients of depolarization and repolarizations, to maintain the normal electro-mechanical activation sequence for the pumping heart functions. The dominant determiner of these spatial gradients is the regional differences in repolarizing K^+ channels. These include channel density variations, kinetics and cycling traffic between membrane and cytoplasm. The substrate for reentry is created by disturbances in these gradients, which may permit depolarized regions to reexcite polarized areas [59]. Transmural gradients alterations correlated with arrhythmogenic tendencies in a number of both pharmacological canine and genetic murine models for LQTS and BrS. The reexcitation may occur when the epicardial action potential duration is much shorter than the endocardial, potentially leading to new AP (**Figure 2C**).

This new environment of electrical dispersion within the cardiac tissue was proved to be arrhythmogenic in cardiomyopathies. This spatial heterogeneity was linked to T wave alternans (TWA) and ventricular tachycardia [62]. Reentry created by epicardial dispersion of repolarization was seen to be the trigger for ventricular tachycardia in preparation of canine right ventricular wedge [63] and the $Scn5a^{+/-}$ mouse model [64]. Source of arrhythmia in Brugada syndrome is thought to be secondary to AP duration differences between left ventricle and right ventricle. This is reflected in Brugada patients as ST elevation in right precordial leads and right epicardial AP changes [65].

3.3 Temporal electrophysiological heterogeneity

Electrical dispersion may also affect activation sequence. Temporal beat-to-beat variation in the AP amplitude or duration, a phenomenon known as alternant (**Figure 2D**), has been associated with arrhythmogenesis in both clinical and experimental studies [66, 67]. This can have significant consequences on the spatial organization of repolarization across the ventricle, amplifying the heterogeneities of repolarization present at baseline into pathophysiological heterogeneities of sufficient magnitude to produce conduction block and reentrant excitation. Regions which alternate out of phase generate a line of block called the nodal line between them. This has the potential to act as a focus for reentrant circuits following the addition of a triggered beat.

3.4 The channelopathies

3.4.1 Long QT syndromes

LQTS constitute a group of genetic disorders distinguished by long QT interval in the electrocardiogram, representing prolongation of repolarization period associated with the risk of ventricular arrhythmias (in specific torsade de point) and sudden death. In comparison to Brugada syndrome, the genetic mutations in LQTS result in tendency for electrical disturbance, affecting depolarization rather than repolarization. An arrhythmic substrate with prolonged AP duration was implicated in several mouse models [68] (**Figure 3**). Functional block pockets are created by prolonged depolarization phase during which the impulse pathway will be refractory. This functional block will create reentry focus and myocardial excitation. In addition, repolarization potentials dispersion across the myocardium will provide a functional reentry pathway facilitating initiation of torsade de point. Prolonged depolarization may result in EAD with consequent polymorphic VT. Data from transgenic rabbits [69], have recently been instrumental to support a novel view on the arrhythmogenesis in LQTS by Chang et al. [70]. These authors developed an in silico model (i.e. computational modelling, simulation and visualization of the cardiomyocyte electrophysiological behaviour and arrhythmogenesis in a virtual computerized environment) of prolonged repolarization. They were able to demonstrate that arrhythmogenesis is initiated by two types of spiral waves: short cycle and long cycle. The short cycle is mediated through *I*Na (**Figure 4A**) and the long cycle is mediated through slow L-type calcium current (ICa) (**Figure 4B**) [70]. The alteration of those two types of waves gives what resemble torsade de point in the ECG. Arrhythmogenesis in LQT1 was investigated by Kim et al. using transgenic rabbit models. Multiple EAD foci were demonstrated as well as AP bimodal distribution compatible with the concept of two excitation types [70].

3.4.2 Brugada syndrome (BrS)

BrS is clearly distinguished between other channelopathies with its electrocardiographic manifestation in the form of delayed right ventricular activation with posterior T wave manifested mainly in V1 and V2. Clinically it is characterized by episodic history of poly morphic VT and ventricular fibrillation (VF) [59]. Genetic heterogeneity is a hall mark feature of BrS where multiple genetic mutations result in the same phenotype. All mutations end up with imbalance of the currents favouring repolarization over depolarization (in contrast to LQTS). The most famous BrS mutation is the SCN5A gene where there is loss of function encoding the alpha subunit of the Na^+ voltage-gated channel. INa reduction seems to be the underlying mechanism.

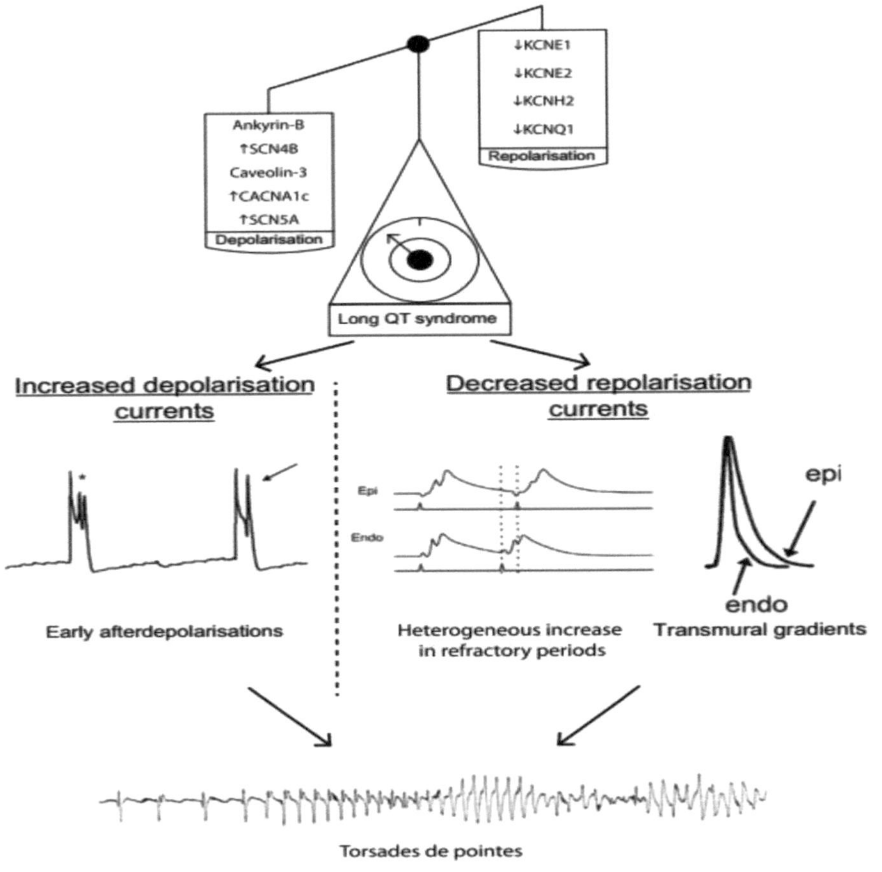

Figure 3.
LQTS mechanistic representation of arrhythmogenesis as understood from animal model. Scales showed genetic mutations can give rise to either gain of depolarization currents or loss of repolarization currents. EAD (triggered activity) will result as well as transmural gradients and refractory pockets formation. The clinical outcome as seen in ECG is represented by the trace at the bottom of the graph (torsade de pointes) [59].

Experimental studies using canine hearts as well as clinical studies support this pathophysiological mechanism underlying BrS [71, 72]. Reduction of Na^+ current can impose its effect represented by the deep notch of phase 1 of the epicedial AP, which is most impressive in RV. This reduction in Na^+ current creates voltage gradient across RV. This state of electrical imbalance in RV epicardium facilitates participation of the proximal myocardium to reactivate RV, ending up with reentry. This type of reentry is called phase 2 reentry (**Figure 5**). Another perspective to interpret the ECG manifestations of BrS is based on right ventricular out flow (RVOT) conduction delay perspective [73]. This perspective was derived from echocardiographic measurements, signal-averaged ECG (SAECG) potentials and mapping of body surface [74, 75]. An ex vivo experiment demonstrating RVOT conduction delay was published [76]. Fractionated late potentials that was amenable for catheter ablation was documented in the anterior aspect of RVOT epicardium. This specific site ablation normalized ECG and prevented VT and VF associated with BrS [77].

3.4.3 Catecholaminergic polymorphic ventricular tachycardia (CPVT)

Surge of catecholamines due to stress or exercise is the substrate fuel of bidirectional VT leading to syncope or SCD. This is creating an important category

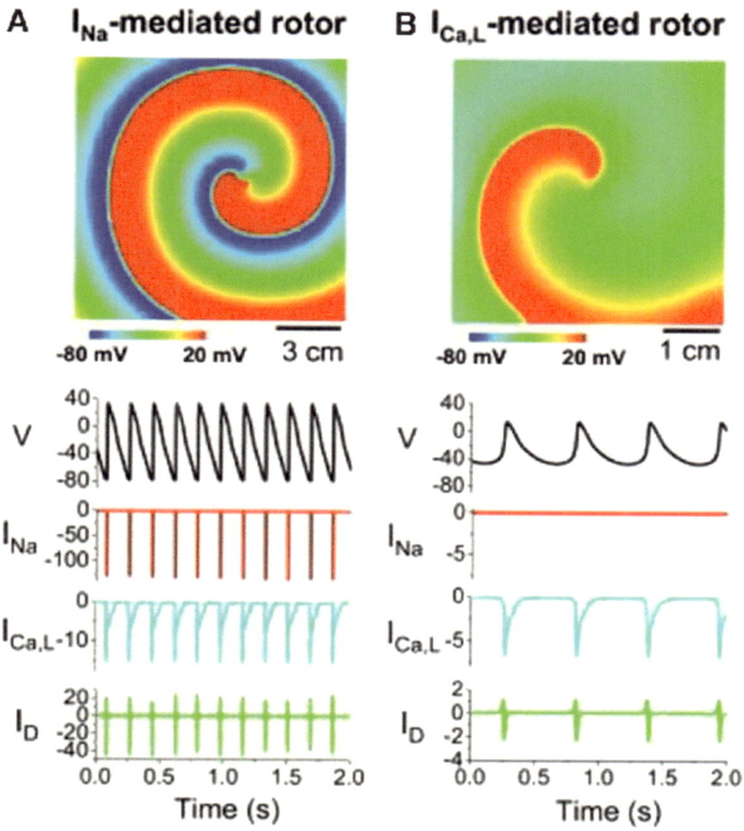

Figure 4.
In silico cardiac tissue model of prolonged repolarization. Arrhythmogenesis is initiated by two types of spiral waves: short cycle and long cycle. The short cycle is mediated through INa (A) and the long cycle is mediated through slow L-type calcium current (ICa) (B) [70].

of channelopathies called CPVT. At cellular level, enhanced Ca^{2+} release from the cellular calcium store organelle called sarcoplasmic reticulum (SR) is the operating mechanism. This enhanced Ca^{2+} release is due to gain of function gene mutation encoding ryanodine receptor 2 (RyR2), which is an important regulator of Ca^{2+} release for myocardial cells excitation contraction coupling [78]. The other important gene mutation results in loss of function affecting calsequestrin (CASQ2) protein, which is in normal situations functioning as SR calcium buffering protein [79]. This Ca^{+} release affects AP in a way favouring DAD as in digitalis toxicity concluded in arrhythmic trigger [36] (**Figure 6**). A net inward current is generated secondary to cytosolic Ca^{+} overload in vitro studies with RyR2 and CASQ2 mutations [61, 80]. RyR2 [81] or in CASQ2 [82] genes deliberately inserted into transgenic animals (mouse in this situation) revealed abnormal Ca^{+} transients and bidirectional VT. This level of evidence is supporting the idea that inward current might be the underlying mechanism of DAD triggering the abnormal beat. RYR2 mutations have also been suggested to be associated with dilated cardiomyopathy [83], hypertrophic cardiomyopathy [84] and arrhythmogenic right ventricular cardiomyopathy [85].

3.4.4 Other syndromes

While a majority of cases of SCD in the absence of structural heart abnormalities are caused by LQTS, BrS and CVVT, other less common syndromes are of

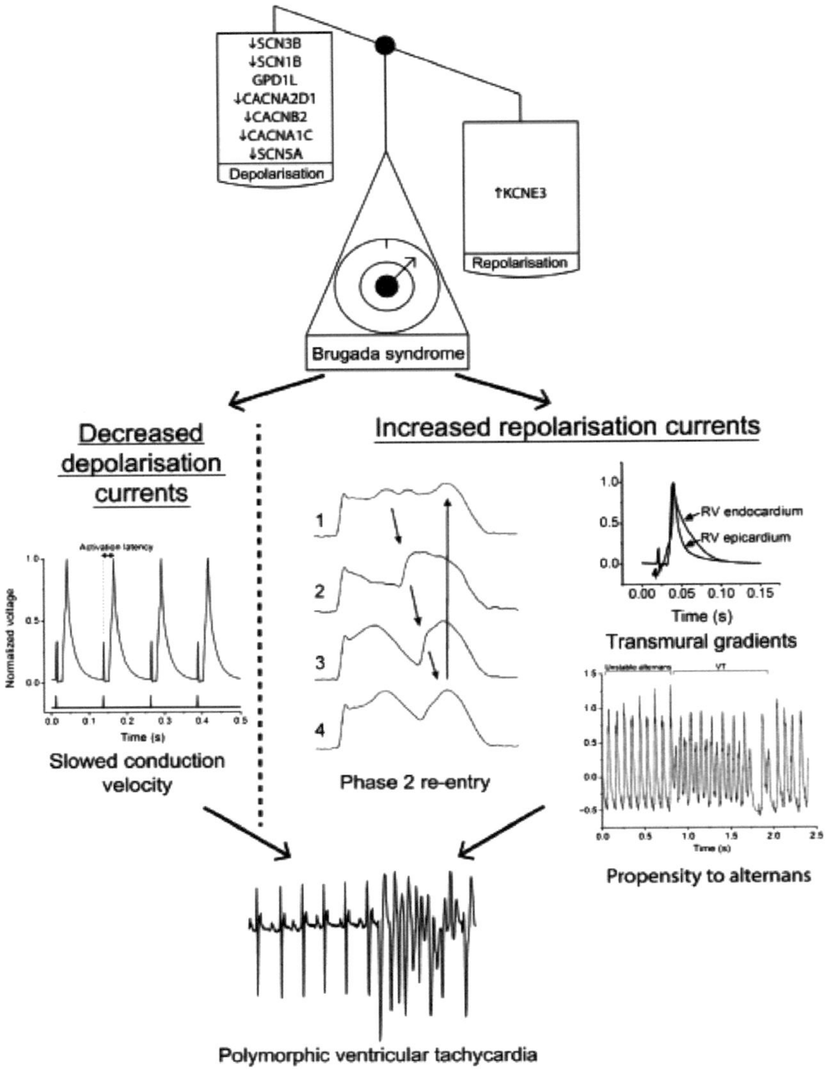

Figure 5.

Brugada syndrome's mechanistic representation of arrhythmogenesis as understood from animal model. Scales showed genetic mutations can give rise to either loss of depolarization currents or gain of repolarization currents. The ultimate outcome of those AP changes is more likelihood for alternans and phase 2 reentry. The clinical outcome as seen in ECG is represented by the trace at the bottom of the graph (polymorphic VT) [59].

importance. Short AP and accordingly QT intervals in short QT syndrome (SQTS) is due to mutations causing gain of function handling K^+ channels [86] or mutations causing loss of function handling Ca^+ channels [87]. An increase in repolarization gradients was seen to be the underlying mechanism [88]. In early repolarization syndrome (ERS), J point elevation with prominent T wave is seen (early repolarization pattern). This electrocardiographic pattern is associated clinically with VT and sudden death [89]. The exact mechanism is still obscure although AP early phase increment in transmural gradients has been suggested in canines hearts [90]. Rarely, reduction in inward Ca^+ current [91] or increment in outward K^+ current mutations [92] has been described, although a majority of cases lack genetic mutations. The weight of evidence nowadays is supporting that the ER pattern is polygenic with an important contribution of epigenetic and environmental factors.

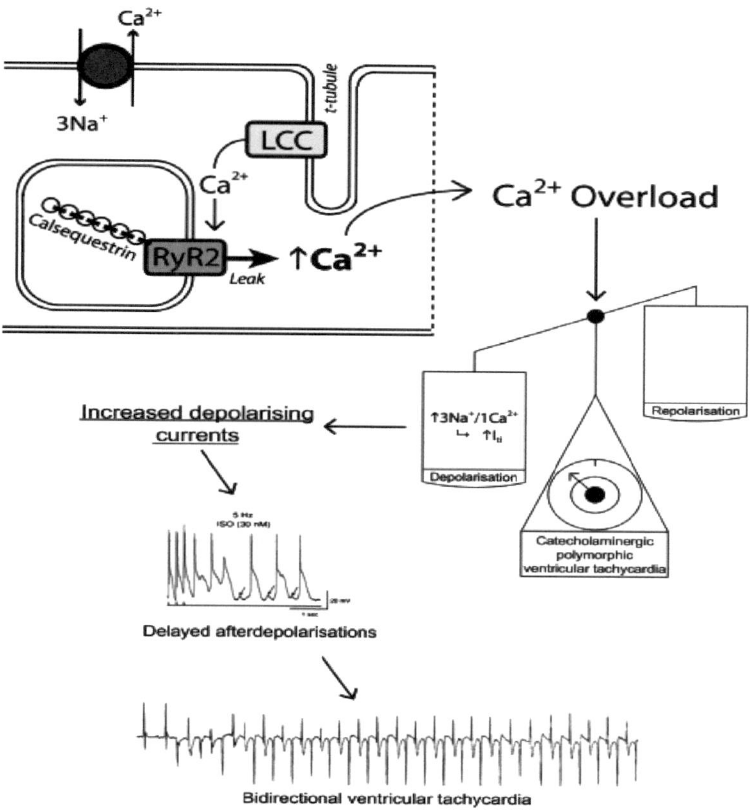

Figure 6.
CPVT mechanistic representation of arrhythmogenesis as understood from animal model. DAD-triggered activity is due to genetic mutation causing rise in cytosolic Ca^+ which in turn will result in depolarization current obeying the electrogenic nature of the Na^+/Ca^{2+} exchanger. The clinical outcome as seen in ECG is represented by the trace at the bottom of the graph (bidirectional VT) [59].

Progressive cardiac conduction disease (PCCD) also known as Lenegre's disease is a rare progressive degenerative disease of the cardiac conduction system with autosomal dominant pattern of inheritance that may end up with widening of QRS complexes, long pauses and bradycardia. It is a cause of SCD. The first gene mutation of PCCD described was SCN5A. This mutation can be associated with complex phenotype of PCCD, Brs and LQT3, sometimes referred as (overlap syndrome) [93]. Recently, PCCD was seen as an association with altered expressions of other gene proteins encoding impulse propagation like Ca^+-activated ion channel and cytoskeletal components. The conclusive phenotype as seen in mouse experiments is thought to be an additive effect of genetic components with environmental modifiers and aging [94].

4. Summary

SCD is extreme, devastating and traumatic life event. Inherited ventricular arrhythmias, which is due to disturbed ionic traffic across cardiac cell membrane (channelopathy), comprised 1/3 of all cases of SUD and 10% of SCD as a whole. Channelopathies occupies strategic location in the basic science as well as clinical and research arenas due to its recalcitrant behaviour and complexity. The discoveries of the genetic mutations of channelopathies heralded in 1995 have expanded drastically, resulting in revolutionary understanding of the disease. The most important described channelopathies up to date are long QT syndromes (LQTS), Brugada syndrome (BrS), catecholaminergic polymorphic ventricular tachycardia (CPVT), short QT syndrome (SQTS), early repolarization syndrome (ERS) and idiopathic VF. New disease entities are expected to be discovered in the near future. LQTS is an inherited genetically heterogeneous group of arrhythmias characterized by a prolonged QTc interval in the 12-lead ECGs (with QTc values >470 ms for males and >480 ms for females, representing approximate 99th percentile values). LQTSs as a whole occurs in 1:2500 of the general population. At least 17 genes were identified contributing to LQTSs with mutations positive in about half of the affected individuals. The incidence of LQTSs in decreasing frequency illustrates LQT1 as the commonest (35%) followed by LQT2 (30%) and then LQT3 (10%). The least frequent but most lethal and more difficult to manage is LQT3. Other rare types of LQTSs account for less than 1%. It seems that the normal range of QTc interval is critical for normal AP and normal heart rhythm. Prolongation or shortening of QTc interval is arrhythmogenic. Short QT syndrome with QTc < 350 ms (reported in 1:3400) is etiologically proven cause of malignant VT and VF. Brugada syndrome diagnosed as coved ST-segment elevation in anterior precordial leads occurs in approximately 0.02% up to 0.20% in general population. It overlaps with some of the genetic and clinical features of LQT3. Catecholaminergic polymorphic ventricular tachycardia (CPVT) is relatively a rarely inherited arrhythmogenic disorder (1;10,000) characterized by polymorphic VT induced by physical or emotional stress without any detectable morphological abnormalities in the heart. The most important mutations causing CPVT are in genes encoding cardiac ryanodine type 2 receptor (RYR2) [autosomal dominant] and calsequestrin 2 (CASQ2) [autosomal recessive]. It is considered as highly malignant heart rhythm if neglected. ERS is characterized by elevation of the QRS-ST junction (J point) and QRS notching or slurring (J wave) in multiple leads, especially the inferior and/or left precordial leads. It seems to be more frequent than ever thought with ranges from approximately 6–13% in the general population. Approaching channelopathies in its broad spectrum is an excellent example of the demand of system biology approach in medicine. Channelopathies involving the heart may overlap with manifestations in the nervous system, gastrointestinal system, hearing, infant death syndrome and others. Fatal ventricular arrhythmias are due primarily to abnormal formation or mutations of trans-membrane pores or its regulatory subunits. Aberrancy of cardiac action potential (AP) formation can be interpreted through three main mechanisms: reentry, triggered activity or automaticity. All the different mechanisms described will end up with anomalous action potential. Spatial as well as temporal electrophysiological heterogeneity are important basic electrophysiological derangements that underline cardiac action potential anomalies. Heterogeneity of AP in time and location between myocardium and epicardium are critical predisposing factors to the fatal cardiac rhythm. In comparison to Brugada syndrome, the genetic mutations in LQTS result in tendency for electrical disturbance affecting depolarization rather than repolarization. Surge of catecholamines due to stress or exercise is the substrate fuel of bidirectional VT leading to syncope or SCD in CPVT. RYR2 mutations have also been suggested to be associated with dilated cardiomyopathy, hypertrophic cardiomyopathy and arrhythmogenic right ventricular cardiomyopathy. ER pattern is thought to be polygenic with an important contribution of epigenetic and environmental factors. Advances in our knowledge and understanding of disease epidemiology and the basic electrophysiological derangements of channelopathies are intelligent directions that should guide all diagnostic and therapeutic approaches.

Acknowledgements

To the spirit of the later crown prince of Saudi Arabia HRH Sultan Bin Abdulaziz Al Saud, who made my dreams in establishing the prestigious Prince Sultan Cardiac Center reality and from which this science and others are introduced to the world.

Conflict of interest

I declare no conflict of interest.

Notes/thanks/other declarations

Showers of mercy to the spirit of my Great Beloved Father who shocked me with his sudden agonizing absences during writing this chapter. Prayers for long peaceful life for my great mother. Both of them fed me the love to all humanity and all biology. Thanks to all my teachers who taught me that sky is not the limit.

Appendices and nomenclature

BrS	Brugada syndrome
CC	cardiac coherence
CPVT	catecholaminergic polymorphic ventricular tachycardia
ERS	early repolarization syndrome
LQTS	long QT syndrome
PCCD	progressive cardiac conduction disease
SCD	sudden cardiac death
SQTS	short-QT syndrome
VF	ventricular fibrillation
VT	ventricular tachycardia

Author details

Abdullah Abdulrhman Al Abdulgader
Senior Congenital Cardiologist and Invasive Electrophysiologist, Prince Sultan Cardiac Center, Alhasa, Hofuf, Saudi Arabia

*Address all correspondence to: kidsecho@yahoo.com

References

[1] Zipes DP, Wellens HJJ. Sudden cardiac death. Circulation. 1998;**98**(21):2334-2351

[2] Fishman GI, Chugh SS, Dimarco JP, Albert CM, Anderson ME, Bonow RO, et al. Sudden cardiac death prediction and prevention. Circulation. 2010;**122**(22):2335-2348

[3] Werf CVD, Langen IMV, Wilde AA. Sudden death in the young. Circulation. Arrhythmia and Electrophysiology. 2010;**3**(1):96-104

[4] Sarquella-Brugada G, Campuzano O, Iglesias A, Sánchez-Malagón J, Guerra-Balic M, Brugada J, et al. Genetics of sudden cardiac death in children and young athletes. Cardiology in the Young. 2013;**23**(2):159-173

[5] Murakoshi N, Aonuma K. Epidemiology of arrhythmias and sudden cardiac death in Asia. Circulation Journal. 2013;**77**(10):2419-2431

[6] Schwartz PJ, Stramba-Badiale M, Crotti L, Pedrazzini M, Besana A, Bosi G, et al. Prevalence of the congenital long-QT syndrome. Circulation. 2009;**120**(18):1761-1767

[7] Earle N, Crawford J, Smith W, Hayes I, Shelling A, Hood M, et al. Community detection of long QT syndrome with a clinical registry: An alternative to ECG screening programs? Heart Rhythm. 2013;**10**(2):233-238

[8] Uhm J-S, Hwang I-U, Oh Y-S, Choi M-S, Jang S-W, Shin W-S, et al. Prevalence of electrocardiographic findings suggestive of sudden cardiac death risk in 10,867 apparently healthy young Korean men. Pacing and Clinical Electrophysiology. 2011;**34**(6):717-723

[9] Hayashi K, Fujino N, Uchiyama K, Ino H, Sakata K, Konno T, et al. Long QT syndrome and associated gene mutation carriers in Japanese children: Results from ECG screening examinations. Clinical Science. 2009;**117**(12):415-424

[10] Mahida S, Hogarth AJ, Cowan C, Tayebjee MH, Graham LN, Pepper CB. Genetics of congenital and drug-induced long QT syndromes: Current evidence and future research perspectives. Journal of Interventional Cardiac Electrophysiology. 2013;**37**(1):9-19

[11] Horigome H, Nagashima M, Sumitomo N, Yoshinaga M, Ushinohama H, Iwamoto M, et al. Clinical characteristics and genetic background of congenital long-QT syndrome diagnosed in fetal, neonatal, and infantile life. Circulation. Arrhythmia and Electrophysiology. 2010;**3**(1):10-17

[12] Zareba W, Moss AJ, Schwartz PJ, Vincent GM, Robinson JL, Priori SG, et al. Influence of the genotype on the clinical course of the long-QT syndrome. The New England Journal of Medicine. 1998;**339**(14):960-965

[13] Skinner JR. Guidelines for the diagnosis and management of familial long QT syndrome. Heart, Lung & Circulation. 2007;**16**(1):22-24

[14] Goldenberg I, Moss AJ, Peterson DR, Mcnitt S, Zareba W, Andrews ML, et al. Risk factors for aborted cardiac arrest and sudden cardiac death in children with the congenital long-QT syndrome. Circulation. 2008;**117**(17):2184-2191

[15] Gaita F, Giustetto C, Bianchi F, Wolpert C, Schimpf R, Riccardi R, et al. Short QT syndrome. Circulation. 2003;**108**(8):965-970

[16] Funada A, Hayashi K, Ino H, Fujino N, Uchiyama K, Sakata K, et al. Assessment of QT intervals and

prevalence of short QT syndrome in Japan. Clinical Cardiology. 2008;**31**(6):270-274

[17] Maury P, Extramiana F, Sbragia P, Giustetto C, Schimpf R, Duparc A, et al. Short QT syndrome. Update on a recent entity. Archives of Cardiovascular Diseases. 2008;**101**(11-12):779-786

[18] Giustetto C, Schimpf R, Mazzanti A, Scrocco C, Maury P, Anttonen O, et al. Long-term follow-up of patients with short QT syndrome. Journal of the American College of Cardiology. 2011;**58**(6):587-595

[19] Chockalingam P, Wilde A. The multifaceted cardiac sodium channel and its clinical implications. Heart. 2012;**98**(17):1318-1324

[20] Amin AS, Asghari-Roodsari A, Tan HL. Cardiac sodium channelopathies. Pflügers Archiv - European Journal of Physiology. 2010;**460**(2):223-237

[21] Gaw AC, Lee B, Gervacio-Domingo G, Antzelevitch C, Divinagracia R, Jocano F Jr. Unraveling the enigma of bangungut. Is sudden unexplained nocturnal death syndrome (SUNDs) in the Philippines a disease allelic to the Brugada syndrome? Philippine Journal of Internal Medicine. 2011;**49**:165-176

[22] Chen Q, Kirsch GE, Zhang D, Brugada R, Brugada J, Brugada P, et al. Genetic basis and molecular mechanism for idiopathic ventricular fibrillation. Nature. 1998;**392**(6673):293-296

[23] Hedley PL, Jørgensen P, Schlamowitz S, Moolman-Smook J, Kanters JK, Corfield VA, et al. The genetic basis of Brugada syndrome: A mutation update. Human Mutation. 2009;**30**(9):1256-1266

[24] Priori SG, Napolitano C, Gasparini M, Pappone C, Bella PD, Brignole M, et al. Clinical and genetic heterogeneity of right bundle branch block and ST-segment elevation syndrome. Circulation. 2000;**102**(20):2509-2515

[25] Brugada J, Brugada R, Antzelevitch C, Towbin J, Nademanee K, Brugada P. Long-term follow-up of individuals with the electrocardiographic pattern of right bundle-branch block and ST-segment elevation in precordial leads V 1 to V 3. Circulation. 2002;**105**(1):73-78

[26] Probst V, Veltmann C, Eckardt L, Meregalli P, Gaita F, Tan H, et al. Long-term prognosis of patients diagnosed with Brugada syndrome. Circulation. 2010;**121**(5):635-643

[27] Kamakura S, Ohe T, Nakazawa K, Aizawa Y, Shimizu A, Horie M, et al. Long-term prognosis of Probands with Brugada-pattern ST-elevation in leads V 1–V 3. Circulation. Arrhythmia and Electrophysiology. 2009;**2**(5):495-503

[28] Antzelevitch C. Genetic, molecular and cellular mechanisms underlying the J wave syndromes. Circulation Journal. 2012;**76**(5):1054-1065

[29] Haïssaguerre M, Derval N, Sacher F, Jesel L, Deisenhofer I, Roy LD, et al. Sudden cardiac arrest associated with early repolarization. New England Journal of Medicine. 2008;**358**(19):2016-2023

[30] Noseworthy P, Porthan K, Tikkanen J, Peloso G, Merchant F, Pietila A, et al. The early repolarization pattern: Clinical correlates and heritability. Journal of the American College of Cardiology. 2011;**57**(14)

[31] Tikkanen JT, Anttonen O, Junttila MJ, Aro AL, Kerola T, Rissanen HA, et al. Long-term outcome associated with early repolarization on electrocardiography. The New England Journal of Medicine. 2009;**361**(26):2529-2537

[32] Kui C, Congxin H, Xi W, Yan-Hong T, Okello E, Salim M, et al. Characteristic of the prevalence of J wave in apparently healthy Chinese adults. Archives of Medical Research. 2008;**39**(2):232-235

[33] Haruta D, Matsuo K, Tsuneto A, Ichimaru S, Hida A, Sera N, et al. Incidence and prognostic value of early repolarization pattern in the 12-Lead electrocardiogram. Circulation. 2011;**123**(25):2931-2937

[34] Obeyesekere MN, Klein GJ, Nattel S, Leong-Sit P, Gula LJ, Skanes AC, et al. A clinical approach to early repolarization. Circulation. 2013;**127**(15):1620-1629

[35] Tikkanen JT, Junttila MJ, Anttonen O, Aro AL, Luttinen S, Kerola T, et al. Early repolarization. Circulation. 2011;**123**(23):2666-2673

[36] Leenhardt A, Lucet V, Denjoy I, Grau F, Ngoc DD, Coumel P. catecholaminergic polymorphic ventricular tachycardia in children. Circulation 1995;91(5):1512-1519.

[37] Priori SG, Napolitano C, Tiso N, Memmi M, Vignati G, Bloise R, et al. Mutations in the cardiac ryanodine receptor gene (hRyR2) underlie catecholaminergic polymorphic ventricular tachycardia. Circulation. 2001;**103**(2):196-200

[38] Lahat H, Pras E, Olender T, Avidan N, Ben-Asher E, Man O, et al. A missense mutation in a highly conserved region of CASQ2 is associated with autosomal recessive catecholamine-induced polymorphic ventricular tachycardia in Bedouin families from Israel. American Journal of Human Genetics. 2001;**69**(6):1378-1384

[39] Vega AL, Tester DJ, Ackerman MJ, Makielski JC. Protein kinase A-dependent biophysical phenotype for V227F-KCNJ2 mutation in catecholaminergic polymorphic ventricular tachycardia. Circulation. Arrhythmia and Electrophysiology. 2009;**2**(5):540-547

[40] Kawamura M, Ohno S, Naiki N, Nagaoka I, Dochi K, Wang Q, et al. Genetic background of catecholaminergic polymorphic ventricular tachycardia in Japan. Circulation Journal. 2013;**77**(7):1705-1713

[41] Hayashi M, Denjoy I, Extramiana F, Maltret A, Buisson NR, Lupoglazoff J-M, et al. Incidence and risk factors of arrhythmic events in catecholaminergic polymorphic ventricular tachycardia. Circulation. 2009;**119**(18):2426-2434

[42] Swan H, Piippo K, Viitasalo M, Heikkilä P, Paavonen T, Kainulainen K, et al. Arrhythmic disorder mapped to chromosome 1q42–q43 causes malignant polymorphic ventricular tachycardia in structurally normal hearts. Journal of the American College of Cardiology. 1999;**34**(7):2035-2042

[43] Behere S, Weindling S. Inherited arrhythmias: The cardiac channelopathies. Annals of Pediatric Cardiology. 2015;**8**(3):210

[44] Niaz A, Rizvi SF, Khurram D. Prevalence of long QT syndrome and other cardiac defects in deaf-mute children. Journal of Ayub Medical College, Abbottabad. 2011;**23**(1):5-8

[45] Chang RK, Lan YT, Silka MJ, Morrow H, Kwong A, Smith-Lang J, et al. Genetic variants for long QT syndrome among infants and children from a statewide newborn hearing screening program cohort. The Journal of Pediatrics. Mar 2014;**164**(3):590-5.e1-3

[46] Partemi S, Cestèle S, Pezzella M, Campuzano O, Paravidino R, Pascali VL, et al. Loss-of-function KCNH2 mutation in a family with long QT syndrome, epilepsy, and sudden death. Epilepsia. Aug 2013;**54**(8):e112-e116

[47] Hazle MA, Shellhaas RA, Bradley DJ, Dick M, Lapage MJ. Arrhythmogenic channelopathy syndromes presenting as refractory epilepsy. Pediatric Neurology. 2013;**49**(2):134-137

[48] Chockalingam P, Rammeloo LA, Postema PG, Hruda J, Clur S-AB, Blom NA, et al. Fever-induced life-threatening arrhythmias in children harboring an SCN5A mutation. Pediatrics. 2010;**127**(1)

[49] Kenny D, Martin R. Drowning and sudden cardiac death. Archives of Disease in Childhood. 2010;**96**(1):5-8

[50] Tester DJ, Medeiros-Domingo A, Will ML, Ackerman MJ. Unexplained drownings and the cardiac channelopathies: A molecular autopsy series. Mayo Clinic Proceedings. 2011;**86**(10):941-947

[51] Beyder A, Mazzone A, Strege PR, Tester DJ, Saito YA, Bernard CE, et al. Loss-of-function of the voltage-gated sodium channel NaV1.5 (channelopathies) in patients with irritable bowel syndrome. Gastroenterology. 2014;**146**(7):1659-1668

[52] Diamant U-B, Jensen SM, Winbo A, Stattin E-L, Rydberg A. Vectorcardiographic recordings of the Q-T interval in a pediatric long Q-T syndrome population. Pediatric Cardiology. 2012;**34**(2):245-249

[53] Rice KS, Dickson G, Lane M, Crawford J, Chung S-K, Rees MI, et al. Elevated serum gastrin levels in Jervell and Lange-Nielsen syndrome: A marker of severe KCNQ1 dysfunction? Heart Rhythm. 2011;**8**(4):551-554

[54] Ramirez AH, Shaffer CM, Delaney JT, Sexton DP, Levy SE, Rieder MJ, et al. Novel rare variants in congenital cardiac arrhythmia genes are frequent in drug-induced torsades de pointes. The Pharmacogenomics Journal. 2012;**13**(4):325-329

[55] Tester DJ, Tan B-H, Medeiros-Domingo A, Song C, Makielski JC, Ackerman MJ. Loss-of-function mutations in the KCNJ8-encoded Kir6.1 K ATP channel and sudden infant death syndrome. Circulation. Cardiovascular Genetics. 2011;**4**(5):510-515

[56] Tan B-H, Pundi KN, Norstrand DWV, Valdivia CR, Tester DJ, Medeiros-Domingo A, et al. Sudden infant death syndrome–associated mutations in the sodium channel beta subunits. Heart Rhythm. 2010;**7**(6):771-778

[57] Yoshinaga M, Ushinohama H, Sato S, Tauchi N, Horigome H, Takahashi H, et al. Electrocardiographic screening of 1-month-old infants for identifying prolonged QT intervals. Circulation. Arrhythmia and Electrophysiology. 2013;**6**(5):932-938

[58] Anuwutnavin S, Wanitpongpan P, Chungsomprasong P, Soongswang J, Srisantiroj N, Wataganara T. Fetal long QT syndrome manifested as atrioventricular block and ventricular tachycardia: A case report and a review of the literature. Pediatric Cardiology. 2012;**34**(8):1955-1962

[59] Martin CA, Matthews GDK, Huang CL-H. Sudden cardiac death and inherited channelopathy: The basic electrophysiology of the myocyte and myocardium in ion channel disease. Heart. 2012;**98**(7):536-543

[60] January CT, Riddle JM, Salata JJ. A model for early afterdepolarizations: Induction with the Ca2 channel agonist bay K 8644. Circulation Research. 1988;**62**(3):563-571

[61] Jiang D, Wang R, Xiao B, Kong H, Hunt DJ, Choi P, et al. Enhanced store overload–induced Ca 2 release and channel sensitivity to luminal Ca 2 activation are common defects of RyR2 mutations linked to

ventricular tachycardia and sudden death. Circulation Research. 2005;**97**(11):1173-1181

[62] Chauhan VS, Downar E, Nanthakumar K, Parker JD, Ross HJ, Chan W, et al. Increased ventricular repolarization heterogeneity in patients with ventricular arrhythmia vulnerability and cardiomyopathy: A human in vivo study. American Journal of Physiology—Heart and Circulatory Physiology. Jan 2006;**290**(1):H79-H86

[63] Morita H, Zipes DP, Fukushima-Kusano K, Nagase S, Nakamura K, Morita ST, et al. Repolarization heterogeneity in the right ventricular outflow tract: Correlation with ventricular arrhythmias in Brugada patients and in an in vitro canine Brugada model. Heart Rhythm. 2008;**5**(5):725-733

[64] Martin CA, Grace AA, Huang CL. Spatial and temporal heterogeneities are localized to the right ventricular outflow tract in a heterozygotic Scn5a mouse model. American Journal of Physiology—Heart and Circulatory Physiology. 2011;**300**(2):H605-16

[65] Kurita T, Shimizu W, Inagaki M, Suyama K, Taguchi A, Satomi K, et al. The electrophysiologic mechanism of ST-segment elevation in Brugada syndrome. Journal of the American College of Cardiology. 2002;**40**(2):330-334

[66] Rosenbaum DS, Jackson LE, Smith JM, Garan H, Ruskin JN, Cohen RJ. Electrical alternans and vulnerability to ventricular arrhythmias. The New England Journal of Medicine. 1994;**330**(4):235-241

[67] Pastore JM, Girouard SD, Laurita KR, Akar FG, Rosenbaum DS. Mechanism linking T-wave alternans to the genesis of cardiac fibrillation. Circulation. 1999;**99**(10):1385-1394

[68] Salama G, London B. Mouse models of long QT syndrome. The Journal of Physiology. 2006;**578**(1):43-53

[69] Kim TY, Kunitomo Y, Pfeiffer Z, Patel D, Hwang J, Harrison K, et al. Complex excitation dynamics underlie polymorphic ventricular tachycardia in a transgenic rabbit model of long QT syndrome type 1. Heart Rhythm. 2015;**12**(1):220-228

[70] Chang MG, Sato D, Lange ED, Lee J-H, Karagueuzian HS, Garfinkel A, et al. Bi-stable wave propagation and early afterdepolarization–mediated cardiac arrhythmias. Heart Rhythm. 2012;**9**(1):115-122

[71] Yan G-X, Antzelevitch C. Cellular basis for the Brugada syndrome and other mechanisms of arrhythmogenesis associated with ST-segment elevation. Circulation. 1999;**100**(15):1660-1666

[72] Shimizu W, Aiba T, Kurita T, Kamakura S. Paradoxic abbreviation of repolarization in epicardium of the right ventricular outflow tract during augmentation of Brugada-type ST segment elevation. Journal of Cardiovascular Electrophysiology. 2001;**12**(12):1418-1421

[73] Meregalli P, Wilde A, Tan H. Pathophysiological mechanisms of Brugada syndrome: Depolarization disorder, repolarization disorder, or more? Cardiovascular Research. 2005;**67**(3):367-378

[74] Tukkie R, Sogaard P, Vleugels J, Groot IKD, Wilde AA, Tan HL. Delay in right ventricular activation contributes to Brugada syndrome. Circulation. 2004;**109**(10):1272-1277

[75] Eckardt L, Bruns H-J, Paul M, Kirchhof P, Schulze-Bahr E, Wichter T, et al. Body surface area of ST elevation and the presence of late potentials correlate to the inducibility of ventricular tachyarrhythmias in Brugada

syndrome. Journal of Cardiovascular Electrophysiology. 2002;**13**(8):742-749

[76] Coronel R, Casini S, Koopmann TT, Wilms-Schopman FJ, Verkerk AO, Groot JRD, et al. Right ventricular fibrosis and conduction delay in a patient with clinical signs of Brugada syndrome. Circulation. 2005;**112**(18):2769-2777

[77] Nademanee K, Veerakul G, Chandanamattha P, Chaothawee L, Ariyachaipanich A, Jirasirirojanakorn K, et al. Prevention of ventricular fibrillation episodes in Brugada syndrome by catheter ablation over the anterior right ventricular outflow tract epicardium. Circulation. 2011;**123**(12):1270-1279

[78] Marks AR, Priori S, Memmi M, Kontula K, Laitinen PIJ. Involvement of the cardiac ryanodine receptor/calcium release channel in catecholaminergic polymorphic ventricular tachycardia. Journal of Cellular Physiology. 2002;**190**(1):1-6

[79] Lahat H, Eldar M, Levy-Nissenbaum E, Bahan T, Friedman E, Khoury A, et al. Autosomal recessive catecholamine- or exercise-induced polymorphic ventricular tachycardia. Circulation. 2001;**103**(23):2822-2827

[80] Lehnart SE, Wehrens XH, Laitinen PJ, Reiken SR, Deng S-X, Cheng Z, et al. Sudden death in familial polymorphic ventricular tachycardia associated with calcium release channel (ryanodine receptor) leak. Circulation. 2004;**109**(25):3208-3214

[81] Liu N, Colombi B, Memmi M, Zissimopoulos S, Rizzi N, Negri S, et al. Arrhythmogenesis in catecholaminergic polymorphic ventricular tachycardia. Circulation Research. 2006;**99**(3):292-298

[82] Knollmann BC, Chopra N, Hlaing T, Akin B, Yang T, Ettensohn K, et al. Casq2 deletion causes sarcoplasmic reticulum volume increase, premature Ca^{2+} release, and catecholaminergic polymorphic ventricular tachycardia. Journal of Clinical Investigation. Sep 2006;**116**(9):2510-2520

[83] Bhuiyan ZA, Berg MPVD, Tintelen JPV, Bink-Boelkens MT, Wiesfeld AC, Alders M, et al. Expanding Spectrum of human RYR2-related disease. Circulation. 2007;**116**(14):1569-1576

[84] Tang Y, Tian X, Wang R, Fill M, Chen SW. Abnormal termination of Ca^{2+} release is a common defect of RyR2 mutations associated with cardiomyopathies. Circulation Research. 2012;**110**(7):968-977

[85] Tiso N. Identification of mutations in the cardiac ryanodine receptor gene in families affected with arrhythmogenic right ventricular cardiomyopathy type 2 (ARVD2). Human Molecular Genetics. 2001

[86] Brugada R, Hong K, Dumaine R, Cordeiro J, Gaita F, Borggrefe M, et al. Sudden death associated with short-QT syndrome linked to mutations in HERG. Circulation. 2004;**109**(1):30-35

[87] Antzelevitch C, Pollevick GD, Cordeiro JM, Casis O, Sanguinetti MC, Aizawa Y, et al. Loss-of-function mutations in the cardiac calcium channel underlie a new clinical entity characterized by ST-segment elevation, short QT intervals, and sudden cardiac death. Circulation. 2007;**115**(4):442-449

[88] Extramiana F, Antzelevitch C. Amplified transmural dispersion of repolarization as the basis for arrhythmogenesis in a canine ventricular-wedge model of short-QT syndrome. Circulation. 2004;**110**(24):3661-3666

[89] Mehta M, Jain AC, Mehta A. Early repolarization. Clinical Cardiology. 1999;**22**(2):59-65

[90] Yan G-X, Antzelevitch C. Cellular basis for the electrocardiographic J wave. Circulation. 1996;**93**(2):372-379

[91] Burashnikov E, Pfeiffer R, Barajas-Martinez H, Delpón E, Hu D, Desai M, et al. Mutations in the cardiac L-type calcium channel associated with inherited J-wave syndromes and sudden cardiac death. Heart Rhythm. 2010;**7**(12):1872-1882

[92] Haïssaguerre M, Chatel S, Sacher F, Weerasooriya R, Probst V, Loussouarn G, et al. Ventricular fibrillation with prominent early repolarization associated with a rare variant of KCNJ8/KATP channel. Journal of Cardiovascular Electrophysiology. 2009;**20**(1):93-98

[93] Grant AO, Carboni MP, Neplioueva V, Starmer CF, Memmi M, Napolitano C, et al. Long QT syndrome, Brugada syndrome, and conduction system disease are linked to a single sodium channel mutation. Journal of Clinical Investigation. 2002;**110**(8):1201-1209

[94] Veen TAV, Stein M, Royer A, Le Quang K, Charpentier F, Colledge WH, et al. Impaired impulse propagation in Scn5a-knockout mice. Circulation. 2005;**112**(13):1927-1935

Chapter 6

Inherited Ventricular Arrhythmias, the Channelopathies and SCD: Current Knowledge and Future Speculations - Risk Stratification, Management Plans and Future Speculations

Abdullah Abdulrhman Al Abdulgader

Abstract

Channelopathy constitutes significant proportion of SCD worldwide (around 10% or 370,000 deaths annually). It was creating a mysterious group of diseases until the second half of the last century when Anton Jervell and Fred Lange-Nielsen described Jervell Lange-Nielsen syndrome in 1957. It was late until 1995 where genetic characterization commenced. Later on, the massive genetic information with the discovery of genetic heterogeneity and allelic het¬erogeneity was a major victory in the field. The basic sciences in cellular electrophysiology and genetics complemented by meticulous clinical detection and the different clinical trials in the field opened a new era of wide therapeutic choices for clinicians. The knowledge obtained from the different experimental platforms especially the induced pluripotent stem cells is promising. The revolutionary move in SCD and channelopathies is described where correlation between the arrhythmogenesis and fluctuation in SGMA is established and must be investigated. The observation of the arrhythmogenicity of SGMA fluctuation and its effect on HRV together with the differential effect of certain sympathovagal tones (more sympathetic innervation is favoring VT/VF in LQTS1, LQTS2 and SQTS but not BrS or ERS) are all future directions to optimize our preventive, diagnostic as well as therapeutic options of SCD and channelopathy in humans.

Keywords: arrhythmia, BrS: Brugada syndrome, CC: cardiac coherence, catecholaminergic polymorphic ventricular tachycardia, ERS: Early repolarization syndrome, heart rate variability, LQTS: Long QT syndrome, progressive cardiac conduction disease, sudden cardiac death, Schumann resonance, solar geomagnetic activity, SNP, SQTS

1. Introduction

One of the most devastating life moments that may impact the whole life of persons, families and societies is the sudden death experience of a close relative

IntechOpen

or a beloved one. The whole medical provision is dedicated to prevent or delay death while maintaining good quality of life (QOL). For this reason, sudden loss of human life is creating the most serious challenge for medical professionals and decision makers. Sudden cardiac death (SCD) is defined as death occurring unexpectedly in the first hour after symptoms commence. In the United States, around 300,000 deaths occur every year because of SCD. It is conspicuous that this huge loss in the world communities is creating a major social impact. This impact is undoubtedly more destructive with the loss of a young member of the family. Sadly, life-threatening arrhythmias and sudden cardiac death can be the first presenting symptom. Scientists and clinicians were racing in the last two decades in a unique complementary scientific effort to reconcile the rapidly growing body of knowledge of the molecular mechanisms and clinical correlates of SCD. In this chapter, we will discuss the available risk stratification for channelopathies and detailed management steps with focus on the different trials for pharmaceutical approach of the different channelopathies. The electrical therapy in the form of ICD is a critical management step but will be prioritized according to channelopathy type and clinical settings. Future speculations of fatal ventricular rhythms are going to be discussed with special reference to solar and geomagnetic activity fluctuation and heart rate variability (HRV) correlations to SCD and the up to the moment knowledge in its impact on channelopathies.

2. Management of ventricular arrhythmias in suspected channelopathies

2.1 The long QT syndromes' risk stratification and management plan

The yield of genetic mutations in LQTS is better than in other channelopathies but still did not exceed 50%. The cutoff numbers for QTc interval before labeling it long is 480 and 470 ms in post pubertal women and men, respectively. In the 12 leads ECG, manual measurement from limb lead 2 or chest lead V5 using Bazzet's formula (**$QTc = QT/\sqrt{RR}$**) is a must. Moss and Schwartz developed a reliable scoring system for better risk stratification of LQTS individuals (**Table 1**) [1, 2]. Goldenburg criteria for risk stratification in long QT are also useful to add in clinical practice (**Table 2**) [3]. There must be no medications affecting ECG.

Schwartz score is more commonly used. The Schwartz score was proposed in 1993 and revised in 2011 by Schwartz and Crotti [4]. Schwartz Moss scoring system comprises clinical, electrocardiographic as well as familial historical data. It is designed for use for the index case but not others. It was found to have high correlation to positive genetic testing with 75% likelihood if the score is more than 4 points. It is not of use for a family member with long QT interval but with no symptoms [5]. T-wave abnormalities are important indicators for electrical instability. The score will count 1 point for positive T-wave alternans in the TWA test and another 1 point for notched T waves that are considered as poor prognostic sign. Poor prognostic factors with more likelihood for SCD are QTc more than 500 ms, LQTS symptoms, genotype of LQT2 or LQT3 and female gender. Male gender with LQT1 refers to lower risk group. The strongest indicator for SCD is the QTc interval [6]. Survival from cardiac arrest before age 7 or development of syncope before puberty carries worse overall prognosis [7]. Risk of recurrence is very high if syncope or cardiac arrest happens in the first year of life [8]. Genetic testing carries important prognostic value as asymptomatic positive mutation individuals below 40 years of age carry 10% higher risk of life-threatening arrhythmia if not treated [9]. Placebo controlled

Risk factor	Points
EKG findings	
A: QTc	
≥480 ms	3
460–479 ms	2
450–459 (men)	1
B: QTc fourth minute of recovery from exercise	1
Stress test ≥480 ms	
C: TdP	2
D: T-wave alternans	1
E: Notched T-wave in 3 leads	1
F: Low heart rate for age (resting heart rate below the second percentile for age)	0.5
Clinical History	
A: Syncope	
With stress	2
Without stress	1
B: Congenital deafness	0.5
Family History	
A: Family members with definite LQTS	1
B: Unexplained SCD at age < 30 years among immediate family members	0.5

Score ≤ 1 point: low probability of LQTS. 1.5–3 points: intermediate probability of LQTS. ≥3.5 points: high probability of LQTS.

Table 1.
Updated Schwartz score: The same family member cannot be counted in A and B.

randomized trials in LQTS management are lacking (except 2019 AHA editorial Published online 2019 May 29. doi: 10.1161/JAHA.119.012833, entitled "Energy Drinks: Another Cause of QT Prolongation?") The assignment of placebo group in LQTS creates difficult ethical choices. Almost all present strategic plans in LQTS management were deduced from registries with beta blockers and cardioverter defibrillator (ICD) therapy [10]. Electrolytes disturbances correction like hypokalemia and hypomagnesaemia is a critical primary step in LQTS management. Magnesium sulfate intravenously proved to be safe and effective for acquired or congenital TdP management [11]. Beta blockers are the first line and the easiest therapeutic choice for both LQT1 and LQT2. In the current medical literature, there is controversy regarding the use of beta blockers in LQT3. For LQT1 and LQT2, propranolol and nadolol seem to be more effective than metoprolol [12]. Nadolol with its longer half life (twice a day) and sustained release propranolol seem to be attractive options. There are data suggesting that propranolol is more effective than atenolol [13]. Disease-specific favorable responses are suggested with nadolol providing the sole significant risk reducer in LQT2, while metoprolol, atenolol, propranolol and

Very high risk (secondary prevention)
Postcardiopulmonary resuscitation
Spontaneous TdP
High risk (primary prevention)
QTc >500 ms
Prior syncope
Low risk
Qtc <500 ms and no prior syncope

Table 2.
Goldenburg criteria for LQTS risk stratification.

nadolol have similar risk reduction in LQT1 [14]. No significant scientific evidence is favoring selective beta blockers over the non-selective group [15]. It is always advised to keep beta blockers as adjunct treatment after ICD implants. The sympathetic surge after delivery of a shock is always a risk for recurrence [16]. There are experimental data supporting the use of beta blockers in LQT3 [17] and others contradicting its use [18]. Analysis of 493 LQT3 patients derived from 9 registries supports the use of beta blockers [19]. There is in the horizon an early evidence suggesting significant therapeutic role of sodium channel blockers like ranolazine, mexiletine and flecainide in LQT3 treatment [20–22]. Mexiletine was proved also of being an effective therapeutic option in LQT3 as well as LQT1 and LQT2 [23].

Rarely, cautious use of mexiletine in LQT3 is needed as it may cause QT interval prolongation [24]. Successful shortening of the QTc interval (565 ± 60 ms to 461 ± 23 ms; $P < 0.04$) was achieved with flecainide. With its potent sodium blockage properties, flecainide was able to normalize QTc in five patients with LQT3 with DKPQ mutation [25]. Ranolazine, a late INa blocker, was seen to be effective to shorten the QT interval as well as suppress TdP as proved by experimental models of LQT3 [26]. Dose-dependent shortening of QT interval was achieved in human patients with DKPQ mutation of LQT3 using ranolazine [27]. What seems to be a therapeutic paradox is the benefit of adrenergic stimulation in cases with acquired LQTS and low heart rate with pauses. In the absence of concomitant gene mutations, epinephrine and isoproterenol were found to be effective in acquired LQTS [28]. In addition, selective effect of β-adrenergic stimulation was reported in the different LQTSs. The effect was seen in canine models as induction of TdP in LQT1 and LQT2 but suppression in LQT3 [29]. This concludes that therapeutic paradox is evident in LQTSs, as beta blockers are therapy of LQT1 and LQT2 but beta adrenergic stimulation is therapy for LQT3. Pause-dependent TdP in case of acquired or congenital LQT can be minimized using temporary pacing [30].

The implantation of an ICD is pivotal secondary prevention in LQTS and a reasonable primary prevention approach in selected cases [31]. Thoughtful ICD programming to prevent inappropriate shocks is important. In our practice, for LQTS secondary prevention, we do not incorporate tiered therapy for this type of patients but program the ICD to VF-only zone (detect rate, >220 beats per minute). ICD is indicated in the following conditions:

1. As secondary prevention after aborted cardiac arrest

2. Failure of optimal medical therapy to control events of cardiac arrest

3. Intolerance to primary pharmacotherapy (β-blockers)

4. Symptomatic patients with QTc of 500 ms or greater, especially women with LQT2

5. LQT3 genotype

Well-accepted treatment option in LQTS patients is left cardiac sympathetic denervation (LCSD). It is an exceptional therapeutic option that can be leaned on in selected cases like LQT1 and LQT2 patients with no proper response to beta blockers, intolerance to beta blockers, or after ICD implant with recurrent arrhythmias [32]. LCSD can be chosen as a primary treatment option or secondary, with what is described as excellent results in selected patients [33]. It seems that there are specific selection criteria to obtain optimal outcome of LCSD. More than half of high-risk patients did not benefit from the procedure. Addition of right cardiac sympathetic denervation to LCSD might be of benefit in selected patients [34]. At all times, LCSD is not a replacement of the beta blockers and/or ICD therapy.

2.2 Brugada syndrome risk stratification and management plan

Any patient that survived a VF arrest or with syncope and an ECG consistent with spontaneous type I pattern should undergo permanent cardiac defibrillator. Other high-risk factors include male gender, atrial fibrillation or a fragmented QRS. There is no consensus on the use of electrophysiologic study to risk stratify patients. Importantly, the programmed electrical stimulation predictive value (PRELUDE) registry showed that the inability to induce arrhythmias does not correlate with a negative predictive value [35]. A family history of SCD and the presence of an SCN5A mutation have proven to be high risk predictors as well. Criteria to diagnose Brugada syndrome [36] in symptomatic patients are as follows: Type I ST segment elevation via drug challenge or spontaneously in at least 1 right precordial lead (V1 or V2). In asymptomatic patients, the situation is little bit guarded. Constellation of strong and concealed electrocardiographic manifestation should be looked for. Attenuation of the ST segment during maximum exercise with subsequent coved ST segment elevation when rested is an important finding, in the setting of absent structural heart disease. StT wave alternans (TWA), development of spontaneous left bundle branch or PVCs are all relevant to alert to BrS diagnosis in the absence of symptoms. Other subtle electrical alerts are first-degree AV block and left axis deviation as well as fragmented QRS. In TWA test, late potentials are additional alerting alarm. During electrophysiological study, a ventricular effective refractory period less than 200 ms is alarming also. Other alerts are the fragmentation of QRS as well as the presence of atrial fibrillation.

BrS is well known to be triggered by febrile illness. This is why meticulous fever management should be carried out in Brugada patients and their families. Pharmaceutical agents inducing Brugada arrhythmias should be avoided. Physicians and public may refer to (www.brugadadrugs.org) for reliable information in this regard. Sympathovagal imbalance with dominant parasympathetic tone predisposes to ventricular arrhythmias in BrS patients. Isoproterenol intravenously is used with success to control VF storms in BrS patients [37]. In a limited study, quinidine was found to be of a role in asymptomatic individuals [38]. In case of frequent ICD shocks, quinidine can be used as adjunct treatment. Quinidine effectiveness was found to be 85% in a follow-up of up to 4 years with a dose of ≤600 mg per day [39]. An empirical quinidine registry for asymptomatic Brugada individuals recommended doses of 600–900 mg per day if tolerated [40]. The decision of ICD implant in asymptomatic Brugada individuals needs true contemplation in view of the rarity of the events. Annual rate of cardiac events in this group is 0.5% versus 7.7%–10.2% in VF patients and 0.6%–1.2% in syncope patients [41]. Many authorities in the field do not recommend ICD implant in asymptomatic Brugada individuals [42]. With a history of VT/VF or arrhythmia-related syncope, in Brugada individuals, ICD must be the first-line management. In contrast to what we have mentioned earlier in LQTS management, tiered therapy is recommended in BrS ICD programming. Fractionated late potentials in the anterior aspect of right ventricular out flow tract (RVOT) were detected in nine patients with VF storm due to Brugada syndrome [43]. Ablation at this site normalized the Brugada ECG findings in majority of patients (with one patient only left with amiodarone) [44]. These electrocardiographic findings and site ablation results were repeated in recent works [45, 46].

2.3 Catecholaminergic PMVT risk stratification and management plan

Catecholaminergic polymorphic VT (CPVT) is a syndrome of exercise- or stress-induced PMVT in the absence of overt structural heart disease or abnormalities on the baseline ECG. CPVT should be suspected in patients with exertional presyncope/syncope and a normal resting QTc interval. The most useful diagnostic test is the stress ECG. The hallmark finding is exertional bidirectional VT, although more commonly exertional ventricular ectopy or short runs of PMVT may occur [47, 48]. The prevalence of CPVT is estimated to be 1 in 10,000, and it is often diagnosed among healthy children or young adults [49]. High doses (nadolol, 3–5 mg/kg) may be necessary to suppress exertional ectopy; doses can be titrated to effect based on inducibility of ventricular arrhythmias with stress testing [50]. Because of the high risk of recurrent events and SCD on β-blockers, adjunctive ICD implantation is recommended in all symptomatic patients.

Pharmaceutical emergency management involves intravenous beta blockers. Anesthetic measures to reduce adrenergic sympathetic surge like conscious sedation or even general anesthesia might be used in emergency situation especially with ICD shock storm. This approach still lacks scientific evidence. In spite of the pivotal role of beta blockers in CPVT management, recurrence of arrhythmic events is still high. Eleven studies have been reviewed comprising 493 patients, and 88% were on beta blockers, with follow-up periods of 20–96 months. The eight-year arrhythmic event rate was 37.2%, with a near-fatal event rate of 15.3% and a fatal event rate of 6.4% [51]. This review alerts the arrhythmia community to very important management alert, where suppression of arrhythmia induced by exercise with beta blockers does not imply long-term effectiveness.

If gene mutation is positive for CPVT, without using beta blockers, SCD may occur even if exercise test is negative [52]. Flecainide is also a promising first-line drug. It might be used as second-line treatment combined with beta blockers regardless of the presence or absence of genetic mutation [53, 54]. It was proved to target the calcium waves inducing arrhythmia as it targets RYR2 channels [55]. Flecainide was shown to be highly effective if combined with beta blockers compared to beta blockers alone ($P < 0.003$) [56]. The recommended daily dose of flecainide is 150–200 mg with maximum dose not exceeding 300 mg/day. In genotype-negative CPVT patients, flecainide was shown to reduce VT during exercise test [57].

Surgical option represented by left cardiac sympathetic denervation (LCSD) is an effective choice as a hybrid therapy to pharmaceutical agents. It was found to be safe and effective and requires minimal endoscopic surgery, although its availability is a problem. LCSD was found to raise the VT threshold and ventricular refractoriness [58]. In high-risk patients, it might be advisable to be done early in the treatment plan. Larger cohort studies are needed for better understanding the role of LCSD in PCVT [59].

ICD, with primary termination, was able to clear VT in 24 young patients with PCVT. In spite of its critical role in management, ICD may act as proarrhythmic due to its induction of adrenergic state [60]. In certain patients with cautious personalities, ICD may act paradoxically to increase arrhythmic events through emotionally higher adrenergic state of fear. This is why reducing negative emotions should be thought of as primary essential non-pharmaceutical measure to inhibit arrhythmic events in any adrenergic-mediated arrhythmia [61]. This should be emphasized more in younger age group and patients with higher shock frequency. It was found that patients younger than 50 years of age might be at higher risk due to life style disruption and distressing social comparisons [62]. Programming ICD in PCVT patients should be tiered therapy with three zones of management (SVT, VT and VF). This is important to avoid inappropriate shocks with its vicious cycle arrhythmic effects. Symptomatic CPVT patients should avoid exercise. Guarded exercise might be allowed to asymptomatic CPVT individuals.

As we emphasized above, suppression of exercise-induced ventricular arrhythmias with β-blocker therapy does not necessarily translate into long-term effectiveness of therapy [63].

2.4 Early repolarization syndrome (ERS) risk stratification and management plan

This is a steep repolarization of transmural AP gradients that was thought to be benign and was proven to be truly arrhythmogenic in 2008 after Haïssaguerre et al.'s landmark study [64]. Because of their similar pathophysiological mechanisms, it is not surprising that the approach to therapy of ERS is similar to that of BrS. β-adrenergic activation with isoproterenol is effective in suppressing ER arrhythmias by enhancing inward calcium current [65]. As cardiac transient outward potassium current (I_{to}) inhibitor, quinidine is also effective [66]. An observational cohort study of 122 patients (age 25–49, 90 male patients) with ERS who implanted ICD was done [67]. Follow-up was done through ICD interrogation. Successful suppression of VF in this cohort was demonstrated using isoproterenol (100% success) in acute cases, while quinidine was shown superior in chronic cases. Quinidine was able to abolish all VF attacks over 2 years. Quinidine success was extraordinarily confirmed as it was able to restore normal ECG. To the surprise, medications like β-blockers, amiodarone, class 1C agents, mexiletine and verapamil were found not to be effective. In another publication of five BrS and two ERS patients, a combination of cilostazol and bepridil was found to suppress VF effectively [68]. Cilostazol inhibits the activity of phosphodiesterase III in the heart. It thereby increases the inward calcium current (ICa) via elevation of the intracellular concentrations of cyclic adenosine monophosphate (cyclic AMP), which shares some pharmacological features with isoproterenol. Cilostazol can cause symptomatic palpitations and its long-term effects have not been reported. Bepridil (calcium antagonist with fast kinetic block of sodium currents) inhibits most types of potassium currents, including (I_{to}) and could decrease the number of sudden VF episodes in patients with idiopathic VF (including those with BrS). The addition of bepridil could attenuate cilostazol-induced palpitations without preventing the suppressive effects of cilostazol on VF [69].

If VT or VF is documented, then ICD is indicated. No available clinical strategy is present for asymptomatic individuals with ERS electrocardiographic manifestation. Syncope correlation to the arrhythmia in ESR is unusual. The presence of syncope in ERS-diagnosed individuals should warrant more investigations.

2.5 Idiopathic VF management plan

Although the exit list of primary arrhythmias from idiopathic VF circle is increasing, it still stands alone as a primary diagnosis. Acute suppression of the VF can be achieved successfully with isoproterenol or quinidine [70, 71]. The mechanism of quinidine effect in idiopathic VF is unknown [72]. The famous Ca++ channel blocker, verapamil, also proves to be successful acutely [73]. Ventricular ectopy mostly originating from the distal Purkinje system is observed in up to 30% of cases of idiopathic ventricular fibrillation VF [74].

Promising publications report the successful ablation of the triggering PVC with cure rate of 89% [75]. After ablation rate of recurrence is low (18%), there is a possibility that the recurrence is due to another site of triggering PVC [76]. For patients who were lucky to be retrieved after VF, ICD implant is a MUST.

2.6 Progressive cardiac conduction disease (PCCD) and inherited sinus node dysfunction (SND) management plan

Both PCCD and SND contain channelopathy elements and overlap with channelopathy syndromes in some cases. Until the research in genetic engineering and tissue engineering reaches to revolutionary solutions for those two conductions, device therapy with pacemakers and ICDs will be the standard management. ICD (which carries pacer capabilities) will be the choice in rare cases of the overlap nature with other tachyarrhythmias. In this condition, hybrid pharmaceutical agent might be used.

3. Future speculations on the approach to channelopathy

The explosive medical informatics that we have obtained as human species about SCD in the last three decades are landmarks in human history. In addition to continuation of the gracious efforts in the arena of cardiovascular genetics, epigenetics and molecular genetics, it is always advisable to dive more into the microperspective, as well as macroperspective. It is a way of interpreting facts with the true spectrum of the creature and biology from genes to galaxies. This is a visionary way of thinking that we and our team adopted since 2006 in the King of Organs series for advanced cardiac sciences conferences (2006, 2008, 2010, 2012 and 2019). Channelopathy and its related experimental research especially exploring the secrets of SCD are creating an ideal example of scientific incorporation of this new visionary understanding. Induced pluripotent stem cell–derived cardiomyocytes provide a new platform for studying arrhythmic disorders leading to sudden cardiac death. Cellular transfection models, which are the most commonly used cellular models, are able to mimic the expression of a single-ion channel. Both are amenable for the weak electromagnetic currents that are in common between genes and cosmos.

3.1 Future speculations in the genetic arena

Tremendous progress has been made in the discovery of putative mutations and genes responsible for different channelopathies. In the way of advances to scrutinize the pathogenic mutations comes the growing number of variants of unknown significance (VUS). It is an allele, or variant form of a gene, that has been identified through genetic testing but whose significance to the function or health of an organism is not identified. Researchers continue to work on better understanding how to stratify the risk of life-threatening arrhythmia based on the genotype and phenotype of the individual. Giustetto and his colleagues reported finding on a study of 53 patients from the European Short QT Registry. They found that A familial or personal history of cardiac arrest was present in 89%. Sudden death was the clinical presentation in 32%. The average QTc was 314 ± 23 ms. A mutation in genes related to SQTS was found in 23% of the probands; most of them had a gain of function mutation in HERG (SQTS1). Almost 43(45%) of patients received an implantable cardioverter defibrillator, and 12(23%) patients received long-term prophylaxis with hydroquinidine. Patients with a HERG mutation had shorter QTc at baseline and a greater QTc prolongation after treatment with HQ. During follow-up, 2(4%) already symptomatic patients received appropriate implantable cardioverter defibrillator shocks and 1(2%) had syncope. The event rate was 4.9% per year in the patients without antiarrhythmic therapy. No arrhythmic events occurred in patients receiving HQ [77]. The delta T50 is a measure of the variability of ventricular repolarization (at 50% of the T-wave downslope). It has been used to identify patients with LQTS in combination with QT interval cutoffs, as well as to identify patients at higher risk for cardiac events [78]. Rest and exercise QT interval measurements have been used to create a validated algorithm for diagnosing LQTS [79]. End-recovery QT interval measurements have also been used and, in combination with clinical history and mutation-specific information, can aid in understanding the pathogenicity of VUS [80]. Copy number variations (CNV) are a form of genetic abnormality that may explain the genetic basis of channelopathies in cases where there is no identifiable point mutation [81]. It is conceivable that in the future CNV may be added to genetic screens. Despite our increasingly sophisticated knowledge of the underlying pathophysiology, novel medical therapies tailored specifically for these syndromes have yet emerged in the clinical setting. Novel forms of treatment that specifically address the aberrant molecular pathophysiology defining these conditions will be our immediate priority step in order to effectively suppress arrhythmic events and to ultimately obviate the need for ICD implants.

3.2 Decoding the channelopathies' mysteries using induced pluripotent stem cell-derived cardiomyocyte research

The available platforms, shaping the future, to develop and investigate pharmaceutical therapeutic mechanisms for successful channelopathies treatment can be classified into different levels. First is at the organism level including clinical as well as animal models. Second is at the tissue and organ level (Purkinje fibers). Third is at cellular and molecular level (cardiac ions, induced pluripotent stem cells) [82]. Since the first report in 2006, bench researchers have made use of "induced pluripotent stem cell" (iPS) systems to study the electrophysiological and pharmacological characteristics of cardiomyocyte cells that are specific to an individual patient and his/her mutation and channelopathy. This technology has huge potential to promote our understanding of individual channelopathies and further steer the management of channelopathies in an individualistic, genotype-specific manner in the future [83, 84]. It provides a robust platform to advance the science and clinical care of sudden cardiac death. Major ion channels of the human heart are expressed in the human induced pluripotent stem cell-derived cardiomyocyte (iPSC-CM). The iPSC-CMs are created by somatic cells reprogramming into pluripotent stem cells using viral transduction or non-viral transfection or soluble proteins to introduce transcriptional factors to the somatic cell [85]. The resulting induced pluripotent stem cell can be differentiated specifically to induced pluripotent stem cell-derived cardiomyocyte (iPSC-CM) [86]. The iPSC-CMs can express encoded genes of the heart that might be absent in the original donor somatic cell. An ion channel disease can be expressed and recapitulated electrophysiologically so clinical diagnosis can be identified as well as genetic screening in the family. Variant of uncertain significance (VUS) can be developed where electrophysiological testing can be examined in the produced iPSC-CMs. Then comparison to the index case can be done. As the case in genetic testing, iPSC-CM may miss identifying the arrhythmia. In this situation, we will rely on clinical evaluation and family screening. Induced pluripotent stem of human cardiomyocyte (iPSC-CM) is superior to animal models or heterologous transfection models for channelopathies research (**Figure 1**) [87]. Its capabilities to create specific therapeutic options and its abilities to define disease-specific drug toxicity are unique.

This level of research is expected to illuminate our understanding of the true pathophysiology of channelopathies and their targeted therapies.

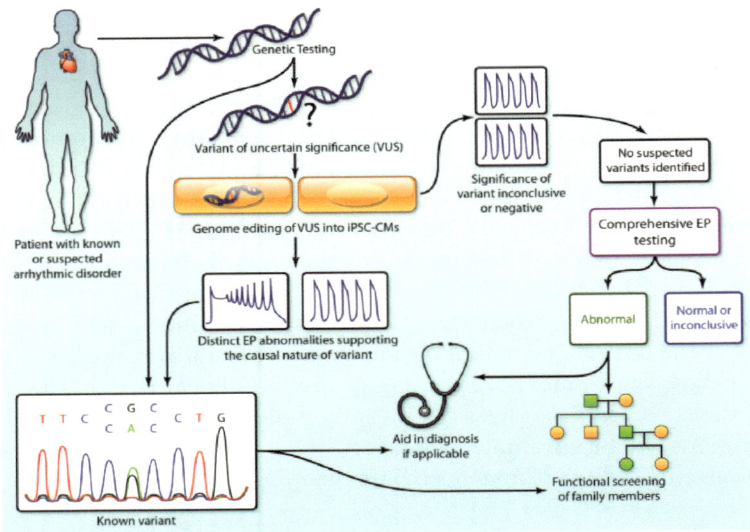

Figure 1.
Potential role for iPSC-CMs in the evaluation of patients with known or at risk for arrhythmic disorders. Clinical genetic testing attempts to identify a rare variant in genes commonly associated with arrhythmic disorders. (illustration credit: Ben smith) [87].

3.3 Fine-tuning the sympathovagal balance

Since the early 1990s, ICD have become a standard therapeutic option for VT/VF in channelopathy subjects and in most of the times the first therapeutic choice to defibrillate the fatal rhythms. As time passed, we gained the knowledge of how to fine-tune our ICD subjects to minimize or abolish shocks without using medications as much as possible. Despite the effectiveness of the ICD in preventing sudden death, anxiety, depression and post-traumatic stress disorder (PTSD) plays a contributing role in the high 1-year mortality rate observed after ICD implantation. ICD patients are at higher risk of having arrhythmias and therefore of receiving shocks, because of their fear of receiving shocks. Negative emotions lead to an increased incidence of disorders in heart rhythms and in the autonomic nervous system functioning. On the other hand, the positive psychophysiological state, called heart coherence, is associated with high performance, stress reduction and greater emotional stability, and less arrhythmic events. Heart rate variability (HRV) is considered a measure of neurocardiac function that reflects heart-brain interactions and autonomic nervous system (ANS) dynamics. HRV pattern with cardiac coherence (CC) is seen as sine wave highly regular pattern compared to the chaotic pattern seen with anger, frustration and other negative emotions. The HeartMath Institute (California, Boulder Creek) developed a heart rhythm monitoring and feedback system that enables physiological coherence to be objectively monitored and quantified.

Training ICD patients' to self-regulate emotions can produce broad improvements in increasing or strengthening self-regulatory capacity, making them less vulnerable to depletions and fear of and consequently less rhythmic events. Resilience is defined by the HeartMath researchers as the capacity to prepare for, recover from and adapt in the face of stress, adversity, trauma or challenge. It reflects the state of sympathovagal balance where the ion travel across the cellular membrane channels is in true physiological homeostasis. Teaching how to improve self-resilience is especially important for highly potential subjects for PTSD like ICD patients. In view of the role of the effects of negative emotions on induction of T-wave alternans (TWA) and repolarization instability and its relation to future ventricular arrhythmias in patients with ICDs, we postulate that teaching the importance of positive emotional states and building a heart coherent pattern are excellent life choices that can interrupt the negative emotion, fatal rhythm and shock continuum for ICD patients [88, 89].

3.4 Earth geomagnetic activity orchestrating autonomic nervous system, arrhythmogenesis and SCD

New perspective is evident disclosing the scientific background of historical and philosophical dilemmas. The human heart rate variability as a measure of the autonomic nervous system (ANS) functions is in delicate resonance with planetary magnetic field. Statistically significant correlations have been established linking earth's magnetic activity to psychophysiological well-being including arrhythmias and sudden cardiac death. Different pathomechanisms are operating through which ANS induces the fatal heart rhythms. Andrew Armor, the pioneer of neurocardiology, elaborates in this direction as well as heart brain communications [90]. The state of cardiac coherence (CC) where HRV-dominant frequency peak is in the 0.04–0.26 Hz range and more peculiarly around 0.1 Hz carries the secrets of psychophysiological well-being and planetary resonance [91–93]. Daily autonomic nervous system activity not only responds to changes in solar and geomagnetic activity (SGMA), but it is also synchronized with the time-varying magnetic fields associated with geomagnetic field-line resonances and Schumann resonances [94, 95]. The great planetary frequency around 0.1 Hz acts also indirectly toward normal heart rhythm by reducing systemic blood pressure in hypertensive subjects [96, 97]. SCD and cerebral strokes and increase in emergency calls were linked to periods of geomagnetic disturbances (low level) and higher level of cosmic rays. This is suggesting biophysical cause effect relationship between cosmic rays and medical events of elderly humans [98, 99]. Daily autonomic nervous system activity not only responds to changes in solar and geomagnetic activity, but it is also synchronized with the time-varying magnetic fields associated with geomagnetic field-line resonances and Schumann resonances [100].

In this direction, the longest record of human heart activity synchronized to solar wind indices as well as Schumann resonances and the cosmic rays has been done by our group. A total of 97,000 hours of records were managed statistically. We have satisfying scientific evidence illustrating daily changes of the ANS in response to solar as well as geomagnetic activity. Those ANS responses are initiated after different times of the changes of the solar and planetary activities and when it occurs and it persists for varying times. Increasing heart rate was correlated to increase in solar wind intensity. This is explained as biological stress response of solar winds on human heart through sophisticated mechanisms. The rise of Schumann resonance power, solar radio flux and cosmic rays are all reflected in the increase of parasympathetic tone and HRV. The degree of effect of those energetic environmental stressors on human cardiovascular system affects different people differently depending on their health, sensitivity and self-regulation capabilities [101]. The scientific community in the field is active to establish the effect of SGMA on heart rhythm at cellular level. Laboratory findings demonstrate the effect of ion cyclotron mechanism on extracted myocardial cell regulation [102]. It seems that Schumann resonance is a major interlayer in the SGMA effect on ion channels and the ion transport in cardiac cells and accordingly in the susceptibility of channelopathic subjects to the fatal rhythms. The influence of extremely weak magnetic field in the Schumann resonances (ScR) on the creatine kinase (CK) release, calcium transients as well as spontaneous contractions of rat cardiac cell cultures was examined. The application of 7.8 Hz, magnetic field of 90 nT was associated with gradual reduction in the spontaneous Ca++ transient amplitude. After 40 minutes of magnetic field application, 28% of the initial amplitude was reached. This reduction was associated with the calcium transient time gradually reduced. The effect is frequency dependent. The described changes occurred only in the 7.6–8 Hz. The frequency of 7.8 Hz is frequency of both central nervous system and cardiovascular system. It is the basic frequency responsible for the resonance between us humans as well as the biology on one hand and the cosmic environment on the other hand. The application of 7.8 Hz, magnetic field of 90 nT for 90 minutes results in the reduction of creatine kinase (CK) release to the buffer. This result was obtained during normal conditions, hypoxic environment and use of 80 μM H_2O_2 to induce oxidative stress. It sees that the first range of ScR has an effect on cardiac cell characterized by CK release reduction as a stress response and this effect is of a protective effect [103]. Magnetic field dynamics could add to our future understanding of the SGMA interaction with human heart in health and disease. The known transmembrane pacemaker protein CHN4, present in both sinoatrial and AV nodal cells, could interact with field information to provide specificity in an electronic key-to-lock mechanism interaction [104]. It is conspicuous that the near future is carrying more details to disclose the true pathomechanism of how modulation of HRV with fluctuation of SGMA can trigger the fatal rhythms and sudden death. More intelligent preventive as well as therapeutic strategies will be then available.

4. Summary

Risk stratification for LQTSs is available with high correlation to positive genetic testing with 75% likelihood if the score is more than 4 points. Half of LQTS cases prove positive mutation. This is not the case with other channelopathies where paucity of positive mutations is the role. Beta blockers (propranolol and nadolol than metoprolol) are the first-line and easiest therapeutic choice for both LQT1 and LQT2. There is no scientific evidence favoring selective over non-selective beta blockers. It is always advised to keep beta blockers as adjunct treatment after ICD implants. In the current medical literature, there is controversy regarding the use of beta blockers in LQT3. Scientific evidence is suggesting significant therapeutic role of sodium channel blockers like ranolazine, mexiletine and flecainide in LQT3 treatment. Mexiletine was proved also of being an effective therapeutic option in LQT3 as well as LQT1 and LQT2. In the absence of concomitant gene mutations, epinephrine and isoproterenol were found to be effective in acquired LQTS. The implantation of an ICD is pivotal secondary prevention in LQTS and a reasonable primary prevention approach in selected cases. Surgical therapy in the form of left cardiac sympathetic denervation (LCSD) is a well-accepted treatment option in LQTS patients. It is an option in selected cases like LQT1 and LQT2 patients with no proper response to beta blockers, intolerance to beta blockers, or after ICD implant with recurrent arrhythmias. Aggressive management of febrile illnesses as well as avoidance of drugs inducing VT/VF is critical in BrS arrhythmia patients. Isoproterenol intravenously is used with success to control VF storms in BrS. ICD implant is a must for secondary prevention but is guarded in primary prevention especially in asymptomatic individuals. In case of frequent ICD shocks, quinidine can be used as adjunct treatment (up to 600 mg a day). Ablation of the anterior aspect of RVOT seems a promising and successful option in BrS patients. In PCVT, high doses of nadolol (3–5 mg/kg) may be necessary to suppress exertional ectopy. Because of the high risk of recurrent events and SCD on β-blockers, adjunctive ICD implantation is recommended in all PCVT symptomatic patients. Physicians must never rely on exercise test result for PCVT management. Flecainide (150–200 mg a day) is a promising first-line drug or as adjunct with beta blockers. Surgical option for PCVT represented by LCSD is an effective choice as a hybrid therapy to pharmaceutical agents. ICD, with primary termination, is the golden choice. Due to the role of emotional upset to induce attacks of VT/VF in PCVT, emotional management is of paramount importance. ER pattern was proven to be truly arrhythmogenic in 2008. Pathophysiological mechanism, as well as therapeutic approaches of ERS, is similar to that of BrS. Enhancing inward calcium current with β-adrenergic activation using isoproterenol is effective in suppressing ER arrhythmias in acute cases. Inhibiting cardiac transient outward potassium current (I_{to}) using quinidine is also effective to suppress ER arrhythmias and was of proven superiority in chronic cases. A combination of cilostazol and bepridil was found to suppress VF in ERS and BrS effectively. In idiopathic VF (IVF) secondary prevention; immediate ICD implantation is a must. Acute suppression of the VF can be achieved successfully with isoproterenol or quinidine. Verapamil was found to be also successful acutely. Ablation of the triggering PVC seems to be a very promising choice. For PCCD and SND with channelopathy elements, ICD with pacemaker capabilities is the standard choice. Toward the discovery of putative mutations and genes comes *variants of unknown significance (VUS)* (looking for functional significance of allele or gene variant). The delta T50 (a measure of the variability of ventricular repolarization at 50% of the T-wave downslope) is a new tool to improve our diagnostic accuracy of channelopathies. In the absence of identifiable point mutation, *copy number variation (CNV)* is a form of genetic abnormality, which may explain the genetic basis of channelopathies. The psychophysiological well-being associated with positive emotional state orchestrates the sympathovagal tone favorably. Cardiac coherence (CC) (where heart frequencies dominate in the range of 0.04–0.26 Hz) is a state of recruiting positive emotion by special training resulting in homogeneity between all body functions and systems. It is seen as sine wave appearance of HRV. Training ICD patients to self-regulate emotions with cardiac coherence can increase self-regulatory capacity, making them less vulnerable to depletions and fear of and consequently less rhythmic events. In view of the complexity of the different channelopathies and its variable responses to different treatment modalities, it is believed that comprehensive global perspective is highly needed. We adopted new universal perspective for diseases management extending from genes to galaxies. Experimental research on channelopathies is a model in this direction. Induced pluripotent stem cell–derived cardiomyocytes provide a new platform for studying arrhythmic disorders leading to sudden cardiac death. Cellular transfection models are able to mimic the expression of a single-ion channel. Both are amenable for the weak electromagnetic currents that are common between genes and cosmos. The rise of Schumann resonance power, solar radio flux and cosmic rays are all reflected in the increase of parasympathetic tone and HRV. The degree of effect of those energetic environmental stressors on human cardiovascular system affects different people differently depending on their health, sensitivity and self-regulation capabilities. The protective effect of simulated weak magnetic field in the range of the first Schumann resonance (7.8 Hz) is proven at cellular level. The future in this direction is promising to revolutionize our interventional capabilities to treat and prevent channelopathies in the human kind.

Acknowledgements

The author acknowledges his great parents the late Abdulrhman Alabdulgader and Mariam Almulhim (with a blessing for her for a long peaceful life) who taught him the mercy and gratitude to his society, human species and all biology in large. The author's special praise goes to his brother Khalid who shared his scientific life journey until dreams became reality.

Conflict of interest

The author declares no conflict of interest.

Thanks

Showers of mercy to the spirit of my great beloved father who shocked me with his sudden agonizing absences during writing this chapter. The author prays for a long peaceful life for his great mother. Both of them fed the author to love all humanity and all biology. The author thanks all his teachers who taught him that the sky is not the limit.

Appendices and nomenclature

BrS	Brugada syndrome
CC	cardiac coherence
CPVT	catecholaminergic polymorphic ventricular tachycardia
ERS	early repolarization syndrome
HRV	heart rate variability
LQTS	long QT syndrome
PCCD	progressive cardiac conduction disease
SCD	sudden cardiac death
ScR	Schumann resonance
SGMA	solar geomagnetic activity
SNP	single-nucleotide polymorphism
SQTS	short-QT syndrome
VF	ventricular fibrillation
VT	ventricular tachycardia

Author details

Abdullah Abdulrhman Al Abdulgader
Senior Congenital Cardiologist and Invasive Electrophysiologist, Prince Sultan Cardiac Center, Alhasa, Hofuf, Saudi Arabia

*Address all correspondence to: kidsecho@yahoo.com

References

[1] Chockalingam P, Rammeloo LA, Postema PG, Hruda J, Clur S-AB, Blom NA, et al. Fever-induced life-threatening arrhythmias in children harboring an SCN5A mutation. Pediatrics. 2011 Jan;**127**(1):e239-e244

[2] Schwartz PJ, Moss AJ, Vincent GM, Crampton RS. Diagnostic criteria for the long QT syndrome. An update. Circulation. 1993;**88**(2):782-784

[3] Sarquella-Brugada G, Campuzano O, sssIglesias A, Sánchez-Malagón J, Guerra-Balic M, Brugada J, et al. Genetics of sudden cardiac death in children and young athletes. Cardiology in the Young. 2013;**23**(2):159-173

[4] Schwartz PJ, Crotti L. QTc behavior during exercise and genetic testing for the long-QT syndrome. Circulation. 2011;**124**(20):2181-2184

[5] Zipes DP, Camm AJ, Borggrefe M, Buxton AE, Chaitman B, Fromer M, et al. ACC/AHA/ESC 2006 guidelines for management of patients with ventricular arrhythmias and the prevention of sudden cardiac death. Circulation. 2006;**114**:1088-1113

[6] Kamakura S, Ohe T, Nakazawa K, Aizawa Y, Shimizu A, Horie M, et al. Long-term prognosis of Probands with Brugada-pattern ST-elevation in leads V 1 –V 3. Circulation. Arrhythmia and Electrophysiology. 2009;**2**(5):495-503

[7] Antzelevitch C. Genetic, molecular and cellular mechanisms underlying the J wave syndromes. Circulation Journal. 2012;**76**(5):1054-1065

[8] Priori SG. Association of Long QT syndrome loci and cardiac events among patients treated with β-blockers. Journal of the American Medical Association. 2004;**292**(11):1341

[9] Schwartz PJ, Priori SG, Spazzolini C, Moss AJ, Vincent GM, Napolitano C, et al. Genotype-phenotype correlation in the long-QT syndrome. Circulation. 2001;**103**(1):89-95

[10] Spazzolini C, Mullally J, Moss AJ, Schwartz PJ, Mcnitt S, Ouellet G, et al. Clinical implications for patients with long QT syndrome who experience a cardiac event during infancy. Journal of the American College of Cardiology. 2009;**54**(9):832-837

[11] Priori SG, Schwartz PJ, Napolitano C, Bloise R, Ronchetti E, Grillo M, et al. Risk stratification in the long-QT syndrome. New England Journal of Medicine. 2003;**348**(19):1866-1874

[12] Kline J, Costantini O. Inherited cardiac arrhythmias and channel-opathies. The Medical Clinics of North America. 2019;**103**(5):809-820

[13] Hoshino K, Ogawa K, Hishitani T, Isobe T, Etoh Y. Successful uses of magnesium sulfate for torsades de pointes in children with long QT syndrome. Pediatrics International. 2006;**48**(2):112-117

[14] Chockalingam P, Crotti L, Girardengo G, Johnson JN, Harris KM, Heijden JFVD, et al. Not all Beta-blockers are equal in the management of long QT syndrome types 1 and 2. Journal of the American College of Cardiology. 2012;**60**(20):2092-2099

[15] Chatrath R, Bell CM, Ackerman MJ. β-blocker therapy failures in symptomatic probands with genotyped long-QT syndrome. Pediatric Cardiology. 2004;**25**(5):459-465

[16] Abu-Zeitone A, Peterson DR, Polonsky B, Mcnitt S, Moss AJ. Efficacy of different Beta-blockers in the treatment of long QT syndrome. Journal of the American College of Cardiology. 2014;**64**(13):1352-1358

[17] Obeyesekere MN, Antzelevitch C, Krahn AD. Management of ventricular arrhythmias in suspected channelopathies. Circulation. Arrhythmia and Electrophysiology. 2015;**8**(1):221-231

[18] Calvillo L, Spazzolini C, Vullo E, Insolia R, Crotti L, Schwartz PJ. Propranolol prevents life-threatening arrhythmias in LQT3 transgenic mice: Implications for the clinical management of LQT3 patients. Heart Rhythm. 2014;**11**(1):126-132

[19] Shimizu W, Antzelevitch C. Differential effects of beta-adrenergic agonists and antagonists in LQT1, LQT2 and LQT3 models of the long QT syndrome. Journal of the American College of Cardiology. 2000;**35**(3):778-786

[20] Wilde AA, Kaufman ES, Shimizu W, Moss AJ, Benhorin J, Lopes CM, et al. Clinical aspects of type 3 long-QT syndrome: An international multicenter study. Circulation. 2016;**134**(12):872-882

[21] Windle JR, Geletka RC, Moss AJ, Zareba W, Atkins DL. Normalization of ventricular repolarization with Flecainide in long QT syndrome patients with SCN5A:?KPQ mutation. Annals of Noninvasive Electrocardiology. 2001;**6**(2):153-158

[22] Roden D. Pharmacogenetics and drug-induced arrhythmias. Cardiovascular Research. 2001;**50**(2): 224-231

[23] Antzelevitch C, Belardinelli L, Zygmunt AC, Burashnikov A, Diego José M, Di Fish JM, et al. Electrophysiological effects of Ranolazine, a novel antianginal agent with antiarrhythmic properties. Circulation. 2004;**110**(8):904-910

[24] Shimizu W, Antzelevitch C. Sodium Channel block with Mexiletine is effective in reducing dispersion of repolarization and preventing torsade de pointes in LQT2 and LQT3 models of the long-QT syndrome. Circulation. 1997;**96**(6):2038-2047

[25] Ruan Y, Denegri M, Liu N, Bachetti T, Seregni M, Morotti S, et al. Trafficking defects and gating abnormalities of a novel SCN5A mutation question gene-specific therapy in long QT syndrome type 3. Circulation Research. 2010;**106**(8):1374-1383

[26] Moss AJ, Zareba W, Schwarz KQ, Rosero S, Mcnitt S, Robinson JL. Ranolazine shortens repolarization in patients with sustained inward sodium current due to Type-3 long-QT syndrome. Journal of Cardiovascular Electrophysiology. 2008;**19**(12):1289-1293

[27] Raviña T, Raviña M, Gutierrez J. Isoproterenol enhancement of IKs current in Amiodarone-induced long QT syndrome. International Journal of Cardiology. 2009;**133**(3):402-406

[28] Shimizu W, Antzelevitch C. Differential effects of beta-adrenergic agonists and antagonists in LQT1, LQT2 and LQT3 models of the long QT syndrome. Journal of the American College of Cardiology. 2000;**35**(3):778-786

[29] Viskin S. Cardiac pacing in the long QT syndrome. Journal of Cardiovascular Electrophysiology. 2000;**11**(5):593-599

[30] Priori SG, Wilde AA, Horie M, Cho Y, Behr ER, Berul C, et al. Executive summary: HRS/EHRA/APHRS expert consensus statement on the diagnosis and management of patients with inherited primary arrhythmia syndromes. Heart Rhythm. Dec 2013;**10**(12):e85-108

[31] Collura CA, Johnson JN, Moir C, Ackerman MJ. Left cardiac sympathetic

denervation for the treatment of long QT syndrome and catecholaminergic polymorphic ventricular tachycardia using video-assisted thoracic surgery. Heart Rhythm. 2009;**6**(6):752-759

[32] Bos JM, Bos KM, Johnson JN, Moir C, Ackerman MJ. Left cardiac sympathetic denervation in long QT syndrome. Circulation. Arrhythmia and Electrophysiology. 2013;**6**(4):705-711

[33] Priori SG, Gasparini M, Napolitano C, et al. Risk stratification in Brugada syndrome: Results of the PRELUDE (PRogrammed ELectrical stimUlation predictive valuE) registry. Journal of the American College of Cardiology. 2012;**59**:37-45

[34] Ohgo T, Okamura H, Noda T, Satomi K, Suyama K, Kurita T, et al. Acute and chronic management in patients with Brugada syndrome associated with electrical storm of ventricular fibrillation. Heart Rhythm. 2007;**4**(6):695-700

[35] Viskin S, Wilde AA, Tan HL, Antzelevitch C, Shimizu W, Belhassen B. Empiric quinidine therapy for asymptomatic Brugada syndrome: Time for a prospective registry. Heart Rhythm. 2009;**6**(3):401-404

[36] Hermida J-S, Denjoy I, Clerc J, Extramiana F, Jarry G, Milliez P, et al. Hydroquinidine therapy in Brugada syndrome. Journal of the American College of Cardiology. 2004;**43**(10): 1853-1860

[37] Márquez MF, Bonny A, Hernández-Castillo E, Sisti AD, Gómez-Flores J, Nava S, et al. Long-term efficacy of low doses of quinidine on malignant arrhythmias in Brugada syndrome with an implantable cardioverter-defibrillator: A case series and literature review. Heart Rhythm. 2012;**9**(12):1995-2000

[38] Mizusawa Y, Wilde AAM. Brugada syndrome. Circulation. Arrhythmia and Electrophysiology. 2012;**5**:606-616

[39] Nademanee K, Veerakul G, Chandanamattha P, Chaothawee L, Ariyachaipanich A, Jirasirirojanakorn K, et al. Prevention of ventricular fibrillation episodes in Brugada syndrome by catheter ablation over the anterior right ventricular outflow tract Epicardium. Circulation. 2011;**123**(12):1270-1279

[40] Sunsaneewitayakul B, Yao Y, Thamaree S, Zhang S. Endocardial mapping and catheter ablation for ventricular fibrillation prevention in Brugada syndrome. Journal of Cardiovascular Electrophysiology. Nov 2012;**23**(Suppl 1):S10-S16

[41] Priori SG, Napolitano C, Tiso N, Memmi M, Vignati G, Bloise R, et al. Mutations in the cardiac ryanodine receptor gene (hRyR2) underlie catecholaminergic polymorphic ventricular tachycardia. Circulation. 2001;**103**(2):196-200

[42] Laitinen PJ, Brown KM, Piippo K, Swan H, Devaney JM, Brahmbhatt B, et al. Mutations of the cardiac ryanodine receptor (RyR2) gene in familial polymorphic ventricular tachycardia. Circulation. 2001;**103**(4):485-490

[43] Napolitano C, Priori SG, Bloise R. Catecholaminergic polymorphic ventricular tachycardia. In: Adam MP, Ardinger HH, Pagon RA, Wallace SE, LJH B, Stephens K, Amemiya A, editors. GeneReviews®. Seattle (WA): University of Washington, Seattle; 1993-2020

[44] Werf CVD, Zwinderman AH, Wilde AAM. Therapeutic approach for patients with catecholaminergic polymorphic ventricular tachycardia: State of the art and future developments. Europace. 2011;**14**(2): 175-183

[45] Werf CVD, Kannankeril PJ, Sacher F, Krahn AD, Viskin S, Leenhardt A, et al. Flecainide therapy reduces exercise-induced ventricular arrhythmias in patients with catecholaminergic polymorphic ventricular tachycardia. Journal of the American College of Cardiology. 2011;**57**(22):2244-2254

[46] Hayashi M, Denjoy I, Extramiana F, Maltret A, Buisson NR, Lupoglazoff J-M, et al. Incidence and risk factors of arrhythmic events in catecholaminergic polymorphic ventricular tachycardia. Circulation. 2009;**119**(18):2426-2434

[47] Watanabe H, Werf CVD, Roses-Noguer F, Adler A, Sumitomo N, Veltmann C, et al. Effects of flecainide on exercise-induced ventricular arrhythmias and recurrences in genotype-negative patients with catecholaminergic polymorphic ventricular tachycardia. Heart Rhythm. 2013;**10**(4):542-547

[48] Watanabe H, Chopra N, Laver D, Hwang HS, Davies SS, Roach DE, et al. Flecainide prevents catecholaminergic polymorphic ventricular tachycardia in mice and humans. Nature Medicine. 2009;**15**(4):380-383

[49] Wilde AA, Bhuiyan ZA, Crotti L, Facchini M, Ferrari GMD, Paul T, et al. Left cardiac sympathetic denervation for catecholaminergic polymorphic ventricular tachycardia. New England Journal of Medicine. 2008;**358**(19):2024-2029

[50] Moray A, Kirk EP, Grant P, Camphausen C. Prophylactic left thoracic sympathectomy to prevent electrical storms in CPVT patients needing ICD placement. Heart, Lung & Circulation. 2011;**20**(11):731-733

[51] Haruta D, Matsuo K, Tsuneto A, Ichimaru S, Hida A, Sera N, et al. Incidence and prognostic value of early repolarization pattern in the 12-Lead electrocardiogram. Circulation. 2011;**123**(25):2931-2937

[52] Tikkanen JT, Junttila MJ, Anttonen O, Aro AL, Luttinen S, Kerola T, et al. Early repolarization. Circulation. 2011;**123**(23):2666-2673

[53] Leenhardt A, Lucet V, Denjoy I, Grau F, Ngoc DD, Coumel P. Catecholaminergic polymorphic ventricular tachycardia in children. Circulation. 1995;**91**(5):1512-1519

[54] Priori SG, Napolitano C, Tiso N, Memmi M, Vignati G, Bloise R, et al. Mutations in the cardiac ryanodine receptor gene (hRyR2) underlie catecholaminergic polymorphic ventricular tachycardia. Circulation. 2001;**103**(2):196-200

[55] Vega AL, Tester DJ, Ackerman MJ, Makielski JC. Protein kinase A-dependent biophysical phenotype for V227F-KCNJ2 mutation in catecholaminergic polymorphic ventricular tachycardia. Circulation. Arrhythmia and Electrophysiology. Oct 2009;**2**(5):540-547

[56] Mohamed U, Gollob MH, Gow RM, Krahn AD. Sudden cardiac death despite an implantable cardioverter-defibrillator in a young female with catecholaminergic ventricular tachycardia. Heart Rhythm. 2006;**3**(12): 1486-1489

[57] Alabdulgader A. Neuropsychological functioning after implantable cardioverter-defibrillator surgery. In : Proietti R, Manzoni GM, Pietrabiss G, Castelnuovo G, editors. Psychological, Emotional, Social and Cognitive Aspects of Implantable Cardiac Devices. Springer; 2017. pp. 13-46. DOI: 10.1007/978-3-319-55721-2

[58] Alabdulgader A. ICD in children and youth. In: Proietti R, Manzoni GM, Pietrabiss G, Castelnuovo G, editors. Psychological, Emotional, Social and Cognitive Aspects of Implantable Cardiac Devices.

Springer; 2017. pp. 149-179. DOI: 10.1007/978-3-319-55721-2

[59] Haugaa KH, Leren IS, Berge KE, Bathen J, Loennechen JP, Anfinsen O-G, et al. High prevalence of exercise-induced arrhythmias in catecholaminergic polymorphic ventricular tachycardia mutation-positive family members diagnosed by cascade genetic screening. Europace. 2010;**12**(3):417-423

[60] Haïssaguerre M, Derval N, Sacher F, Jesel L, Deisenhofer I, Roy LD, et al. Sudden cardiac arrest associated with early repolarization. New England Journal of Medicine. 2008;**358**(19): 2016-2023

[61] Benito B, Guasch E, Rivard L, Nattel S. Clinical and mechanistic issues in early repolarization. Journal of the American College of Cardiology. 2010;**56**(15):1177-1186

[62] Haïssaguerre M, Sacher F, Nogami A, Komiya N, Bernard A, Probst V, et al. Characteristics of recurrent ventricular fibrillation associated with inferolateral early repolarization. Journal of the American College of Cardiology. 2009;**53**(7):612-619

[63] Shinohara T, Ebata Y, Ayabe R, Fukui A, Okada N, Yufu K, et al. Combination therapy of cilostazol and bepridil suppresses recurrent ventricular fibrillation related to J-wave syndromes. Heart Rhythm. 2014;**11**(8):1441-1445

[64] Belhassen B, Glick A, Viskin S. Excellent long-term reproducibility of the electrophysiologic efficacy of quinidine in patients with idiopathic ventricular fibrillation and Brugada syndrome. Pacing and Clinical Electrophysiology. 2009;**32**(3): 294-301

[65] Leenhardt A, Glaser E, Burguera M, Nürnberg M, Maison-Blanche P, Coumel P. Short-coupled variant of torsade de pointes. A new electrocardiographic entity in the spectrum of idiopathic ventricular tachyarrhythmias. Circulation. 1994;**89**(1):206-215

[66] Haïssaguerre M, Hocini M, Cheniti G, Duchateau J, Sacher F, Puyo S, et al. Localized structural alterations underlying a subset of unexplained sudden cardiac death. Circulation. Arrhythmia and Electrophysiology. Jul 2018;**11**(7):e006120

[67] Michel H, Shoda M, Pierre J, Nogami A, Shah DC, Kautzner J, et al. Mapping and ablation of idiopathic ventricular fibrillation. Circulation. 2002;**106**(8):962-967

[68] Gaw AC, Lee B, Gervacio-Domingo G, Antzelevitch C, Divinagracia R, Jocano F Jr. Unraveling the enigma of bangungut. Is sudden unexplained nocturnal death syndrome (SUNDs) in the Philippines a disease allelic to the Brugada syndrome? The Philippine Journal of Internal Medicine. 2011;**49**:165-176

[69] Chen Q, Kirsch GE, Zhang D, Brugada R, Brugada J, Brugada P, et al. Genetic basis and molecular mechanism for idiopathic ventricular fibrillation. Nature. 1998;**392**(6673):293-296

[70] Hedley PL, Jãrgensen P, Schlamowitz S, Moolman-Smook J, Kanters JK, Corfield VA, et al. The genetic basis of Brugada syndrome: A mutation update. Human Mutation. 2009;**30**(9):1256-1266

[71] Priori SG, Napolitano C, Gasparini M, Pappone C, Bella PD, Brignole M, et al. Clinical and genetic heterogeneity of right bundle branch block and ST-segment elevation syndrome. Circulation. 2000;**102**(20):2509-2515

[72] Probst V, Veltmann C, Eckardt L, Meregalli P, Gaita F, Tan H,

et al. Long-term prognosis of patients diagnosed with Brugada syndrome. Circulation. 2010;**121**(5):635-643

[73] Knecht S, Sacher F, Wright M, Hocini M, Nogami A, Arentz T, et al. Long-term follow-up of idiopathic ventricular fibrillation ablation. Journal of the American College of Cardiology. 2009;**54**(6):522-528

[74] Sy RW, Werf CVD, Chattha IS, Chockalingam P, Adler A, Healey JS, et al. Derivation and validation of a simple exercise-based algorithm for prediction of genetic testing in relatives of LQTS probands. Circulation. 2011;**124**(20):2187-2194

[75] Funada A, Hayashi K, Ino H, Fujino N, Uchiyama K, Sakata K, et al. Assessment of QT intervals and prevalence of short QT syndrome in Japan. Clinical Cardiology. 2008;**31**(6):270-274

[76] Maury P, Extramiana F, Sbragia P, Giustetto C, Schimpf R, Duparc A, et al. Short QT syndrome. Update on a recent entity. Archives of Cardiovascular Diseases. 2008;**101**(11-12):779-786

[77] Giustetto C, Schimpf R, Mazzanti A, Scrocco C, Maury P, Anttonen O, et al. Long-term follow-up of patients with short QT syndrome. Journal of the American College of Cardiology. 2011;**58**(6):587-595

[78] Chockalingam P, Wilde A. The multifaceted cardiac sodium channel and its clinical implications. Heart. 2012;**98**(17):1318-1324

[79] Amin AS, Asghari-Roodsari A, Tan HL. Cardiac sodium channelopathies. Pflügers Archiv - European Journal of Physiology. 2010;**460**(2):223-237

[80] Obeyesekere MN, Sy RW, Klein GJ, Gula LJ, Modi S, Conacher S, et al. End-recovery QTc: A useful metric for assessing genetic variants of unknown significance in long-QT syndrome. Journal of Cardiovascular Electrophysiology. 2012;**23**(6):637-642

[81] Barc J, Briec F, Schmitt S, Kyndt F, Cunff ML, Baron E, et al. Screening for copy number variation in genes associated with the long QT syndrome. Journal of the American College of Cardiology. 2011;**57**(1):40-47

[82] Sallam K, Li Y, Sager PT, Houser SR, Wu JC. Finding the rhythm of sudden cardiac death. Circulation research. 2015;**116**(12):1989-2004

[83] Noseworthy P, Porthan K, Tikkanen J, Peloso G, Merchant F, Pietila A, et al. The early repolarization pattern: Clinical correlates and heritability. Journal of the American College of Cardiology. 31 May 2011;**57**(22):2284-2289

[84] Tikkanen JT, Anttonen O, Junttila MJ, Aro AL, Kerola T, Rissanen HA, et al. Long-term outcome associated with early repolarization on electrocardiography. New England Journal of Medicine. 2009;**361**(26):2529-2537

[85] Kui C, Congxin H, Xi W, Yan-Hong T, Okello E, Salim M, et al. Characteristic of the prevalence of J wave in apparently healthy Chinese adults. Archives of Medical Research. 2008;**39**(2):232-235

[86] Rice KS, Dickson G, Lane M, Crawford J, Chung S-K, Rees MI, et al. Elevated serum gastrin levels in Jervell and Lange-Nielsen syndrome: A marker of severe KCNQ1 dysfunction? Heart Rhythm. 2011;**8**(4):551-554

[87] Terrenoire C, Wang K, Tung KWC, Chung WK, Pass RH, Lu JT, et al. Induced pluripotent stem cells used to reveal drug actions in a long QT syndrome family with complex genetics.

The Journal of General Physiology. 2012;**141**(1):61-72

[88] Matsa E, Burridge PW, Wu JC. Human stem cells for modeling heart disease and for drug discovery. Science Translational Medicine. 4 Jun 2014;**6**(239):239ps6

[89] Sanchez-Freire V, Lee AS, Hu S, Abilez OJ, Liang P, Lan F, et al. Effect of human donor cell source on differentiation and function of cardiac induced pluripotent stem cells. Journal of the American College of Cardiology. 2014;**64**(5):436-448

[90] Armour JA. Anatomy and function of the intrathoracic neurons regulating the mammalian heart. In: Zucker IH, Gilmore JP, editors. Reflex Control of the Circulation. Boca Raton, Ann Arbor, Boston: CRC Press; 1991. pp. 1-37. Available from: http://www.oalib.com/references/10512297

[91] McCraty R, Deyhle A. Science of Interconnectivity [Internet]. HeartMath Institute. 2020. Available from: https://www.heartmath.org/resources/downloads/science-of-interconnectivity/

[92] Alabdulgader MC, Atkinson M, Vainoras K, et al. Human heart rhythm sensitivity to earth local magnetic field fluctuations. Journal of Vibroengineering. 2015;**17**(6):3271-3278

[93] Halberg F, Cornelissen G, McCraty R, Czaplicki J, Alabdulgader A. Time Structures (Chronomes) of the Blood Circulation, Populations' Health, Human Affairs And Space Weather [Internet]. HeartMath Institute. 2020. Available from: https://www.heartmath.org/research/research-library/clinical/time-structures-chronomes-of-blood-circulation-health-human-affairs-space-weather/

[94] McCraty R, Atkinson M, Stolc V, Alabdulgader A, Vainoras A, Ragulskis M. Synchronization of human autonomic nervous system rhythms with geomagnetic activity in human subjects. International Journal of Environmental Research and Public Health. 13 July 2017;**14**(7)

[95] Alabdulgader AA. Coherence: a novel nonpharmacological modality for lowering blood pressure in hypertensive patients [Internet]. Global advances in health and medicine. Global Advances in Health and Medicine. 2012. Available from: https://www.ncbi.nlm.nih.gov/pmc/articles/PMC3833499/

[96] Alabdulgader AA. Modulation of heart rate variability: A novel non-pharmacological modality for lowering blood pressure in hypertensive patients [Internet]. Modulation Of Heart Rate Variability: A Novel Non-pharmacological Modality For Lowering Blood Pressure In Hypertensive Patients | 47609. OMICS International. 2016. Available from: https://www.omicsonline.org/proceedings/modulation-of-heart-rate-variability-a-novel-nonpharmacological-modality-for-lowering-blood-pressure-in-hypertensive-pat-47609.html

[97] Alabdulgader A, Guillaume G, Halberg F. Vascular variability disorders in the middle east: Case reports. [Internet]. World Heart Journal. 2011. Available from: https://www.researchgate.net/publication/289223333_Vascular_variability_disorders_in_the_middle_east_Case_reports

[98] Stoupel E, Babayev E, Abramson E, Sulkes J. Days of Zero level geomagnetic activity accompanied by the [Internet]. 2013. Available from: https://file.scirp.org/pdf/Health_2013052714384830.pdf

[99] Stoupel E, Kalediene R, Petrauskiene J, Starkuviene S, Abramson E, Israelevich P, et al. Twenty years study of solar, geomagnetic,

cosmic ray [Internet]. 2020. Available from: https://file.scirp.org/pdf/JBiSE20110600002_88324954.pdf

[100] McCraty R, Atkinson M, Timofejeva I, Joffe R, Alabdulgader A, Vainoras A, et al. The Influence of Heart Coherence on Synchronization ... [Internet]. 2020. Available from: https://www.heartmath.org/research/research-library/coherence/influence-of-heart-coherence-on-synchronization-human-hrv-and-geomagnetic-activity/

[101] Alabdulgader A, McCraty R, Atkinson M, Dobyns Y, Vainoras A, Ragulskis M, et al. Long-Term Study of Heart Rate Variability Responses to Changes in the Solar and Geomagnetic Environment [Internet]. Nature News. Nature Publishing Group. 2018. Available from: https://www.nature.com/articles/s41598-018-20932-x

[102] Gaetani R, Ledda M, Barile L, et al. Differentiation of human adult cardiac stem cells exposed to extremely low-frequency electromagnetic fields [Internet]. OUP Academic. Oxford University Press. 2009. Available from: https://academic.oup.com/cardiovascres/article/82/3/411/475221

[103] Elhalel G, Price C, Fixler D, Shainberg A. Cardioprotection from stress conditions by weak magnetic fields in the Schumann resonance band. Scientific Reports. 2019;**9**(1)

[104] Ballester-Rodés M, Carreras-Costa F, Versyp-Ducaju T, Ballester-Rodés M, Mehta D. Field dynamics in atrioventricular activation. Clinical evidence of a specific field to-protein interaction. Med Hypotheses. Mar 2019;**124**:56-59

Chapter 7

Mechanisms of Diabetes Mellitus-Induced Sudden Cardiac Death

Manal M.A. Smail, Frank C. Howarth, Jaipaul Singh, Sunil Rupee, Khemraj Rupee, Carlin Hanoman, Abla Mohammed Ismail, Farah Ahmed Sleiman, Samar Abdulkhalek and Keshore Bidasee

Abstract

More than 450 million people worldwide have diabetes mellitus (DM), a metabolic disorder characterized by an increase in blood glucose level (hyperglycemia) that arises from insufficient insulin secretion or resistance to insulin's action. More than 70% of individuals with chronic DM will develop cardiovascular diseases (CVDs) including atherosclerosis and coronary artery diseases (CADs), hypertension, cardiac arrhythmias, cardiomyopathy (heart failure), stroke, and chronic kidney disease. A significant number of these individuals will also succumb to sudden cardiac death (SCD). SCD usually occurs in early morning from abnormal heart rhythms or arrhythmias and ventricular fibrillation. When the pumping action of the heart becomes erratic, a reduction in oxygenated blood to the brain leads to unconsciousness and brain damage. SCD is independent of age and sex and positively correlates with impairment in cardiac metabolism, muscle damage, fibrosis, apoptosis, hypertrophy, ischemia, and deranged cation signaling. This review centers on mechanisms by which intracellular cations (Na+, K+, and Ca^{2+}) handling, inflammation, and oxidative and carbonyl stresses due to diabetes-induced hyperglycemia can lead to the deterioration of excitation/contraction coupling (ECC), impaired contractility, arrhythmias, and SCD in DM patients. It also discusses the beneficial effects of exercise training to attenuate the risk of SCD.

Keywords: arrhythmias, cardiomyopathy, diabetes, exercise, heart, hyperglycemia, patients, sudden cardiac death

1. Introduction

Sudden cardiac death (SCD) remains a major global public health problem, especially in developed countries such as the United States of America (USA), United Kingdom (UK), Germany and other countries. Moreover, SCD is also the most common cause of death worldwide, accounting for >50% of all cardiovascular disease (CVD)-related deaths. SCD is characterized by unexpected loss of the pumping action of the heart due to a disturbance in its electrical system that results in irregular and dangerously fast beating of the heart [1]. The ventricles may flutter or quiver (ventricular fibrillation), disrupting the pumping action of the myocardium, thereby stopping blood flow to the body. The blood flow to the brain is a matter of grave concern for the patients since reduced oxygenated blood supply to the brain can lead to unconsciousness and permanent damage to the brain. As such, death can follow unless the patient receives emergency treatment [2, 3]. Therefore, time is extremely critical when someone or a clinician is helping an unconscious person whose heart is not pumping (no pulse). SCD represents a major challenge for the clinician especially in individuals without a previous history of cardiac diseases. Early prediction of individuals at risk of SCD can be life-saving. Currently, most individuals experiencing SCD may not be identified as being a high risk and as such, the patients do not have ready access to a defibrillator. As a result, there must be community-based public access to defibrillation programmes in order to save the lives of the potential victims. SCD seems to occur most frequently in adults in their mid-30s to mid-40s and during working age, affecting both men and women. With SCD, some patients experience tachycardia, dizziness and fainting while in some cases there are no prior symptoms [4, 5].

2. Risk factors

The two major risk factors are previous myocardial infarction and coronary artery disease (CAD). However, there are other risk factors which include age, gender (predominant in males), ethnicity, reduced ejection fraction, a previous sudden cardiac arrest, familial predisposition to SCD, bradycardia, ventricular fibrillation, heart defects at birth, coronary artery abnormalities due to atherosclerosis, dilated cardiomyopathy, hypertrophic cardiomyopathy, significant changes in blood levels of potassium and magnesium, obesity, diabetes, recreational drug abuse and taking drugs that are "pro-arrhythmic" which may increase the risk for life-threatening arrhythmias [4].

3. Management of SCD

In order to prevent SCD, it is imperative to impose an aggressive management of cardiovascular risk factors at all levels including schools, universities, clinics, workplace and others. These include performing moderate exercise regularly, educating patients about the dangers of CVDs, promoting a healthy diet, restricting stress, reducing consumption of sugar, saturated fat and salt and stop smoking to promote a heart healthy behavior to all, particularly in young children and adolescents.

Finally, a preclinical prediction of patients at risk of SCD and early detection of the disease is crucial for early intervention and definitely these will reduce the incidence of SCD dramatically [4, 5]. Screening of family members who are susceptible to arrhythmias and SCD can help with early diagnosis and also and managing the arrhythmias [6].

4. Epidemiology of diabetes-induced sudden cardiac death

SCD is responsible for more than 100,000 deaths annually in the UK and 400,000 in the USA, far more than cancer and other individual non-communicable disease. It is estimated that 27,000 patients in the UK and 80,000 patients in the USA die annually from diabetes-induced SCD. Globally, SCD is responsible for half of all deaths due to heart disease [7]. Most cases of SCD are related to undetected cardiovascular diseases. SCD are directly linked to DM and CVDs are responsible for over 80% of the mortality in the diabetic population [8]. Epidemiological data show that macro-vascular complications including coronary artery disease (CAD), peripheral vascular disease (PVD) and SCD are 2–4 times more common among diabetic patients when compared with nondiabetic people [9]. According to the Framingham study, the frequency of CAD is twice more common in diabetic patients of both sexes than nondiabetic individuals [10]. This review will now focus on the mechanisms of diabetes-induced SCD, but first it is of paramount importance to understand the structure and function of the heart.

5. Anatomy and physiology of the heart

The mammalian heart is a four-chambered muscular organ, which is located in the anterior mediastinum, posterior to the sternum and encapsulated by the pericardium. The pumping action of the heart is central to the functioning of the circulatory system. The CVS composed of the blood, the heart and blood vessels [11]. The heart is a strong muscular organ, which continues to pump blood to different parts of the body throughout our lives. It beats continuously using up a vast amount of energy daily [12]. The structure of the heart is depicted in **Figure 1** and it is composed mainly of three layers of muscles, namely the epicardium or the external layer, the middle layer or myocardium and the inner most layer or endocardium. Damage to these muscles and other conduction tissues in the heart due to diabetes and other diseases is responsible for SCD.

The larger and strong muscular tissue of the myocardium is responsible for ventricular contraction, and it is also divided into left and right sides by a septal wall. Each side of the heart is made up of two chambers consisting of the upper atria and the lower ventricles [12]. The left side of the heart pumps oxygen-rich blood to the different parts of the body via the aortic valve to the aorta (systemic circulation), while the right side delivers blood to lungs via the pulmonary valve and the pulmonary artery for oxygen replenishment in the lungs (pulmonary circulation). The heart has four valves which allow for unidirectional flow of blood thereby

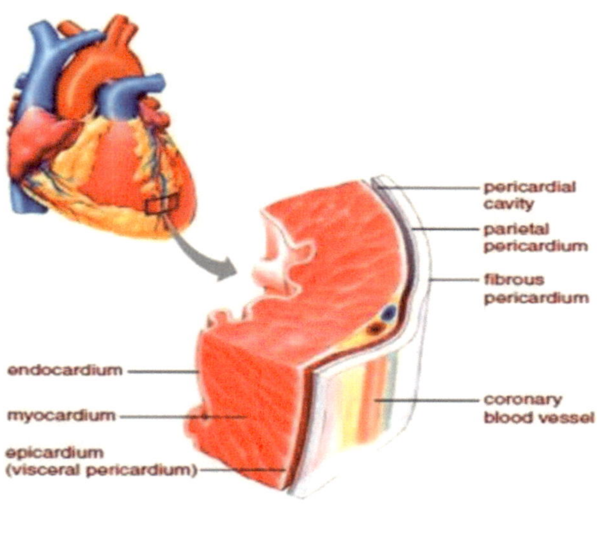

Figure 1.
The mammalian heart. Components are described in the text (image courtesy www.beyondbiology.org).

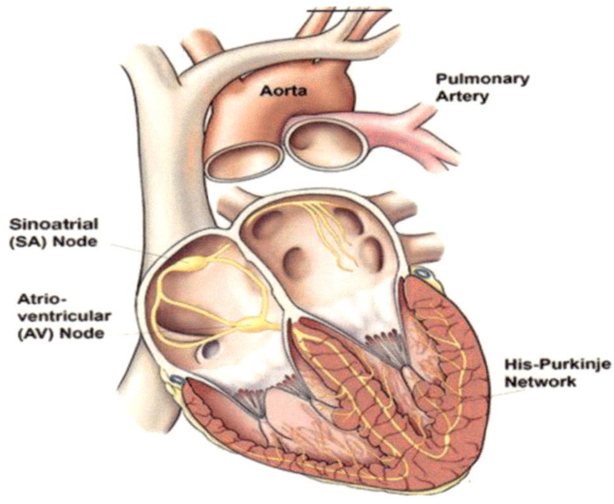

Figure 2.
Diagram showing the electrical system of the mammalian heart with the conducting tissues including the SA node, AV node and Purkinje fiber network. SCD is usually caused by abnormal heart rhythms called arrhythmias and the most common life-threatening arrhythmia is ventricular fibrillation, which is an erratic, disorganized firing of impulses from the ventricles (see lower chambers with Purkinje network of fibers). When this occurs, the heart is unable to pump blood, and death will occur within minutes, if left untreated (image courtesy www.beyondbiology.org).

preventing backflow. In turn, the right atrium receives retuning deoxygenated blood from the body through the superior and inferior vena cavae, while the left atrium receives oxygenated blood from the lungs through pulmonary vein. The heart itself needs a good supply of blood via the coronary arteries. These include the left anterior descending coronary artery, the left circumflex artery and the right coronary artery supplying the myocardium with oxygen-rich blood. The apex of the heart is the pointed end and the other end is called the base of the heart [13].

The orderly events that take place during the cardiac cycle are controlled by the electrical conduction system of the heart (**Figure 2**). An impulse is initiated at the sinoatrial node (SA-node) and then passes on to the atrioventricular node (AV-node) via conducting fibers via the atria. From the AV node, the impulse is conducted throughout the ventricles via the Purkinje fibers resulting in depolarization of the heart. Damage to the conducting tissues can result in sudden arrhythmias and possible SCD. Blood is pumped by the right ventricle into the pulmonary circulation at a lower pressure than blood pumped by the left ventricle into the systemic circulation. It follows that the haemodynamic stresses in the right and left side of the heart are very different. Even within the ventricles, the electro-mechanical properties of ventricular cardiac myocytes vary trans-murally [14].

6. SCD due to diabetes-induced autonomic system neuropathy and brady-arrhythmias

The heart is innervated by the nerves of the autonomic nervous system (ANS) [15]. The ANS consists of sympathetic and parasympathetic nerves which innervate the heart. The parasympathetic or vagus nerve originates from the inhibitory center in medulla of the brainstem. The vagal nerve innervates mainly the atria (sinoatrial node) and the atrio-ventricular node (see **Figure 2**). Upon stimulation, it releases the neurotransmitter, acetylcholine (ACh). The main function of ACh is to activate cholinergic muscarinic receptors in the heart muscles leading to reductions in conduction of impulse (negative dromotropic effect), rate (negative chronotropic effect), contraction (negative inotropic effect) and metabolism of the myocardium. On the other hand, the sympathetic nerve originates from the thoracic region of the spinal cord and it innervates the whole heart. It releases the neurotransmitter noradrenaline (norepinephrine) (NA) which activates beta-1–adrenergic receptors in the heart leading to increases in conduction of impulse (positive dromotropic effect), rate (positive chronotropic effect), contraction (positive inotropic effect) and enhanced metabolism of the myocardium. The two nerves of the ANS work in tandem to maintain the neural homeostasis of the heart [16].

Figure 3 illustrates the relationship between diabetes-induced cardiac autonomic system neuropathy and brady-arrhythmias in SCD. In diabetes-induced cardiac autonomic neuropathy, the sympathetic nerve to the heart is damaged and its activity is reduced leading to slowing of the heart or brady-arrhythmias, heart rhythm disturbances and even SCD. Moreover, diabetes can also downregulate the beta-adrenergic receptor in the myocardium which in turn synergizes the brady-arrhythmias leading to cessation of the heart or SCD. There is new evidence that diabetes-induced cardiomyopathy is common and there is an increased risk of arrhythmias as a result of dysfunction of the cardiac conduction system (CCS) [17, 18]. This is due mainly to hyperglycemia-induced fibrosis which results in

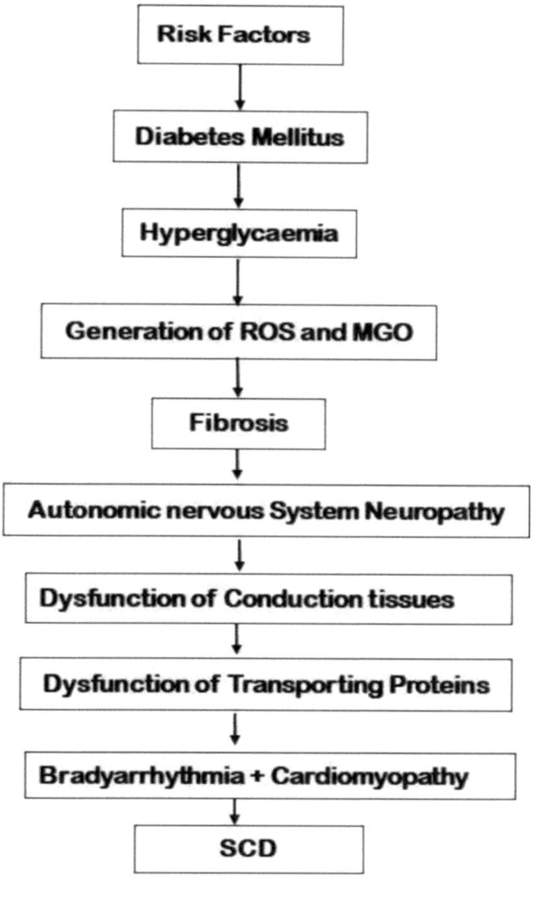

Figure 3.
Flow diagram showing the cellular and molecular events in the myocardium due to diabetes-induced hyperglycemia culminating in Brady-arrhythmias and subsequently SCD. ROS = reactive oxygen species; MGO = methylglyoxal, a reactive carbonyl species.

dysfunction of the CCS in the diabetic heart (see **Figure 2**). Moreover, it was demonstrated by Zhang et al. [18] that diabetes-induced fibrosis of the heart was associated with the reduction of potassium channel (HCN4), $Ca_v1.3$, $Ca_v3.1$ (calcium channel), NCX1, (sodium-calcium exchanger) and connexin (Cx45) protein expression in the sinoatrial node of the heart which in turn resulted in brady-arrhythmia and possibly SCD [18]. Moreover, reduced ryanodine (RyR2) and sodium-calcium exchanger (NCX1) protein expression in the atrio-ventricular junction of the heart (AVJ) is believed to contribute in part to the prolongation of the PR interval. Similarly, reduced protein expressions of RyR2, NCX1, Cx40, Cx43, and Cx45 in the Purkinje fibers (PFs) are responsible for the prolongation of QRS complex. The downregulation of neuro-filament M sub-unit (NF-M) and β_1-adrenergic receptor could also be linked to the reduced autonomic nervous control of the heart [17, 18]. All these cellular and molecular processes subsequently result in cardiac arrhythmias, QT interval prolongation and SCD of diabetic patients [19].

7. Cardiac muscle

In order to appreciate how diabetes-induced hyperglycemia is inducing fibrosis and cardiomyopathy, it is paramount importance to understand first, the structure of the cardiac cell or cardiomyocyte. Cardiac muscle, at the microscopic level, can be described as a composite tissue. It is made of various cell types, mainly myocytes and fibroblasts which are supported by extracellular matrix (ECM), all of which are permeated by fluids [15]. The myocardial ECM is made of macro-molecules which are produced by local fibroblasts. They consist of a fibrillar collagen network, a basement membrane and proteoglycans [20]. The function of the fibrillar collagen network is to strengthen the matrix, thereby giving strong structural support of the adjoining cardiomyocytes and the means by which they shorten to exert their contractile effect efficiently during ventricular pump action and thus, contributes to myocardial diastolic stiffness [21]. The heart is composed of different types of collagens including fibrillar collagen type I with the tensile strength of steel and fibrillary collagen type III which is the most abundant phenotypes [21]. Secondly, the basement membrane which surrounds the myocyte is attached to the sarcolemma and to the fibrillar collagen network. The myocyte adherence to basement membrane is a major determinant in maintaining cell shape and positional integrity within the ventricular wall [22]. Thirdly, the proteoglycans are composed of a protein core to which polysaccharide chains called glycosaminoglycans are covalently bound. These negatively charged molecules possess significant osmotic activity helping to trap and to store growth factors within ECM. Proteoglycan molecules in the connective tissue form a highly hydrated, gel-like "ground substance" in which the fibrous proteins are embedded. [22, 23]. The function of the polysaccharide gel is to prevent any compressive forces on the matrix thereby allowing the rapid diffusion of nutrients, metabolites and hormones between the blood and the cardiac tissue cell [23].

8. Sudden cardiac death due to diabetes-induced cardiomyopathy

Figure 4 illustrates the various pathways and events leading to diabetes-induced cardiomyopathy, arrhythmias and SCD due to the diabetes-induced hyperglycemia. These pathways include structural changes to cardiac muscles as well as apoptosis, altered calcium handling, insulin resistance in the heart, increased lipid uptake into the heart, glucotoxicity, metabolic disturbances, fibrosis, hypertrophy and the renin-angiotensin-aldosterone system (RAAS). DM can also affect cardiac structure

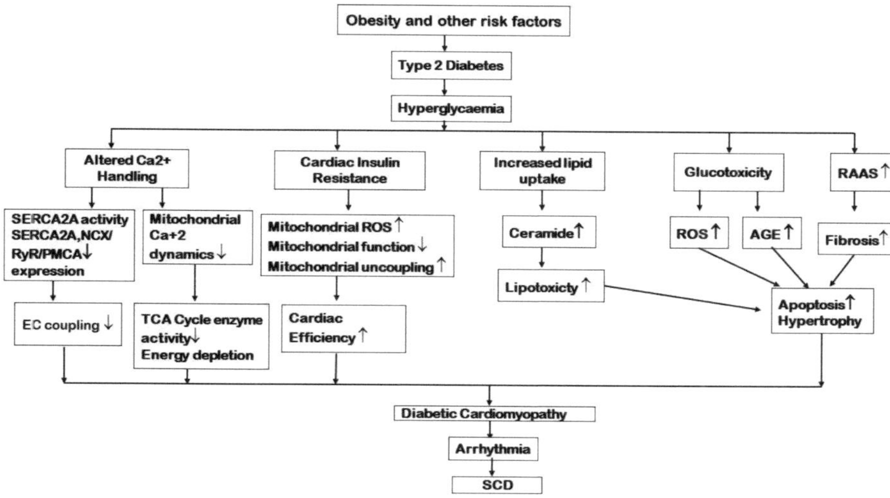

Figure 4.
Flow diagram showing the relationship between obesity and other risk factors-induced diabetes and sudden cardiac death (SCD) in the myocardium. Diabetes-induced hyperglycemia elicits structural, functional, and biochemical changes via different cellular pathways in the heart leading to diabetic cardiomyopathy, arrhythmias, and sudden cardiac death (SCD).

and function without causing changes in either high blood pressure (HBP) or CAD resulting in a debilitating condition called diabetic cardiomyopathy (DC) [24]. This term was first described by cardiac clinicians in 1972 after the examination of patients with DM and HF but without the appearance of HBP or CAD [25]. It is now well established that DC is responsible for mortality and morbidity among diabetics [26]. DC generally refers to the dysfunction of the left ventricle due to an enlarged weak heart in diabetic patients independent of CAD or HBP. The onset of DC is triggered by the diabetes–induced hyperglycemia leading to the production of a number of insults in the myocardium including TGF-beta 1, reactive oxygen species and reactive carbonyl species which in turn induce cellular structural damage to the heart. As a consequence, the initial effect is diastolic dysfunction in which the heart is unable to relax properly due to a derangement in cellular calcium homeostasis or elevated diastolic calcium due to impairment in cellular calcium regulatory transporting proteins in the myocardium. Following this, systolic dysfunction develops in which the heart is unable to pump blood efficiently to meet the demand of the body or heart failure. The final effect over time is arrhythmias and subsequently SCD. The most common contributors to DC onset and progression are left ventricular hypertrophy, metabolic abnormalities, extracellular matrix changes, small vessel disease, cardiac autonomic neuropathy, insulin resistance, oxidative stress and apoptosis, all leading to cardiac remodeling [27].

As DC was first reported in 1972, considerable data on its pathogenesis and clinical feature have been collected. DC affects the heart by enhancing fatty acid metabolism, suppresses glucose oxidation and modifies intracellular signaling, all of which lead to alteration in multiple steps of excitation-contraction coupling process, inefficient energy production, increased susceptibility to ischemia and contractile dysfunction [28, 29].

DM leads to structural and functional changes in the heart. The structural changes are manifested by left ventricular muscle disarray and hypertrophy, interstitial fibrosis, increased cell death (apoptosis) and oxidative stress, all of which result in diastolic and systolic dysfunctions as well as impaired contractile reserve [30]. In DM, the mass of the left ventricle is an independent marker for

SDC, and it often occurs independent of blood pressure in the atria. As such, DM is an independent risk factor which is responsible for enlargement of the left ventricle and generally stiffness of the heart [31].

It is particularly noteworthy that at cellular electrical level in the diabetic heart, the cardiac action potential duration (CAP) is consistently prolonged due to elevated intracellular calcium which is essential for the myocardium contraction [32]. It is now evident that DC-induced abnormalities during cardiac muscle contractility correlate closely with alterations in intracellular free Ca^{2+}concentration $[Ca^{2+}]_i$. It was previously reported that diabetic cardiac dysfunction arises as a result of changes in the expression and/or activity of transporting proteins that regulate Ca^{2+} during the cardiac cycle [33]. Thus, DC results in changes in biomechanical, contractile, and hypertrophic properties of the cardiac myocytes leading subsequently to arrhythmias and SCD.

9. Metabolic disturbances and sudden cardiac death

Metabolic disturbances such as altered lipid handling and substrate utilization, decreased mechanical efficiency, mitochondrial dysfunction, disturbances in non oxidative glucose pathways and increased oxidative stress are all hallmarks of DM [34]. Chronic hyperglycemia leads to non-enzymatic glycation of vascular and membrane proteins, producing advanced glycation end products (AGEs) and reactive oxygen species (ROS) and reactive carbonyl species (RCS) [35]. One major RCS is methylglyoxal (MGO) which is generated during glycolysis and the breakdown of lipids and glucose. In a previous study, it was reported that diabetes was associated with a large amount of collagen deposition around blood vessel and between the myofibers of heart biopsies taken from patients. Moreover, lipofuscins which are brown pigment granules that composed of lipid-containing residues were found to be deposited in left ventricular transmural biopsies. Similarly, myocardial triglyceride and cholesterol were also reported in these biopsies in large amount [36].

Insulin has a vital role to play in the regulation of cardiac metabolism and function [37]. Alterations of myocardial substrate and energy metabolism are considered as significant factors for the development of DC [38]. DM is characterized by reduced glucose and lactate metabolism and increased fatty acid (FA) metabolism [39]. In 1988, the glucose transporter GLUT family was discovered [40] and later, it was reported that glucose transport in the myocardium was impaired during diabetes because of decreased expression of GLUT1 and GLUT4 proteins and mRNA levels [41]. Likewise, glucose oxidation is reduced via the inhibitory effect of FA oxidation on pyruvate dehydrogenase complex due to high circulating FFA [42]. Insulin exerts its effect on glucose uptake in heart muscles by binding to insulin tyrosine kinase receptor (ITKR) via auto-transphosphorylation. In turn, this process initiates a signaling cascade mechanism which is accompanied by phosphorylation of phosphatidyl-inositol-3 kinase (PI3K), phosphoinositide-dependent kinase 1 (PDK1), Akt and protein kinase C (PKC). All these events allow for the translocation of GLUT1 and GLUT4 to the membrane facilitating glucose uptake into cardiac muscle cell. Contraction-evoked GLUT4 translocation represents the major mechanism that regulates glucose uptake by the myocardium heart, with only a small role by GLUT1 [43].

Both insulin resistance (IR) and hyperinsulinemia are risk factors for DC [44]. They seem to disturb insulin-induced glucose metabolism thereby significantly worsen the metabolic efficiency in cardiac and skeletal muscles. Insulin exerts its insulting effect in the diabetic heart via two processes involving the abnormalities of systemic metabolism and insulin signaling pathways, both of which are intrinsic to the cardiac tissue [45]. In the evolution of IR, the initial change that develops in the hearts of animal models is the impairment in the ability of insulin to increase glucose transport [46]. IR is also associated with cardiac contractile dysfunction and SCD [47]. Moreover, IR is associated with metabolic alteration and the development of DC [45]. Circulating FAs and triglyceride (TG) are increased by enhanced lipolysis in adipose tissue and lipoprotein synthesis in liver as a result of hyperglycemia and IR. It is now known that the FAs are converted to a lipid- like TG or ceramide when the FAs exceed the oxidative capacity of the heart leading to lipotoxicity and cell apoptosis [48]. As a result, DM subsequently leads to an increase in the rate of FA oxidation which is accompanied by a concurrent decrease in the rate of glucose oxidation.

10. Relationship between fibrosis and sudden cardiac death

Diabetes is well known to induce severe structural changes in the heart including replacement of apoptotic myocytes with fibrotic tissue and myocyte enlargement and disarray. These changes can affect electrical and mechanical activities of the heart [47]. Fibrosis can result in stiffness of the heart, remodeling, conduction abnormalities, arrhythmias and even SCD [12, 13, 17, 18]. Moreover, increased interstitial deposits of collagen filaments leading to fibrosis can act as insulating barriers, promoting not only impulse conduction slowing, but also conduction block [17, 18]. Recent experimental findings in isolated whole-heart studies indicate that fibrosis may also modulate the formation and propagation of cardiac-after potentials which can trigger electrical activity of the heart resulting in ventricular tachycardia and ventricular fibrillation (VT/VF). Since the infiltration of the myocardium with fibrosis can induce cardiovascular events as well as impairing cardiac diastolic and systolic function, it is now possible to assess the extent of myocardial fibrosis using cardiac magnetic resonance (CMR). CMR is of paramount importance as a prognostic tool in determining the different types of cardiomyopathies, especially when it is combined with myocardial T_1 mapping [49].

In addition, the replacement of myocytes with fibrotic tissue can reduce the number of force generating sarcomeres leading to a reduction in contractile function and subsequently arrhythmias and SCD [50]. Interstitial and perivascular fibrosis is a histological symptom of DC [25] and the extent of fibrosis correlates closely with the weight of the myocardium. The pathogenesis of fibrosis in the diabetic heart is proposed to be due to diabetic micro-angiopathy. When the diabetic heart is affected by either hypertension or CAD, there may be additive micro-angiopathy and large vessel-induced ischemia, all leading to diffuse myocardial scarring. Generalized fibrosis can result in increased wall stiffness and diastolic dysfunction [18, 51]. It is now well recognized that activation of the renin-angiotensin system (RAS) has an important biochemical role to play in the development of DC [42]. In diabetic heart, Angiotensin II (AngII) receptor density and mRNA expression are elevated [52]. It has been reported that DM can enhance the activation of RAS resulting in an increase in oxidative damage, fibrosis and cell apoptosis [53].

In contrast, the inhibition of the RAS can lead to a reduction in reactive oxygen species (ROS) level, similar to the effect observed with antioxidant treatment in streptozotocin-induced diabetic rat model [54]. One example of an ROS generating endogenous molecule is the RCS, methylglyoxal (MGO). Its accumulation to toxic levels during diabetes is due to a decrease in the activity of the enzyme (glyoxylase-1), the primary enzyme responsible for degrading MGO [55]. AngII, given exogenously to rodents, has been shown to cause cellular changes within the myocardium leading to hypertrophy and fibrosis and even SCD [56].

Mitochondria are the powerhouse of cells, and they play a major role in energy production. They are also involved with a number of cellular processes including homeostasis, free radical production and cell death [57]. Mitochondria exert marked biochemical effect on FA and glucose metabolism. However, diabetes can induce mitochondrial dysfunction leading to impaired cellular metabolism. A previous study reported ultrastructural and functional changes, as well as protein composition, in cardiac muscle mitochondria following diabetes [58]. In streptozotocin-induced type 1 diabetic mice, impaired function and ultrastructure abnormalities of cardiac muscles were associated with damage to the mitochondria. The impairment of the mitochondria was accompanied by increases in 11 specific mitochondrial proteins. These include an elevation of mRNA for the mitochondrial regulatory protein and increased total mitochondrial DNA area as well as number. These findings clearly indicate that the mitochondria are the major targets of diabetes-induced damage to the heart [59]. Moreover, a recent study has shown a reduction of ATP production by the mitochondria following diabetes. Another study [60] examined the relationship between impaired insulin signaling and altered mitochondrial energetics in a mouse model of type 1 diabetes with a cardiac-specific deletion of the insulin receptor. The results reveal impaired insulin signaling in the heart and this in turn promotes oxidative stress and mitochondrial uncoupling. These processes were associated with reduced fatty acid oxidative capacity and impaired mitochondrial energetics [61]. It is now well established that mitochondria from the diabetic heart can produce more reactive oxygen species (ROS) and reactive carbonyl species (RCS) than normal mitochondria [62]. According to the molecular theory of DC, hyperglycemia (HG) is the main pathogenic factor or insult resulting in arrhythmias and SCD [60].

11. Obesity and sudden cardiac death

DC is also accompanied by other comorbidities such as obesity and hypertension and these two complications often precede the development of fibrosis, apoptosis, hypertrophy, remodeling of the myocardium, diastolic and systolic dysfunctions, CAD, arrhythmias and SCD [63]. SCD in the young obese population normally happens in individuals without a known cardiac history [64]. More recently, chronic obese patients have been reported to be more susceptible to increased risk of SCD. As such, this is becoming a major concern and challenge for clinicians and health services globally, especially since the prevalence of obesity has been increasing steadily in both developed and developing countries around the world. Both obesity and DM share the main risk factors including inactivity, smoking and diets rich in sugar and fats. Most obese patients are hypertensive, pre-diabetic, as well as having fully blown diabetes, experiencing obstructive sleep apnea due to their excessive weight and metabolic syndrome. All of these pathological parameters are well-known risk factors for CVDs, including SCD. It is now evident that structural, functional and metabolic factors modulate and influence the risk of SCD in the obese population [65]. Obesity exerts numerous haemodynamic changes on the CVS such as increased cardiac output and diastolic filling pressures, both of which result in LV hypertrophy and dilatation. In addition, obesity can induce adverse electrical changes in the myocardium including prolongation of the QRS and increase in QT intervals on the ECG, as well as an increase in QT dispersion. Moreover, the late potentials on signal averaged ECG are also more common in obese compared with lean individuals. These obese-induced adverse structural and electrical insults on the heart seem to create a substrate that is susceptible to SCD [66].

Obesity-induced pathogenesis of the myocardium is associated with the production of lipids, oxidized LDL particles and free FAs which activate the inflammatory process in the body and thus, trigger the development of cardiac dysfunction. Inflammation is responsible for the steps toward the development of atherosclerosis, from early endothelial cell dysfunction to the late atherosclerotic plaque formation causing complications. All these pathological processes are related to obesity, IR and diabetes. During diseased processes in the heart, fatty tissue releases adipocytokines which in turn induce IR, endothelial cell dysfunction, hypercoagulability and systemic inflammation, thereby facilitating the atherosclerotic process. Likewise, the inflammatory adipocytokine such as TNF-α also rises to higher levels in visceral obesity. As a result, the heart releases an increased level of C-reactive protein (CRP) which is associated with an enhanced risk of ischaemia, myocardial infarction and peripheral vascular disease, all of which can facilitate arrhythmias and SCD [67].

12. Impaired calcium and potassium homeostasis and sudden cardiac death

Calcium (Ca^{2+}) is a major trigger, a modulator, a second messenger and a regulator of cardiac contractility [24, 68, 69]. It is well known that most of the Ca^{2+} that activates contraction is released from sarcoplasmic reticulum (SR) through ryanodine receptors (RyRs). RyRs are themselves activated by Ca^{2+} which enters the myocyte via voltage-dependent L- type Ca^{2+} channels and this mechanism is known as Ca^{2+}-induced Ca^{2+} release (CICR) [68]. The cytosolic Ca^{2+} in turn interacts with cardiac contractile proteins. By binding to troponin C, the Ca^{2+} triggers the sliding of thin and thick filaments, which results in cardiac contraction. Ca^{2+} then returns to diastolic levels mainly by the uptake of Ca^{2+} into the SR via the SR Ca^{2+} pump (SERCA2a) and extrusion of Ca^{2+} from the cell via the sarcolemmal Na^+-Ca^{2+} exchanger and the sarcolemma Ca^{2+}-ATPase pump [24]. DM leads to mitochondrial dysfunction which contributes to the development of DC by altering ATP generation and Ca^{2+} mobilization [69]. A previous study has shown that diabetes-induced HG plays an integral role in altering the expression and function of RyRs, Na^+-Ca^{2+} exchanger and SERCA. Failure of these three major calcium transporting proteins to function efficiently in cardiac muscles is the pivotal factor which is responsible the impairment of myocardial systolic and diastolic functions [30]. In such situations, Ca^{2+} homeostasis is altered during DC thereby affecting the ability of SR to take up Ca^{2+} and the Na^+-Ca^{2+} exchanger, and the sarcolemma Ca^{2+} ATPase to move Ca^{2+} out of the cell leading to elevated diastolic $[Ca^{2+}]_i$. Second, in diabetes, channel proteins within RyRs undergo carbonylation leading to asynchronous release of calcium into the cytoplasm from the SR [57]; (see **Figure 4**).

Like cellular calcium, potassium homeostasis is of crucial importance for normal cellular function and it is regulated by ion-exchange pumps, co–transporters and channels. Normal plasma potassium values range between 3.8 to5.1 mmol/l [70]. The deviations to both extremes (hypo- and hyperkalaemia) are associated with increased risk of arrhythmias and SCD especially in diabetes-induced chronic kidney failure. Moreover, diabetic patients are at high risks when the failing kidneys are unable to remove potassium from the plasma and as such it builds up in the body leading to hyperkalaemia. Potassium levels below 3.0 mmol/l cause significant Q-T interval prolongation with subsequent risk of torsade des pointes, ventricular fibrillation and SCD. Potassium levels above 6.0 mmol/l cause peaked T waves, wider QRS komplexes and may result in bradycardia, asystole and SCD [70]. Tight regulation of serum potassium levels is necessary for many physiologic processes, including normal cardiac conduction and function [71].

13. Beneficial effect of daily exercise in sudden cardiac death

The beneficial cardiac protection, following regular exercise training (ET) in diabetic patients, has been reported in both clinical and experimental animal studies. It is now known that acute endurance ET is accompanied with significant increase in maximum oxygen consumption and enhanced cardiac output, stroke volume and systolic blood pressure which are all associated with decreased peripheral vascular resistance. On the other hand, long-term cardiovascular adaptation to dynamic training results in increased maximal oxygen uptake due to increased cardiac output and arteriovenous oxygen difference. In contrast, strength exercise training induces little or no increase in oxygen uptake. Thus, endurance exercise predominantly produces volume load on the left ventricle (LV), and strength exercise causes largely a pressure load [72]. It is now well established that LV physiological hypertrophy due to daily endurance exercise training can result in a proportional increase in myocardial cell length and width without evidence of myocardial hyperplasia in the majority of cases. This beneficial process is mediated via an increase in the expression of cardiac insulin-like growth factor-1 (IGF-1) and a concurrent activation of phophoinositide-3 kinase (PI3K) [73].

Both physiological and pathological cardiac enlargement (hypertrophy) is caused by different stimuli and both are functionally distinguishable. A pathological stimulus is normally caused by a pressure overload due to either aortic stenosis or hypertension producing an increase in systolic wall stress. In turn, this results in a concentric type of hypertrophy. This process occurs when the heart develops a thick wall with relatively small cavities. [74]. ET can also induce an adaptation of the coronary artery circulation which is divided into two main processes. Firstly, angiogenesis is initiated leading to an expansion of the capillary network by the formation of new blood vessels which occur at the level of capillaries and resistance arterioles, but not in large coronary arteries [75]. The cellular and subcellular mechanisms underlying ET-induced angiogenesis are still unknown. A number of studies [76–78] have demonstrated that growth factors including vascular endothelial growth factor (VEGF), fibroblast growth factor (FGF) and angiopoietins (AQP) and their corresponding receptors are involved in the angiogenesis process. Studies have also shown that sprouting angiogenesis is associated with a number of proteases which are relevant for the breakdown of the capillary basement membrane. These functional proteins include matrix metalloproteinases (MMPs), urokinase, tissue plasminogen activator and plasminogen [76–79]. Cardiac muscle function is highly dependent on an adequate coronary blood flow due to high metabolic demand. Thus, coronary artery dysfunction can have a direct impact on myocardial function. It was demonstrated that an eight-week moderate-intensity exercise training regime in individuals with T2DM can significantly enhance endothelial cell function in the brachial coronary artery. This was associated with a significant improved blood flow-mediated dilation [76].

It is now known that repetitive exercise training sessions can stimulate other adaptive changes in the myocardium contributing to both improved insulin sensitivity and metabolic health of the organ. A previous study has revealed that increased oxidative capacity and capillary density were observed in skeletal muscle in response to aerobic exercise [77]. Similarly, insulin sensitivity in adipose tissue is increased within 72-hours after completion of a 6-week exercise intervention [78]. Likewise, calcium homeostasis has a major role in the excitation contracting-coupling process of the heart and ET has been shown to improve significantly cardiac myocytes contractility during diabetes due to an improvement of Ca^{2+} homeostasis. It was reported that ET can also prevent the development of SCD and the dysregulation of SR protein content in an inducible animal model of T2DM [80]. It is now well established that most athletes have a low resting heart rate (brady-arrhythmias), typical of 40–60 beats per minute due to high vagal tone in the heart.

14. Treatment of sudden cardiac death

Therapy of SCD includes non-pharmacological and pharmacological interventions. There are a number of therapeutic options, but the main non-pharmacological therapy is the use of defibrillators [5, 6, 81–83]. However, there must be more community-based public access to defibrillation programs in order to save the lives of those patients who are more impacted. Other factors include screening of family members who are susceptible to arrhythmias and SCD and this in turn will help with early diagnosis and also and managing the arrhythmias. Generally, potential patients have to change their lifestyle habits by reducing their stress level, avoid smoking and drinking alcohol, eat a heart healthy Mediterranean diet and participate in moderate daily exercise. Moreover, potential patients should also education themselves about the signs and symptoms of SCD and how to obtain early treatment. Likewise, public health services globally should introduce health education on SCD to students, workers, patients and others. In terms of pharmacological intervention, SCD patients are treated mainly with beta blockers, ACE inhibitors, anti-arrhythmic drugs and in some cases, amiodarone. These drugs exert their beneficial effects via different cellular and subcellular mechanisms by slowing the rate and force of contraction of the myocardium [81].

It is now the general consensus that the implantable cardioverter-defibrillators (ICD) which was first implanted in patients in the 1980 is the mainstay life-saving and cost-effective clinical device in treating cardiac patients with dangerous abnormal life-threatening arrhythmias and also in the treatment of resuscitated survivors of sudden cardiac arrest substantially and with increased life expectancy compared to pharmacological therapies, including amiodarone [82]. ICD is also employed for primary prevention in high-risk patients, and in biventricular pacing of patients at high risk for arrhythmic events. More recent studies have reported that subcutaneous implantable cardioverter defibrillator (SIDC) is both safe and effective instead of the ICD as an alternative to prevent SCD [83]. The indications and use of the ICDs and SIDCs will continue to grow, resulting in increasing discussions about costs compared to other forms of therapy and the necessity of better selection of ICD/SIDC recipients depending on age, duration of the illness, risks and others [84]. Improvement of results of resuscitation from out-of-hospital cardiac arrest remains an important challenge. Both better methods to recognize asymptomatic patients at risk including genetic screening and development of new technologies to shorten the time interval between cardiac arrest and the resuscitation effort are urgently needed [84]. Further information can be found in the 2017 AHA/ACC/HRS guideline for management of patients with ventricular arrhythmias and prevention of sudden cardiac death [85].

15. Conclusion

Figure 5 summarizes the major events leading to SCD during the development of DM as a result of the various risk factors. It is proposed that during elevated or uncontrolled level of blood glucose (hyperglycemia) due to DM, the body produces a number of endogenous pathological compounds called oxidants, which are classified either as reactive oxygen species (ROS such as $2O^-$, H_2O_2, and others) or RCS. One particular RCS is methylglyoxal (MGO), which is elevated to toxic levels.

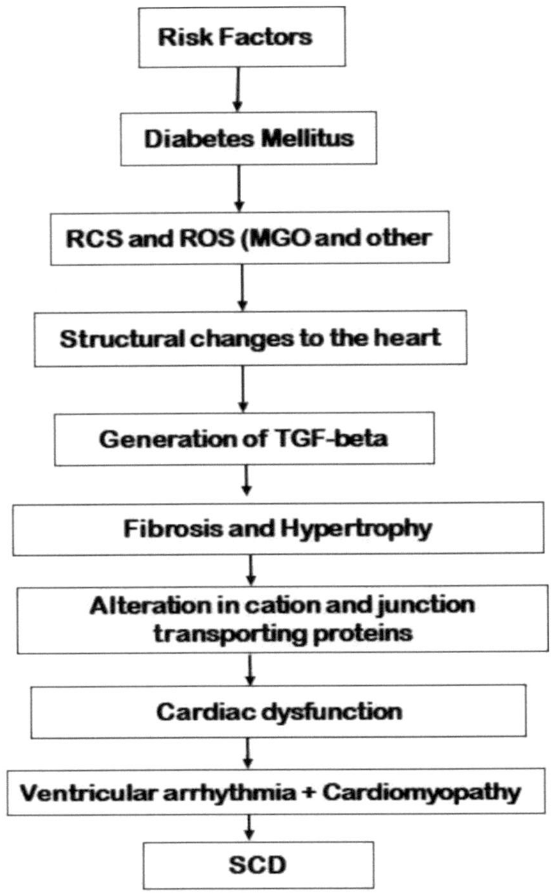

Figure 5.
A flow diagram illustrating the events, starting from the risk factors that lead to sudden cardiac death in diabetes mellitus. ROS, reactive oxygen species; MGO, methylglyoxal; TGF-beta, transforming growth factor-beta; SCD, sudden cardiac death.

This is due to increased synthesis and a decrease in the activity of glyoxylase-1, the enzyme that metabolizes MGO in the different organs of the body [55]. In the heart, MGO exerts a deleterious effect resulting in death of some cells (apoptosis), enlargement and disarray of the structure of cardiac muscles and other tissues which are associated with an elevation of transforming growth factor beta-1 (TGF-beta-1), which in turn elicits hypertrophy of the heart and infiltration of fibrosis [86]. These processes lead to a derangement in cellular calcium homeostasis (elevated diastolic calcium) followed by DC. The resulting effect is remodeling of the heart so that it can maintain its function to pump blood around the body but not at physiological level [87]. Thus, the pathogenesis of diabetic cardiomyopathy in diabetic patients is multifactorial and complex, eventually leading to an energetically compromised heart with reduced working capacity or heart failure, arrhythmias, and SCD. Luckily, patients now have a number of therapies including non-pharmacological and pharmacological interventions to treat SCD.

Author details

Manal M.A. Smail[1,2], Frank C. Howarth[1], Jaipaul Singh[2], Sunil Rupee[3], Khemraj Rupee[3], Carlin Hanoman[2,3], Abla Mohammed Ismail[4], Farah Ahmed Sleiman[4], Samar Abdulkhalek[5] and Keshore Bidasee[6]*

1 Department of Physiology, College of Medicine and Health Sciences, United Arab Emirates University, United Arab Emirates

2 School of Natural Sciences, University of Central Lancashire, Preston, England, United Kingdom

3 School of Medicine, Faculty of Health Sciences, University of Guyana, Turkeyen, Georgetown, Guyana

4 Corniche Hospital, United Arab Emirates

5 Fatima College for Health Science, United Arab Emirates

6 Department of Pharmacology and Neurosciences, University of Omaha Medical Centre, Omaha, NE, USA

*Address all correspondence to: kbidasee@unmc.edu

References

[1] Walker AM, Cubbon RM. Sudden cardiac death in patients with diabetes mellitus and chronic heart failure. Diabetes & Vascular Disease Research. 2015;**12**:228-233

[2] Maron BJ. Clinical course and management of hypertrophic cardiomyopathy. The New England Journal of Medicine. 2018;**16**(379):655-668

[3] Jameson JL. Cardiovascular collapse, cardiac arrest, and sudden cardiac death: Harrison's principles of internal medicine. 20th ed. New York, N.Y.: The McGraw-Hill Companies; 2018

[4] Elkilany GASEMSJSRBEYNC. Updates regarding prediction and prevention of sudden cardiac death. EC Cardiology. 2019;**6**(11):103-121

[5] Elkalany GSRAESJBKSOAHK. Sudden cardiac death. World Heart Journal. 2017;**9**(1):51-62

[6] Neil T, Richard JS. Sudden cardiac death and arrhythmias. Arrhythmia & Electrophysiology Review. 2018;**7**(2):111-117

[7] Wong CX, Brown A, Lau DH, Chugh SS, Albert CM, Kalman JM, et al. Epidemiology of sudden cardiac death: Global and regional perspectives. Heart, Lung & Circulation. 2019;**28**:6-14

[8] Voulgari C, Papadogiannis D, Tentolouris N. Diabetic cardiomyopathy: From the pathophysiology of the cardiac myocytes to current diagnosis and management strategies. Vascular Health and Risk Management. 2010;**21**(6):883-903

[9] Zimmet P, Alberti KG, Shaw J. Global and societal implications of the diabetes epidemic. Nature. 2001;**414**(6865):782-787

[10] Kannel WB, McGee DL. Diabetes and cardiovascular disease: The Framingham study. JAMA. 1979;**241**(19):2035-2038

[11] Sherwood DE. Electromyographic control of movement time in a rapid aiming movement. Perceptual and Motor Skills. 2008;**16**(8):946-954

[12] Lockhart MM, Phelp AL, Van den Hoff MJB, Wessels A. The Epicardium and the development of the atrioventricular junction in the murine heart. Developmental Biology. 2014;**2**:1-17

[13] Parashar K, Starling SK. Daibtese:-history and traditional medication. Sientific Research. 2015;**4**(9):337-342

[14] Greyson CR. The right ventricle and pulmonary circulation: Basic concepts. Revista Española de Cardiología. 2010;**63**(1):81-95

[15] Clayton RH, Bernus O, Cherry EM, Dierckx H, Fenton FH, Mirabella L, et al. Models of cardiac tissue electrophysiology: Progress, challenges and open questions. Progress in Biophysics and Molecular Biology. 2011;**104**(1-3):22-48

[16] Cordeiro JM, Green L, Heilmann C, Antzelevich D, Antzelevich C. Transmural heterogeneity of calcium activity and mechanical function in the canine left ventricle. American Journal of Physiology. Heart and Circulatory Physiology. 2004;**286**(4):H1471-H1479

[17] Anderson RH, Boyett MR, Dobrzynski H, Moorman AF. The anatomy of the conduction system: Implications for the clinical cardiologist. Journal of Cardiovascular Translational Research. 2013;**6**(2):187-196

[18] Kharche S, Zhang H, Holden AV. Hypertrophy in rat virtual left ventricular cells and tissue. LNCS. 2005;**3504**:153-161

[19] Sovari AA, Li Yi-G. Cardiac arrhythmias: Update on mechanisms and clinical managements, Cardiology Research and Practice. 2016;**2016**:9656078-15

[20] Weber KT. Cardiac interstitium in health and disease: The fibrillar collagen network. Journal of the American College of Cardiology. 1989;**13**(7):1637-1652

[21] Cleutjens JPM. Mini-review. The role of matrix metalloproteinases in heart disease. Cardiovascular Research. 1996;**32**:816-821

[22] Briest W. The role of extracellular matrix in the development of experimental cardiac hypertrophy. Carl-Ludwig Institute of Physiology. 2007;**1**:830-838

[23] Cattaruzza S, Perris R. Approaching the proteoglycome: Molecular interactions of proteoglycans and their functional output. Macromolecular Bioscience. 2006;**6**(8):667-680

[24] Boudina S, Abel ED. Diabetic cardiomyopathy revisited. Circulation. 2007;**115**(25):3213-3223

[25] Rubler S, Dlugash J, Yuceoglu YZ, Kumral T, Branwood AW, Grishman A. New type of cardiomyopathy associated with diabetic glomerulosclerosis. The American Journal of Cardiology. 1972;**30**(6):595-602

[26] Abe T, Ohga Y, Tabayashi N, Kobayashi S, Sakata S, Misawa H, et al. Left ventricular diastolic dysfunction in type 2 diabetes mellitus model rats. American Journal of Physiology. Heart and Circulatory Physiology. 2002;**282**(1):138-148

[27] Falcao-Pires I, Leite-Moreira AF. Diabeticcardiomyopathy:Understanding the molecular and cellular basis to progress in diagnosis and treatment. Heart Failure Reviews. 2012;**17**(3):325-344

[28] Miki T, Yuda S, Kouzu H, Miura T. Diabetic cardiomyopathy: Pathophysiology and clinical features. Heart Failure Reviews. 2013;**12**(2):149-166

[29] Spector KS. Diabetic cardiomyopathy. Clinical Cardiology. 1998; **21**(12):885-887

[30] Poornima IG, Parikh P, Shannon RP. Diabetic cardiomyopathy: The search for a unifying hypothesis. Circulation Research. 2006;**98**(5):596-605

[31] Jia G, Demarco VG, Sowers JR. Insulin resistance and hyperinsulinaemia in diabetic cardiomyopathy. Nature Reviews. Endocrinology. 2016;**12**(3):144-153

[32] Shimoni Y, Severson D, Giles W. Thyroid status and diabetes modulate regional differences in potassium currents in rat ventricle. The Journal of Physiology. 1995;**488**(Pt 3):673-688

[33] Lindsey ML, Borg TK. Understanding the role of the extracellular matrix in cardiovascular development and disease: Where do we go from here? Journal of Molecular and Cellular Cardiology. 2009;**48**(3):431-432

[34] Hafstad AD, Boardman N, Aasum E. Exercise training represents nowadays a useful nonpharmacological strategy for the treatment of cardiovascular diseases. Antioxidants & Redox Signaling. 2015;**22**(17):1587-1605

[35] Poirier P, Bogaty P, Philippon F, GarneauC,FortinC.Diastolicdysfunction in normotensive men with well-controlled type 2 diabetes:Importance of manoeuvres in echocardiographic screening for preclinical diabetic cardiomyopathy. Diabetes Care. 2001;**24**:5-10

[36] Boudina S, Abel ED. Diabetic cardiomyopathy, causes and effects. Reviews in Endocrine & Metabolic Disorders. 2010;**11**(1):31-39

[37] Bertrand L, Horman S, Beauloye C, Vanoverschelde JL. Insulin signalling in the heart. Cardiovascular Research. 2008;**79**(2):238-248

[38] Lopaschuk GD. Metabolic abnormalities in the diabetic heart. Heart Failure Reviews. 2002;7(2):149-159

[39] Stanley WC, Lopaschuk GD, McCormack JG. Regulation of energy substrate metabolism in the diabetic heart. Cardiovascular Research. 1997;**34**(1):25-33

[40] Fukumoto H, Kayano T, Buse JB, Edwards Y, Pilch PF, Bell GI, et al. Cloning and characterization of the major insulin-responsive glucose transporter expressed in human skeletal muscle and other insulin-responsive tissues. The Journal of Biological Chemistry. 1988;**264**(14):7776-7779

[41] Camps M, Castello A, Munoz P, Monfar M, Testar X, Palacin M, et al. Effect of diabetes and fasting on GLUT-4 (muscle/fat) glucose-transporter expression in insulin-sensitive tissues. Heterogeneous response in heart, red and white muscle. The Biochemical Journal. 1992;**282**(Pt 3):765-772

[42] Fang ZY, Prins JB, Marwick TH. Diabetic cardiomyopathy: Evidence, mechanisms, and therapeutic implications. Endocrine Reviews. 2004;**25**(4):543-567

[43] Dale Abel E, O'Shea KM, Ramasamy R. Insulin resistance: Metabolic mechanisms and consequences in the heart. Arteriosclerosis, Thrombosis, and Vascular Biology. 2012;**32**(9):2068-2076

[44] Despres JP, Lamarche B, Mauriege P, Cantin B, Dagenais GR, Moorjani S, et al. Hyperinsulinemia as an independent risk factor for ischemic heart disease [see comments]. The New England Journal of Medicine. 1996;**334**(15):952-957

[45] Huang JP, Huang LM. Insulin Resistance and Cardiomyopathy, Cardiomyopathies. Taiwan: Chang Gung University; 2012

[46] Wright JJ, Kim J, Buchanan J, Boudina S, Sena S, Bakirtzi K, et al. Mechanisms for increased myocardial fatty acid utilization following short-term high-fat feeding. Cardiovascular Research. 2009;**82**(2):351-360

[47] Baum J, Duffy HS. Fibroblasts and Myofibroblasts: What are we talking about? Journal of Cardiovascular Pharmacology. 2011;**57**(4):376-379

[48] Zhou YT, Grayburn P, Karim A, Shimabukuro M, Higa M, Baetens D, et al. Lipotoxic heart disease in obese rats: Implications for human obesity. Proceedings of the National Academy of Sciences of the United States of America. 2000;**97**(4):1784-1789

[49] Sovari AA, Karagueuzian HS. Myocardial fibrosis as a riskstratifier for sudden arrhythmic death. Expert Review of Cardiovascular Therapy. 2011;**9**(8):951-953

[50] de Bakker JM, van Rijen HM. Continuous and discontinuous propagation in heart muscle. Journal of Cardiovascular Electrophysiology. 2006;**17**(5):567-573

[51] van Hoeven KH, Factor SM. A comparison of the pathological spectrum of hypertensive, diabetic, and hypertensive-diabetic heart disease [see comments]. Circulation. 1990;**82**(3):848-855

[52] Fiordaliso F, Li B, Latini R, Sonnenblick EH, Anversa P, Leri A, et al. Myocyte death in

streptozotocin-induced diabetes in rats in angiotensin II- dependent. Laboratory Investigation. 2000;**80**(4):513-527

[53] Frustaci A, Kajstura J, Chimenti C, Jakoniuk I, Leri A, Maseri A, et al. Myocardial cell death in human diabetes. Circulation Research. 2000;**87**(12):1123-1132

[54] Cai L, Wang Y, Zhou G, Chen T, Song Y, Li X, et al. Attenuation by metallothionein of early cardiac cell death via suppression of mitochondrial oxidative stress results in a prevention of diabetic cardiomyopathy. Journal of the American College of Cardiology. 2006;**48**(8):1688-1697

[55] D'Souza A, Hussain M, Howarth FC, Woods NM, Bidasee K, Singh J. Pathogenesis and pathophysiology of accelerated atherosclerosis in the diabetic heart. Cellular Biochem. 2009;**331**:89-116

[56] Billet S, Aguilar F, Baudry C, Clauser E. Role of angiotensin II AT1 receptor activation in cardiovascular diseases. Kidney International. 2008;**74**(11):1379-1384

[57] Piquereau J, Caffin F, Novotova M, Lemaire C, Veksler V, Garnier A, et al. Mitochondrial dynamics in the adult cardiomyocytes: Which roles for a highly specialized cell? Frontiers in Physiology. 2013;**4**(102):1-12

[58] Duncan JG. Mitochondrial dysfunction in diabetic cardiomyopathy. Molecular Cell Research. 2011;**1813**(7):1351-1359

[59] Shen X, Zheng S, Thongboonkerd V, Xu M, Pierce WM Jr, Klein JB, et al. Cardiac mitochondrial damage and biogenesis in a chronic model of type I diabetes. American Journal of Physiology. Endocrinology and Metabolism. 2004;**287**(5):896-905

[60] Tarquini R, Lazzeri C, Pala L, Rotella C, Gensini GF. The diabetic cardiomyopathy. Acta Diabetologica. 2016;**48**(3):173-181

[61] Boudina S, Bugger H, Sena S, O'Neill BT, Zaha VG, Ilkun O, et al. Contribution of impaired myocardial insulin signaling to mitochondrial dysfunction and oxidative stress in the heart. Circulation. 2009;**119**(9):1272-1283

[62] Ye G, Metreveli NS, Donthi RV, Xia S, Xu M, Carlson EC, et al. Catalase protects cardiomyocyte function in models of type 1 and type 2 diabetes. Diabetes. 2004;**53**(5):1336-1343

[63] Novoa U, Arauna D, Moran M, Nuñez M, Zagmutt S, Saldivia S, et al. High-intensity exercise reduces cardiac fibrosis and hypertrophy but does not restore the nitroso-redox imbalance in diabetic cardiomyopathy. Oxidative Medicine and Cellular Longevity. 2017;**2017**:1-11

[64] Vishal Go, etal . Obesity and sudden cardiac death in the young: A nationwide retrospective study. Journal of the American College of Cardiology 2020;**75**(11):1-10

[65] Plourde B et al. Sudden cardiac death and obesity. Expert Review of Cardiovascular Therapy. 2014;**12**(9): 1099-1110

[66] Adabag S et al. Obesity related risk of sudden cardiac death in the atherosclerosis risk in communities study. Heart. 2015;**101**:215-221

[67] Csige I, Ujvárosy D, Szabó Z, Lorincz I, Paragh G, Harangi M, et al. The impact of obesity on the cardiovascular system. Journal of Daibetes Research. 2018;**218**(1):12

[68] Wier WG, Balke W. Ca2+ release mechanisms, Ca2+ Sparks, and local control of excitation-contraction coupling in Normal heart muscle. Circulation Research. 1999;**85**:770-776

[69] Sivitz WI, Yorek MA. Mitochondrial dysfunction in diabetes: From molecular mechanisms to functional significance and therapeutic opportunities. Antioxidants & Redox Signaling. 2010;**12**(4):537-577

[70] Widimsky P. Hypokalemia and the heart. e-Journal of Cardiology Practice. 2008;7(9):1-10

[71] Patrick H, Pun BA, John AG, John PM, Laura PS. Serum potassium levels and risk of sudden cardiac death among patients with chronic kidney disease and significant coronary artery disease. Kidney International Reports. 2017;**2**:1122-1131

[72] Maron BJ, Pelliccia A. The heart of trained athletes: Cardiac remodeling and the risks of sports, including sudden death. Circulation. 2006;**114**(15):1633-1644

[73] Galanti G. Increased cardiac sympathetic activity and insulin-like growth factor-I formation are associated with physiological hypertrophy in athletes. Circulation Research. 2001;**89**:977-982

[74] Pluim BM, Zwinderman AH, Van der Laarse, van der Laarse A, van der Wall EE. The athlete's heart. A meta-analysis of cardiac structure and function. Circulation. 2000;**101**:336-344

[75] Leung FP, Yung LM, Laher I, Xiaoqiang Y, Chen Z, Chen ZY, et al. Exercise, vascular wall and cardiovascular diseases: An update (part 1). Sports Medicine. 2008;**38**(12):1009-1024

[76] Okada S, Hiuge A, Makino H, Nagumo A, Takaki H, Konishi H, et al. Effect of exercise intervention on endothelial function and incidence of cardiovascular disease in patients with type 2 diabetes. Atherosclerosis and Thrombosis. 2010;**17**(8):828-833

[77] Dubé JJ, Fleishman KMS, Rousson V, Goodpaster BH, Amati F. Exercise dose and insulin sensitivity: Relevance for diabetes prevention. Medicine and Science in Sports and Exercise. 2012;**44**(5):793-799

[78] Dario A, Gutierrez BS, Michael J, Hasty AH. Impact of increased adipose tissue mass on inflammation, insulin resistance, and dyslipidemia. Current Diabetes Reports. 2009;**9**(1):26-32

[79] Rehman J, Li J, Parvathaneni L, Karlsson G, Panchal VR, Temm CJ, et al. Exercise acutely increases circulating endothelial progenitor cells and monocyte–/macrophage-derived angiogenic cells. Journal of the American College of Cardiology. 2004;**43**(12):2314-2318

[80] Epp R, Susser S, Morissette M, Kehler D, Jassal DS, Duhamel T. Exercise training prevents the development of cardiac dysfunction in the low-dose streptozotocin diabetic rats fed a high-fat diet. Canadian Journal of Physiology and Pharmacology. 2016;**91**(1):80-89

[81] Goldberger JJ. Treatment and prevention of sudden cardiac death:Effect of recent clinical trials. Archives of Internal Medicine. 1999;**159**:1281-1287

[82] Larsen GC, Manolis AS, Sonnenbery FM, Beshansky JR, Estes NA, Pauker SG. Cost effectiveness of the implantable cardoiverter defibrillator: Effect of improved battery life and comparison with amiodarone. Journal of American College of Cardiology. 1992;**19**(6):223-234

[83] Westerman SB, EL-Chami M. The subcutaneous. Implantable cardoiverter defibrillator: Review on recent data. Journal of Geriatric Cardiology. 2018;**15**(3):222-228.199

[84] Josephson M, Hein J, Wellens J. Implantable defibrillators and sudden cardiac death. Circulation. 2004;**109**(22):2685-2691

[85] Al-Khatib SM et al. AHA/ACC/HRS guideline for management of patients with ventricular arrhythmias and prevention of sudden cardiac death: Executive summary. Circulation. 2018;**138**:e210-e271

[86] Alomar F et al. Smooth muscle-generated methylglyoxal impairs endothelial cell-mediated vasodilatation of cerebral micro-vessels in type 1 diabetic rats. British Journal of Pharmacology. 2016;**173**(23):1-10

[87] Iqbal T et al. Effects of diabetes-induced Hyperglycaemia on the heart: Biochemical and structural alterations. In: Textbook of Heart Failure. India: Springer; 2013. pp. 120-142

Chapter 8

Sudden Cardiac Death in Hereditary Dilated Cardiomyopathy

Marianna Leopoulou, Jo Ann LeQuang, Joseph V. Pergolizzi and Peter Magnusson

Abstract

Dilated cardiomyopathy (DCM) is characterized by the phenotype of a dilated left ventricle with systolic dysfunction. It is classified as hereditary when it is deemed of genetic origin; more than 50 genes are reported to be related to the condition. Symptoms include, among others, dyspnea, fatigue, arrhythmias, and syncope. Unfortunately, sudden cardiac death may be the first manifestation of the disease. Risk stratification regarding sudden death in hereditary DCM as well as preventive management poses a challenge due to the heterogeneity of the disease. The purpose of this chapter is to present the epidemiology, risk stratification, and preventive strategies of sudden cardiac death in hereditary DCM.

Keywords: cardiomyopathy, dilated cardiomyopathy, heart failure, implantable cardioverter defibrillator, risk stratification

1. Introduction

Cardiomyopathies are categorized based on their phenotype. In that context, dilated cardiomyopathy (DCM) is characterized by a dilated left ventricle (LV), typically with thin walls, and systolic dysfunction (**Figure 1**). Sometimes the dysfunction is not limited to the left ventricle but also affects the right ventricle. It is estimated that approximately 1 in 2500 people suffer from DCM [1]. The causative pathways are often complex, and several risk factors work together. In the vast majority of patients, there is a history of hypertension. Other well-known etiologies are myocarditis, chemotherapy, toxins, radiation, and coronary artery disease. However, when a causative reason for the dilation of the heart cannot be identified, DCM is considered idiopathic. About 20–50% of idiopathic DCM is considered to be of a genetic origin, being consequently hereditary [2]. Interestingly, only in 30–40% of cases of familial DCM can a specific gene be identified [3].

In hereditary DCM, there is variability among phenotypes, and the manifestation of LV dysfunction is heterogeneous. More than 50 genes are associated with the disease [4] (**Table 1**). Many of the gene mutations responsible for DCM affect the cell structure called sarcomere, which is involved in cardiac contractility. That is why some of those genes may be responsible for the development of hypertrophic cardiomyopathy as well. In 20% of the cases of hereditary DCM, mutations of the titin (TTN) gene are found, which encodes the protein titin found in the sarcomere [5].

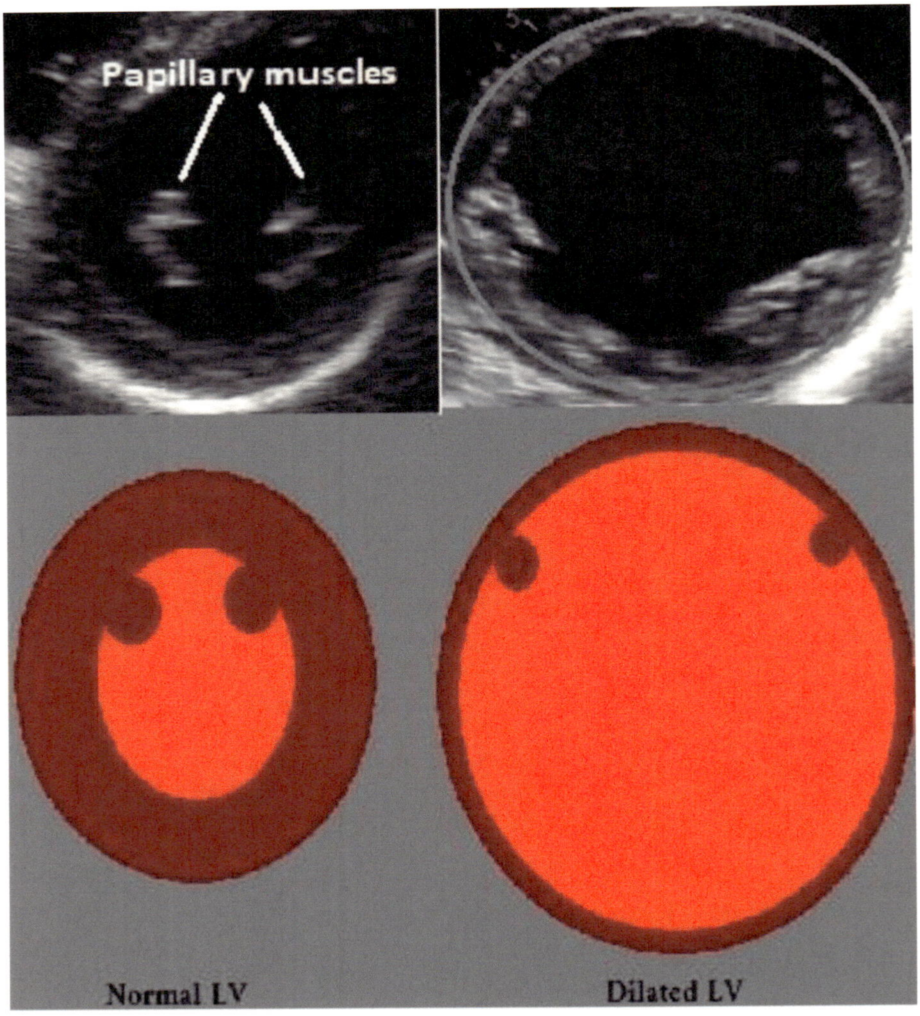

Figure 1.
Normal and dilated left ventricle in parasternal short-axis view.

The inheritance pattern is autosomal dominant in the vast majority of the cases, which means that an individual has a 50% chance to inherit the gene if one of the parents carries it. In other cases, the pattern is autosomal recessive, which means that if both parents are affected, there is a 25% chance of inheriting the disease genotype. X-linked patterns, in which the gene is inherited through an X chromosome, have also been reported. In some cases, it is possible that the carrier may not develop the phenotype of the disease due to variable penetrance of the disease.

Inherited DCM is defined by (a) the presence of two or more affected individuals in a single family who fulfill DCM criteria; fractional shortening <25% and/or ejection fraction <45% and left ventricular end diastolic diameter > 117% of the upper reference level corrected for age and body surface area based on Henry's formula or (b) the presence of a first-degree relative with unexplained sudden death before the age of 35 years [6].

Symptoms of DCM are due to ventricular dysfunction and compensatory left ventricular remodeling as well as the involvement of the electrical conduction system of the heart [7]. Symptoms vary among patients, even if they are members of

Gene	Cellular structure
ABCC9	Calcium/sodium handling
ACTC1	Sarcomere and cytoskeleton
ACTN2	Sarcomere and cytoskeleton
ANKRD1	Sarcomere and transcription factor
BAG3	Sarcomere
CRYAB	Cytoskeleton
CSRP3	Sarcomere and cytoskeleton
DES	Cytoskeleton
DMD	Cytoskeleton
DSG2	Desmosome
EYA4	Other
FLNC	Cytoskeleton
GATAD1	Other
LAMA4	Extracellular matrix proteins
LCB3	Cytoskeleton
LMNA	Nuclear envelope
MYBPC3	Sarcomere
MYH6	Sarcomere
MYH7	Sarcomere
MYPN	Cytoskeleton
PLN	Calcium/sodium handling
PSEN1	Other
PSEN2	Other
RBM20	Other
SCN5A	Calcium/sodium handling
SGCD	Cytoskeleton
TAZ	Other
TCAP	Sarcomere and cytoskeleton
TMPO	Nuclear envelope
TNNC1	Sarcomere
TNNI3	Sarcomere
TNNT2	Sarcomere
TPM1	Sarcomere
TTN	Sarcomere
VCL	Sarcomere and cytoskeleton

Table 1.
The main genes associated with hereditary dilated cardiomyopathy and the cellular structure that they regulate.

the same family [5]. Symptoms can occur at any age; typically, they first appear in mid-adulthood. Patients often report breathlessness, swelling of the legs, fatigue, chest pain, and arrhythmias, ranging from palpitations and syncope to fatal arrhythmias that cause SCD. Unfortunately, SCD is sometimes the first manifestation of the disease.

2. Sudden cardiac death in hereditary DCM

2.1 Definition of sudden cardiac death

Sudden cardiac death (SCD) is defined as the sudden and unexpected death of a person who was otherwise stable prior to the event [8]. If the death is witnessed and occurs within 1 hour of onset of symptoms, it is classified as SCD. If the sudden and unexpected death is not witnessed, then SCD is declared if it occurs within 24 hours of the person last being seen alive and well.

2.2 Mechanisms

In the case of hereditary cardiomyopathies, such as DCM, SCD occurs due to the development of fatal ventricular arrhythmias: ventricular tachycardia (VT) and ventricular fibrillation (VF) are most common, but prolonged bradycardia does occur. Possible underlying mechanisms for the initiation of a fatal re-entry arrhythmia in a DCM patient may include: (a) conduction block caused by a reduction of myocytes and hypertrophy and (b) continuous re-entry regeneration due to increased fibrosis, interstitial, and perivascular as well as post-necrosis fibrosis [9, 10]. Non re-entry mechanisms, such as focal automaticity, electrolyte disturbances, and stretch-induced arrhythmias, also contribute to the presentation of arrhythmias [10]. In particular, focal automaticity predisposes a patient to nonsustained VT (NSVT) [11].

2.3 Epidemiology

DCM ranks third as the cause of SCD among cardiomyopathies, after arrhythmogenic right ventricular cardiomyopathy (ARVC) and hypertrophic cardiomyopathy. SCD accounts for roughly a third of all-cause mortality among hereditary DCM patients. Rates of SCD vary among the patients in regard to their New York Heart Association (NYHA) functional status (**Table 2**). Notably, in patients with NYHA class I and II, 50–60% of deaths are classified as sudden, while in NYHA class IV patients, only 20–30% of deaths are sudden [10]. This is explained by the fact that in NYHA class IV, most patients die from progressive heart failure [12]. In most cases, potentially fatal arrhythmias present in a setting of systolic ventricular dysfunction, although the proportion of SCD is higher among patients with lower NYHA status. However, there is a subset of patients (reported to vary from 2% to one third of the DCM population) who present early in the disease course with

NYHA	Risk of SCD
Class I	50–60%
Class II	50–60%
Class III	20–30%
Class IV	20–30%

Table 2.
Risk of sudden cardiac death as a proportion of overall mortality according to New York Heart Association classification.

Factors associated with a high risk of arrhythmias	
Clinical	Low LVEF (<25–30%) Absence of beta-blockers AR-DCM Family history of SCD
Ambulatory	QRS duration QT dynamicity T-wave alternans NSVT on Holter monitoring
Imaging	Midwall late gadolinium enhancement Impaired global longitudinal strain Mechanical dispersion
Genetic	Desmosomal mutations LMNA mutation SCN5A mutation FLNC mutation RBM20 mutation PLN mutation

Table 3.
Factors associated with a high risk of life-threatening arrhythmias.

life-threatening arrhythmias (**Table 3**) or unexplained syncope that are not related to the severity of LV dysfunction [13, 14]. This specific entity is referred to as arrhythmogenic DCM (AR-DCM). Patients who suffer from AR-DCM, compared to other DCM patients, have a higher risk of experiencing major arrhythmic events and SCD. Thus, a family history of SCD in an AR-DCM patient results in a higher burden of life-threatening arrhythmias and a higher risk of SCD [7]. It is important to mention that DCM patients, due to their high incidence of atrial fibrillation, also have a higher risk for ischemic stroke. However, it should be noted that if a cause of death other than arrhythmia is confirmed, the death will not be classified as sudden.

2.4 Risk stratification

It is crucial to identify patients at high risk of a fatal arrhythmia. There are clues in the clinical history, electrocardiographic, imaging characteristics, and specific genetic features that need to be taken into account. Factors such as QRS duration, QT-interval dispersion, and T-wave alternans have been suggested as risk markers [15]. A considerable burden of ventricular arrhythmias (runs of VT) is usually present in a setting of advanced ventricular dysfunction with left ventricular ejection fraction (LVEF) <25%, which is a validated risk factor. Survived cardiac arrest and sustained ventricular tachycardia with hemodynamic compromise imply a high risk of recurrent arrhythmia and are classified as secondary prevention for an implantable cardioverter defibrillator (ICD) [16]. Unexplained syncope may be secondary to arrhythmia and constitutes a risk factor [15]. In the Marburg Cardiomyopathy study (MACAS), which excluded patients with a history of sustained VT or VF, unexplained syncope within the previous 12 months, and amiodarone therapy, it was shown that a low LVEF (<30%) was the only independent factor for major arrhythmic events. Patients with NSVT and patients who were not on beta-blockers upon enrollment also run a high risk for ventricular arrhythmias. Thus, the combination of documented NSVT on Holter monitoring with a low LVEF (<30%) increased the arrhythmic risk by eight-fold [17]. Family history of SCD, defined as SCD in a first degree relative <40 years of age or SCD in a relative with confirmed DCM at any age, is also an established risk factor.

2.5 Imaging

Imaging can be used to predict arrhythmia risk. In cardiac magnetic resonance imaging, midwall late gadolinium enhancement (LGE) can detect fibrosis. Even if magnetic resonance imaging is not able to detect fibrosis, it may still be found by advanced T1 mapping techniques before and after gadolinium infusion. This is a prominent finding due to the fact that it corresponds to macroscopic midmyocardial fibrosis on postmortem examination [18]. In echocardiography, an impaired global longitudinal strain, a marker of myocardial regional contractility, may reflect myocardial fibrosis [19]. It has been demonstrated that an impaired global longitudinal strain is associated with increased arrhythmic events [20]. A predictor of arrhythmias is also mechanical dispersion, which is defined as the standard deviation of the time to peak negative strain among the different myocardial segments [20].

2.6 Mutations associated with SCD

Regarding genetic factors, DCM patients who carry a desmosomal or LMNA (lamin A/C) mutation run a higher risk of life-threatening ventricular arrhythmias and SCD, regardless of their LVEF. Patients who carry the LMNA gene, which encodes the type V intermediate filament protein, tend to have more life-threatening arrhythmias compared to other variant carriers and variant-negative patients [21, 22]. LMNA mutations are associated with high morbidity and mortality and with a high clinical penetrance [23]. For the LMNA carriers, various risk factors have been identified. These include NSVT during electrocardiogram monitoring, truncating mutations, LVEF <45–50%, and male sex [24, 25]. More recently, 1st degree AV block has been identified as another risk factor in LMNA carriers [26]. Desmosomal gene mutations are present in around 3% of DCM patients. They are also frequent in ARVC patients, creating a genotype overlap between the two cardiomyopathies. They have been associated with a high risk of potentially fatal arrhythmias, independently from the LVEF [21]. The SCN5A (sodium voltage-gated channel alpha subunit 5) gene, which provides instructions for making sodium channels, is also associated with conduction defects and ventricular arrhythmias [10]. Also associated with a higher risk of arrhythmic events are mutations in the FLNC gene, which encodes filamin proteins; the RNA-binding motif protein 20 gene (RBM20 gene), which encodes a protein that regulates splicing and the phospholamban (PLN) gene, which encodes a protein that inhibits a sarcoplasmic ATPase [21, 27]. In a 2019 study, it was demonstrated that RBM20 mutation carriers were more likely to have NSVT and sustained VT than idiopathic DCM cohorts [28]. The AR-DCM phenotype is associated with a high risk of fatal arrhythmias. Spezzacatene et al. identified the AR-DCM phenotype as well as a family history of SCD or sustained VT/VF as the only early significant predictors for SCD or sustained VT/VF in the overall DCM population. Interestingly, the AR-DCM phenotype is associated with a higher risk of arrhythmias, irrespective of LV dilatation and dysfunction, which is in contradiction to the general DCM population, where a low LVEF is associated with a higher arrhythmic risk [14]. However, AR-DCM is not associated with a poorer prognosis due to non-arrhythmic events, including heart failure [14].

2.7 Preventive management

Most DCM patients present with heart failure and are at a high risk of death. The primary management of such patients lies in the stabilization of progressive heart failure. Drugs like renin-angiotensin-aldosterone system (RAAS) antagonists and beta-blockers are first-line management in patients with DCM and reduce the risk of SCD by preventing ventricular remodeling. Angiotensin converting enzyme inhibitors (ACEs)/angiotensin receptor blockers (ARBs), mineralocorticoid receptor antagonists (MRAs), and beta-blockers are recommended, unless contra-indicated or not tolerated. Furthermore, the combination of sacubitril/valsartan has been shown to be superior to ACE inhibitors and tends to replace them in the treatment of patients who are still symptomatic patients despite optimal medical treatment [16]. The anti-diabetic drug, dapagliflozin, seems to reduce the risk of worsening heart failure and death in patients with a reduced LVEF as well, regardless of the presence of diabetes mellitus, as proven in Dapagliflozin in Patients with Heart Failure and Reduced Ejection Fraction (DAPA-HF) study [29]. In NYHA IV patients, asystolic arrest and pulseless electrical activity are a frequent cause of death [10]. Cardiac resynchronization therapy (CRT) and CRT with defibrillator (CRT-D) treatment also has a place in both symptomatic treatment and preventive management of such patients.

Arrhythmia management in hereditary DCM patients follows the general recommendations as SCD prevention in patients with reduced LVEF (<35%) [7]. Thus, patients with diagnosed DCM must be carefully evaluated for ventricular arrhythmias. Regarding drug management, amiodarone has not been proven to further reduce overall mortality or arrhythmic risk in the Amiodarone versus Implantable Defibrillator (AMIOVIRT) study, which showed that DCM patients who were on amiodarone did not have a statistically significant difference in terms of survival, compared to patients who received an ICD [30]. However, in the Sudden Cardiac Death in Heart Failure trial (SCD-HeFT) which enrolled patients with an LVEF <35% and NYHA II or III despite optimal medical therapy and compared ICD insertion vs. amiodarone vs. placebo, ICD therapy conferred a significant benefit in patients in NYHA class II, but not in class III. Furthermore, amiodarone, when compared to placebo therapy, showed no benefit in NYHA Class II patients and decreased survival among NYHA Class III patients. Results varied among NYHA classes but did not vary between heart failure of ischemic or nonischemic origin [31]. The Defibrillator Implantation in Patients with Nonischemic Systolic Heart Failure (DANISH) trial concluded that prophylactic ICD implantation in symptomatic patients with nonischemic heart failure did not offer a significantly lower long-term rate of death from any cause when compared to standard clinical care but decreased the incidence of SCD by 50% [32].

ICD implantation remains the main therapy in preventive management for DCM patients with impaired LV function, who run a high risk of fatal arrhythmias. Guidelines, as well as the Expert Consensus Statement, recommend an ICD implantation in DCM patients with an LMNA gene mutation and risk factors such as NSVT observed during monitoring, male sex, truncating mutations (class IIa, level B), and an LVEF <45%, which is a higher cutoff value than used in heart failure population guidelines [22, 33].

In addition, a primary-prevention ICD should be considered in DCM patients with both an arrhythmogenic phenotype and a family history of SCD or ventricular arrhythmias, irrespective of their LVEF or LV end-diastolic diameter, as they compose a high-risk group for major arrhythmic events and SCD [14]. However, in individual cases, it can be challenging to determine in which particular patients the benefits of ICD implantation would outweigh the risks. The DEFINITE study (Defibrillators in Non-Ischemic Cardiomyopathy Treatment Evaluation) randomized 458 patients with nonischemic DCM (LVEF <36%) and premature ventricular complexes or nonsustained VT, between standard medical therapy and ICD implantation. SCD by arrhythmias during a mean follow-up of 29 months was far fewer in the ICD group, proving the efficacy of defibrillation [34]. Yet, the use of LVEF alone is not always helpful in determining which patients would most benefit from an ICD. This was made clear in the Oregon and Maastricht Registries, in which 80% of SCD victims had an LVEF >35% [35, 36].

CRT is recommended in patients with sinus rhythm, NYHA class III/IV heart failure, LVEF ≤35%, and QRS >120 ms and/or evidence of mechanical dyssynchrony. It has been shown to offer great survival benefits as well as improvement of LV function in DCM patients [37]. This has been observed especially in women, who seem to benefit more than men from CRT [38]. Furthermore, it has been proven that in patients with nonischemic DCM with an LVEF ≤30%, NYHA class II, and QRS duration ≥130 ms, CRT-D device implantation was also beneficial in reducing the risk of death or heart failure when compared with defibrillation only [39]. On the other hand, patients with low LVEF heart failure and permanent atrial fibrillation do not seem to derive extra benefit from a CRT-D device compared with standard ICD treatment, as suggested by the Resynchronization for Ambulatory Heart Failure Trial (RAFT) trial [40]. Of interest in DCM patients, LGE was proven to be a strong, independent predictor of arrhythmic events and was suggested to improve risk stratification for SCD and better identify the need for ICD therapy [41].

Decisions about ICD therapy should incorporate genetic factors. In patients with mutations, i.e. LMNA mutations, the conventional LVEF-threshold based guidelines for ICD do not apply. In fact, an ICD may be considered for a patient with higher LVEF thresholds [26, 42]. Regarding FLNC mutations, 20% of patients with a primary-prevention ICD who carry the mutation had an appropriate ICD shock, much higher than in unselected DCM populations [43]. Appropriate ICD shocks are also more likely in PLN carriers, especially in R14del variant, along with a family history of SCD before the age of 50 years compared to those who do not carry the mutation [44]. These findings support the hypothesis that genetic factors should be considered early in the disease progression.

The CMR-Guide (Cardiac Magnetic Resonance Guided Management of Mild-Moderate Left Ventricular Systolic Dysfunction) trial, which is expected to be completed in 2020, is randomizing ischemic and nonischemic cardiomyopathy patients with an LVEF between 36 and 50% and presence of LGE to either an ICD or an implantable loop recorder in an attempt to determine whether LGE is a sufficient marker alone or whether genetic characterization is also necessary in risk stratification. In general, a polyparametric integration is being introduced in the primary prevention of SCD through ICD implantation in DCM patients that includes family history of SCD, LVEF, late gadolinium enhancement, and possibly genetic parameters [45].

3. Future perspectives

The evaluation and treatment of hereditary DCM constitutes an emerging field. Still, risk stratification regarding SCD is based on general knowledge. Larger registries and long-term follow-up may elucidate more specific risk markers associated with genotypes in addition to phenotype.

4. Conclusion

Hereditary DCM is a heterogeneous condition, which may lead to advanced HF as well as SCD. Risk stratification and preventive management strategies are challenging. Many factors must be considered in the management of patients with hereditary DCM. Gene mutations are surfacing and have already been proven to play a very significant role in clinical decisions. Moreover, based on new data and studies, the profile of each DCM patient tends to be better understood. As a result, both therapy and prevention evolve and ameliorate in a way that will become individualized. ICDs are lifesaving but their role in different genotypic settings remains to be elucidated.

Conflicts of interest

Peter Magnusson has received speaker fees or grants from Abbott, Alnylam, Bayer, AstraZeneca, Boehringer-Ingelheim, Lilly, MSD, Novo Nordisk, Octopus Medical, Pfizer, and Zoll. Joseph Pergolizzi is a principal at Native Cardio, Inc. Marianna Leopoulou and Jo Ann LeQuang have no relevant disclosures.

Acronyms and abbreviations

ACE	angiotensin converting enzyme
ARB	angiotensin receptor blocker
AR-DCM	arrhythmogenic dilated cardiomyopathy
ARVC	arrhythmogenic right ventricular cardiomyopathy
CMR	cardiac magnetic resonance
CRT	cardiac resynchronization therapy
CRT-D	cardiac resynchronization therapy defibrillator
DCM	dilated cardiomyopathy
ICD	implantable cardioverter defibrillator
LGE	late gadolinium enhancement
LMNA	lamin A/C
LV	left ventricle
LVEF	left ventricular ejection fraction
NSVT	nonsustained ventricular tachycardia
NYHA	New York Heart Association
RAAS	renin-angiotensin-aldosterone system
PLN	phospholamban
RBM20	RNA binding motif protein 20
SCD	sudden cardiac death
SCN5A	sodium voltage-gated channel alpha subunit 5
TTN	titin
VF	ventricular fibrillation
VT	ventricular tachycardia

Author details

Marianna Leopoulou[1*], Jo Ann LeQuang[2], Joseph V. Pergolizzi[2,3]
and Peter Magnusson[4,5]

1 Cardiology Clinic, Athens General Hospital "Elpis", Athens, Greece

2 NEMA Research, Inc., USA

3 Native Cardio, Inc., USA

4 Cardiology Research Unit, Department of Medicine, Karolinska Institute, Sweden

5 Centre for Research and Development, Uppsala University, Gävleborg, Sweden

*Address all correspondence to: mariannina.leo@gmail.com

References

[1] Park HY. Hereditary dilated cardiomyopathy: Recent advances in genetic diagnostics. Korean Circulation Journal. 2017;**47**(3):291-298

[2] Bozkurt B, Colvin M, Cook J, Cooper LT, Deswal A, Fonarow GC, et al. Current diagnostic and treatment strategies for specific dilated cardiomyopathies: A scientific statement from the American Heart Association. Circulation. 2016;**134**(23):e579-e646

[3] Ganesh SK, Arnett DK, Assimes TL, Basson CT, Chakravarti A, Ellinor PT, et al. Genetics and genomics for the prevention and treatment of cardiovascular disease: Update: A scientific statement from the American Heart Association. Circulation. 2013;**128**(25):2813-2851

[4] Morales A, Hershberger RE. Genetic evaluation of dilated cardiomyopathy. Current Cardiology Reports. 2013;**15**(7):375

[5] NIH, US National Library of Medicine. Genetics Home Reference. Familial dilated cardiomyopathy. Available from: https://ghr.nlm.nih.gov/condition/familial-dilated-cardiomyopathy [Accessed: 22 December 2019]

[6] Mestroni L, Maisch B, McKenna WJ, Schwartz K, Charron P, Rocco C, et al. Guidelines for the study of familial dilated cardiomyopathies. Collaborative research Group of the European Human and Capital Mobility Project on familial dilated cardiomyopathy. European Heart Journal. 1999;**20**(2):93-102

[7] McNally EM, Mestroni L. Dilated cardiomyopathy: Genetic determinants and mechanisms. Circulation Research. 2017;**121**(7):731-748

[8] Chugh SS, Jui J, Gunson K, Stecker EC, John BT, Thompson B, et al. Current burden of sudden cardiac death: Multiple source surveillance versus retrospective death certificate-based review in a large U.S. community. Journal of the American College of Cardiology. 2004;**44**(6):1268-1275

[9] Wu TJ, Ong JJ, Hwang C, Lee JJ, Fishbein MC, Czer L, et al. Characteristics of wave fronts during ventricular fibrillation in human hearts with dilated cardiomyopathy. role of increased fibrosis in the generation of reentry. Journal of the American College of Cardiology. 1998;**32**:187-196

[10] Sen-Chowdhry S, McKenna WJ. Sudden death from genetic and acquired cardiomyopathies. Circulation. 2012;**125**:1563-1576

[11] Pogwizd SM, McKenzie JP, Cain ME. Mechanisms underlying spontaneous and induced ventricular arrhythmias in patients with idiopathic dilated cardiomyopathy. Circulation. 1998;**98**:2404-2414

[12] Kjekshus J. Arrhythmias and mortality in congestive heart failure. Americal Journal of Cardiology. 1990;**65**:42I-48I

[13] Losurdo P, Stolfo D, Merlo M, Barbati G, Gobbo M, Gigli M, et al. Early arrhythmic events in idiopathic dilated cardiomyopathy. Journal of the American College of Cardiology Clinical Electrophysiology. 2016;**2**:535-543

[14] Spezzacatene A, Sinagra G, Merlo M, Barbati G, Graw SL, Brun F, et al. Arrhythmogenic phenotype in dilated cardiomyopathy: Natural history and predictors of life-threatening arrhythmias. Journal of the American Heart Association. 2015;**4**(10):e002149

[15] Shekha K, Ghosh J, Thekkoott D, Greenberg Y. Risk stratification for sudden cardiac death in patients with

non-ischemic dilated cardiomyopathy. Indian Pacing Electrophysiology Journal. 2005;**5**(2):122-138

[16] Ponikowski P, Voors AA, Anker SD, Bueno H, Cleland JGF, Coats AJS, et al. 2016 ESC guidelines for the diagnosis and treatment of acute and chronic heart failure: The task force for the diagnosis and treatment of acute and chronic heart failure of the European Society of Cardiology (ESC) developed with the special contribution of the heart failure association (HFA) of the ESC. European Heart Journal. 2016;**37**(27):2129-2200

[17] Grimm W, Alter P, Maisch B. Arrhythmia risk stratification with regard to prophylactic implantable defibrillator therapy in patients with dilated cardiomyopathy. Results of MACAS, DEFINITE, and SCD-HeFT. Herz. 2004;**29**(3):348-352

[18] Assomull RG, Prasad SK, Lyne J, Smith G, Burman ED, Khan M, et al. Cardiovascular magnetic resonance, fibrosis, and prognosis in dilated cardiomyopathy. Journal of the American College of Cardiology. 2006;**48**(10):1977-1985

[19] Masarone D, Limongelli G, Ammendola E, Verrengia M, Gravino R, Pacileo G. Risk stratification of sudden cardiac death in patients with heart failure: An update. Journal of Clinical Medicine. 2018;**7**(11)

[20] Haugaa KH, Goebel B, Dahlslett T, Meyer K, Jung C, Lauten A, et al. Risk assessment of ventricular arrhythmias in patients with nonischemic dilated cardiomyopathy by strain echocardiography. Journal of the American Society of Echocardiography. 2012;**25**(6):667-673

[21] Gigli M, Merlo M, Graw SL, Barbati G, Rowland TJ, Slavov DB, et al. Genetic risk of arrhythmic phenotypes in patients with dilated cardiomyopathy. Journal of the American College of Cardiology. 2019;**74**(11):1480-1490

[22] Priori SG, Blomström-Lundqvist C, Mazzanti A, Blom N, Borggrefe M, Camm J, et al. 2015 ESC guidelines for the management of patients with ventricular arrhythmias and the prevention of sudden cardiac death: The task force for the Management of Patients with ventricular arrhythmias and the prevention of sudden cardiac death of the European Society of Cardiology (ESC). European Heart Journal. 2015;**36**(41):2793-2867

[23] Pasotti M, Klersy C, Pilotto A, Marziliano N, Rapezzi C, Serio A, et al. Long-term outcome and risk stratification in dilated cardiolaminopathies. Journal of the American College of Cardiology. 2008;**52**(15):1250-1260

[24] van Rijsingen IA, Arbustini E, Elliott PM, Mogensen J, Hermans-van Ast JF, van der Kooi AJ, et al. Risk factors for malignant ventricular arrhythmias in lamin a/c mutation carriers a European cohort study. Journal of the American College of Cardiology. 2012;**59**(5):493-500

[25] Kumar S, Baldinger SH, Gandjbakhch E, Maury P, Sellal JM, Androulakis AF, et al. Long-term arrhythmic and nonarrhythmic outcomes of lamin a/c mutation carriers. Journal of the American College of Cardiology. 2016;**68**(21):2299-2307

[26] Wahbi K, Ben Yaou R, Gandjbakhch E, Anselme F, Gossios T, Lakdawala NK, et al. Development and validation of a new risk prediction score for life-threatening ventricular tachyarrhythmias in laminopathies. Circulation. 2019;**140**:293-302

[27] Sousa A, Canedo P, Campelo M, Moura B, Leite S, Baixia M, et al. Genetic variants are not rare in ICD candidates with dilated cardiomyopathy:

Time for next-generation sequencing? Cardiology Research and Practice. 2019:2743650

[28] Parikh VN, Caleshu C, Reuter C, Lazzeroni LC, Ingles J, Garcia J, et al. Regional variation in RBM20 causes a highly penetrant arrhythmogenic cardiomyopathy. Circulation: Heart Failure. 2019;**12**(3):e005371

[29] McMurray JJV, Solomon SD, Inzucchi SE, Køber L, Kosiborod MN, Martinez FA, et al. Dapagliflozin in patients with heart failure and reduced ejection fraction. The New England Journal of Medicine. 2019;**381**(21):1995-2008

[30] Wijetunga M, Strickberger SA. Amiodarone versus implantable defibrillator (AMIOVIRT): Background, rationale, design, methods, results and implications. Cardiac Electrophysiology Review. 2003;**7**(4):452-456

[31] Bardy GH, Lee KL, Mark DB, Poole JE, Packer DL, Boineau R, et al. Amiodarone or an implantable cardioverter-defibrillator for congestive heart failure. The New England Journal Medicine. 2005;**352**(3):225-237

[32] Køber L, Thune JJ, Nielsen JC, Haarbo J, Videbæk L, Korup E, et al. Defibrillator implantation in patients with nonischemic systolic heart failure. The New England Journal of Medicine. 2016;**375**(13):1221-1230

[33] Kusumoto FM, Calkins H, Boehmer J, Buxton AE, Chung MK, Gold MR, et al. ACC/AHA expert consensus statement on the use of implantable cardioverter-defibrillator therapy in patients who are not included or not well represented in clinical trials. Circulation. 2014;**130**(1):94-125

[34] Kadish A, Dyer A, Daubert JP, Quigg R, Estes NA, Anderson KP, et al. Prophylactic defibrillator implantation in patients with nonischemic dilated cardiomyopathy. The New England Journal of Medicine. 2004;**350**(21):2151-2158

[35] Stecker EC, Dewland TA. Gradually understanding sudden cardiac death. Journal of the American College of Cardiology. 2016;**67**(18):2116-2117

[36] Gorgels AP, Gijsbers C, de Vreede-Swagemakers J, Lousberg A, Wellens HJ. Out-of-hospital cardiac arrest-the relevance of heart failure. The Maastricht circulatory arrest registry. European Heart Journal. 2003;**24**(13):1204-1209

[37] McLeod CJ, Shen W, Rea RF, Friedman PA, Hayes DL, Wokhlu A, et al. Differential outcome of cardiac resynchronization therapy in ischemic cardiomyopathy and idiopathic dilated cardiomyopathy. Heart Rhythm. 2011;**8**(3):377-382

[38] Arshad A, Moss AJ, Foster E, Padeletti L, Barsheshet A, Goldenberg I, et al. Cardiac resynchronization therapy is more effective in women than in men: The MADIT-CRT (multicenter automatic defibrillator implantation trial with cardiac resynchronization therapy) trial. Journal of the American College of Cardiology. 2011;**57**(7):813-820

[39] Moss AJ, Hall WJ, Cannom DS, Klein H, Brown MW, Daubert JP, et al. Cardiac-resynchronization therapy for the prevention of heart-failure events. The New England Journal of Medicine. 2009;**361**:1329-1338

[40] Healey JS, Hohnloser SH, Exner DV, Birnie DH, Parkash R, Connolly SJ, et al. Cardiac resynchronization therapy in patients with permanent atrial fibrillation: Results from the resynchronization for ambulatory heart failure trial (RAFT). Circulation: Heart Failure. 2012;**5**(5):566-570

[41] Di Marco A, Anguera I, Schmitt M, Klem I, Neilan TG, White JA, et al. Late

gadolinium enhancement and the risk for ventricular arrhythmias or sudden death in dilated cardiomyopathy: Systematic review and meta-analysis. Journal of the American College of Cardiology Heart Failure. 2017;**5**(1):28-38

[42] Akhtar M, Elliott PM. Risk stratification for sudden cardiac death in non-ischaemic dilated cardiomyopathy. Current Cardiology Reports. 2019;**21**(12):155

[43] Ortiz-Genga MF, Cuenca S, Dal Ferro M, Zorio E, Salgado-Aranda R, Climent V, et al. Truncating FLNC mutations are associated with high-risk dilated and arrhythmogenic cardiomyopathies. Journal of the American College of Cardiology. 2016;**68**(22):2440-2451

[44] van der Zwaag PA, van Rijsingen IA, Asimaki A, Jongbloed JD, van Veldhuisen DJ, Wiesfeld AC, et al. Phospholamban R14del mutation in patients diagnosed with dilated cardiomyopathy or arrhythmogenic right ventricular cardiomyopathy: Evidence supporting the concept of arrhythmogenic cardiomyopathy. European Journal of Heart Failure. 2012;**14**(11):1199-1207

[45] Disertori M, Masè M, Rigoni M, Nollo G, Arbustini E, Ravelli F. Implantable cardioverter-defibrillator in dilated cardiomyopathy after the DANISH-trial lesson. A Poly-Parametric Risk Evaluation Is Needed to Improve the Selection of Patients. Frontiers in Physiology. 2017;**8**:873

Chapter 9

Familial Dilated Cardiomyopathy: Risk Stratification for Sudden Cardiac Death

Gustav Mattsson and Peter Magnusson

Abstract

Heart failure implies a considerable burden for patients and resources for the health care system. Dilated cardiomyopathy is defined as left ventricular dilation and reduced systolic function, not solely explained by ischemic heart disease or abnormal loading conditions. Numerous genes have been identified in familial cases of dilated cardiomyopathy. Heart failure with reduced ejection fraction increases the risk for sudden cardiac death. Implantable cardioverter defibrillator therapy can provide a means of preventing sudden cardiac death in those deemed to be at high risk. Health care providers are in need of better tools in order to improve risk stratification. This chapter aims to provide an overview of the current knowledge about risk of arrhythmia and sudden death in patients with familial dilated cardiomyopathy, in particular for those patients with a specific mutation.

Keywords: arrhythmia, cardiology, cardiomyopathy, genetic, heart failure, sudden cardiac death

1. Introduction

The prevalence of heart failure is approximately 1–2% in the adult population and is 10% for those above the age of 70 years [1]. Dilated cardiomyopathy (DCM) is a common form of heart failure defined by dilatation of the left ventricle and reduced ejection fraction [2]. In later phases, dilation of the right ventricle and both atria is often seen, although this is not required for diagnosis. The disease confers a reduction in left ventricular ejection fraction but in early stages dilatation of the left ventricle can be seen with only minimal reduction of systolic function. Definitions vary, sometimes a distinction is made between ischemic and nonischemic DCM; however more often DCM refers to a disease that is not explained by coronary artery disease or abnormal loading conditions due to hypertension or valve defects [2]. With this definition the prevalence is at the least 1 in 2500 in the general population, which is likely an underestimation and some estimates refer the prevalence as high as 1 in 250 [3, 4]. In more than 20% of these patients a known disease causative mutation is found [3, 5]. Mutations in more than 50 different genes have been associated to DCM and some of the most common are the genes encoding for lamin A/C, titin, and desmin [1, 6]. Often the phenotype is the similar regardless of the causative mutation, therefore broad gene panels are used in genetic testing. Some genes however affect the conduction system and have been linked to an increase in sudden cardiac death.

2. Definitions

2.1 Cardiomyopathies

Definitions of cardiomyopathies differ over time and between clinical traditions. While in the future cardiomyopathies might be classified after causative mutations, they have traditionally been classified by phenotype and cardiac morphology, e.g. DCM or hypertrophic cardiomyopathy (HCM). This system of classification has the advantage that the phenotype is most often known prior to the genotype.

Originally, cardiomyopathies were considered distinct primary myocardial disorders of unknown etiology, whereas heart muscle disorders of known etiology or caused by systemic disease were classified as secondary or specific heart muscle disease. In 2006 the American Heart Association proposed a classification that defined cardiomyopathies either as primary or secondary, referring either to a disease were the heart is the sole or primarily affected organ, alternatively where myocardial involvement is part of a systemic disease [7]. However, in 2008, the European Society of Cardiology (ESC) proposed an alternate classification in which a cardiomyopathy is defined as "a myocardial disorder in which the heart muscle is structurally and functionally abnormal in the absence of coronary artery disease, hypertension, valvular disease and congenital heart disease sufficient to cause the observed myocardial abnormality". Furthermore, the ESC subdivides cardiomyopathies depending on morphology and function as well as based upon inheritance pattern; distinguishing between familial or genetic forms versus non-familial or non-genetic forms of cardiomyopathy (**Figure 1**) [2].

2.2 Dilated cardiomyopathy

DCM is a distinct cardiomyopathy and a common cause of heart failure defined by dilatation of the left ventricle and reduced ejection fraction [2]. In later phases dilation of the right ventricle and the atria is often seen, however this is not required for diagnosis. For the diagnosis of DCM, the reduction in global systolic function should not solely be attributable to coronary artery disease or abnormal loading conditions (hypertension, valve disease) [2].

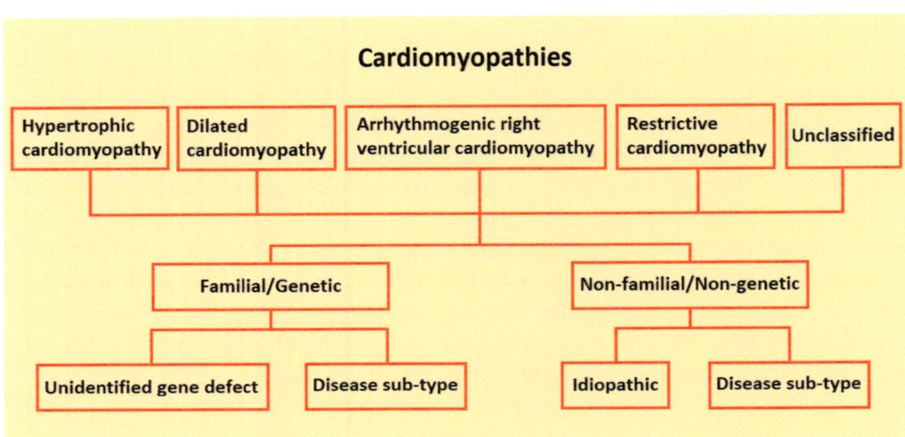

Figure 1.
Classification of cardiomyopathies proposed by the European Society of Cardiology [2]. Cardiomyopathies are primarily classified according to morphology and function, then based on whether the disease is familial or non-familial, and lastly depending on either known disease causing mutation or pathophysiological mechanism.

2.3 Familial dilated cardiomyopathy

Familial DCM is diagnosed when at least two relatives (first-degree or second-degree) meet the diagnostic criteria for DCM [8].

3. Diagnostic evaluation of dilated cardiomyopathy

3.1 Echocardiography

Diagnostic evaluation for suspected heart failure should be managed in accordance with guidelines, such as those of the ESC [1]. Echocardiography constitutes a cornerstone of the evaluation and is readily available. For the diagnosis of DCM both left ventricular systolic dysfunction, as well as dilatation of the left ventricle, needs to be present and not explained by coronary artery disease or abnormal loading conditions (hypertension, valve disease) [9]. Left ventricular systolic dysfunction is defined as abnormal left ventricular systolic ejection fraction measured with any modality, preferentially echocardiography or cardiac magnet resonance tomography. Left ventricular dilatation (**Figure 2**) is defined as left ventricular end-diastolic volumes or diameters >2 standard deviations according to nomograms ($Z > 2$ standard deviations) after correction for body surface area and age, or body surface area and sex [9].

3.2 Cardiac magnetic resonance tomography

Cardiac magnetic resonance tomography is valuable as a complement to echocardiography. It allows for a better evaluation of the whole myocardium including the right ventricle and septum which provides aid in ruling out other cardiomyopathies such as arrhythmogenic right ventricular cardiomyopathy (ARVC) and HCM. Myocarditis has been identified as a cause of acquired forms of DCM [10]. Cardiac magnetic resonance can be used to assess the presence of active myocarditis as well as scar tissue that could indicate previous episodes of myocarditis. Cardiac magnetic resonance imaging is, according to the ESC, indicative of active myocarditis if it, in the setting of clinically suspected myocarditis, fulfills 2 out of 3 Lake Louise criteria [11]. These criteria include; high signaling on T2-weighted images (indicative of edema), early gadolinium enhancement (indicative of increased blood flow), and late gadolinium enhancement (indicative of scar tissue) [11].

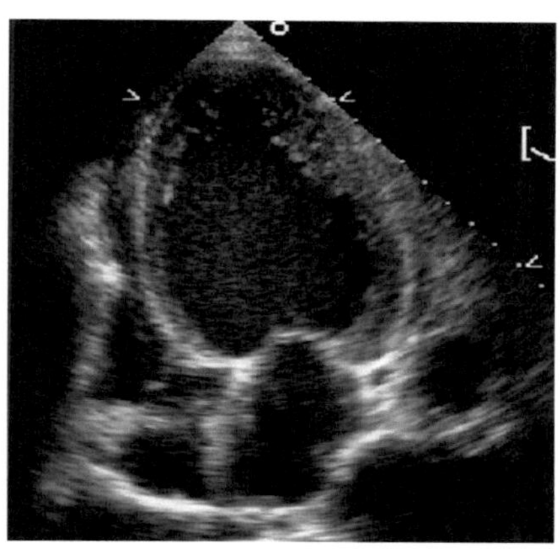

Figure 2.
Echocardiography with apical four chamber view showing spherical dilatation of the left ventricle. Image adapted from Jamil et al. [12]. Published by IntechOpen under open access https://creativecommons.org/licenses/by/3.0/.

3.3 Family history

Of particular importance is a family history of cardiomyopathy, arrhythmia or sudden cardiac death. If another family member also fulfills the criteria for DCM the patient can be said to have familial DCM [8]. A pedigree, a family tree, could be drawn to visualize what family members are affected by the disease or certain symptoms as well as how they are related to each other. By doing this the type of inheritance pattern can often be discerned, see Section 5.1. Inheritance patterns.

3.4 Genetic testing

Genetic testing requires knowledge about genetics, the disease in question, as well as legal and ethical considerations. It is important that the patient is the one who makes an informed decision about if a gene test should be performed [13]. It is also important to be aware of what the benefits and potential detriments of a genetic test are. The current ESC Heart failure guidelines from 2016 recommend that genetic testing should be performed in accordance with the ESC position statement on genetic counseling and testing in cardiomyopathies from 2010 [1, 13]. Most genotypes cannot be distinguished from each other by evaluation of the phenotype. Due to this broad gene panels are required that incorporate most known definite and putative DCM genes. The ESC states that the main role of genetic testing is in patients with an already confirmed diagnosis of idiopathic DCM (where acquired causes has been ruled out) to enable genetic testing of first degree-relatives and possibly cascade screening, see Section 5.2. Family screening. They caution against the use of genetic testing to establish the diagnosis of a cardiomyopathy in borderline cases except for in the setting of expert teams after detailed clinical and family assessment. In definite DCM most often, the exact gene affected do not change the clinical management of that individual patient. However, in some cases of DCM with red flags such as simultaneous conductions disorders indicative of a specific phenotype, genetic testing can be used to establish a specific genetic diagnosis. In patients with mutations in LMNA that causes DCM, genetic diagnosis might affect the clinical management. It should be noted that negative genetic tests do not rule out that the cardiomyopathy is familial or genetic. The interpretation of genetic tests is time consuming, complicated, and often not conclusive. When the ESC position statement was written in 2010 genetic tests had been mainly used for research purposes and had recently become available for clinicians. Genetic tests have today become more affordable and available. The current trend is towards more genetic evaluations being conducted and it is our opinion that this trend should continue. More patients with DCM receiving a genetic diagnosis will over time improve knowledge of the different genotypes. In order to offer equal health care genetic testing must be conducted even outside the setting of tertiary centers.

4. Clinical management of dilated cardiomyopathy

4.1 Heart failure

Heart failure management should be in accordance with guidelines, such as those of the ESC, which are summarized below [1]. An angiotensin converting enzyme inhibitor (ACEi) or angiotensin receptor blocker (ARB) is indicated in left ventricular systolic dysfunction. If symptomatic, i.e. New York Heart Association functional classification (NYHA-class) 2 or above, a beta-blocker should be added to treatment with the ACEi/ARB. In patients who remain symptomatic with systolic ejection fraction ≤35% despite the highest tolerable evidence-based doses of ACEi or ARB as well as a beta-blocker, a mineral receptor antagonist is recommended with maximum tolerated evidence-based dose. If the patient is still symptomatic with systolic ejection fraction ≤35% it is recommended to initiate treatment with an angiotensin receptor neprilysin inhibitor that replaces the ACEi/ARB [1]. Further treatment modalities that should be considered include the addition of ivabradine in patients with sinus rhythm ≥70 beats per minute, or the implantation of a cardiac device to allow for cardiac resynchronization therapy in those with left bundle branch block and QRS ≥130 ms or without left bundle branch block but QRS ≥150 ms. These mentioned treatment modalities have shown increased survival in randomized controlled trials [1]. Digoxin could be considered if symptoms remain, however reduced mortality has not been shown but rather reduced need for hospitalization. The small therapeutic window of digoxin should be kept in mind, most commonly digoxin is used for rate control in atrial fibrillation that is common in heart failure. Loop-diuretics such as furosemide should be considered in patients with heart failure to relieve symptoms and signs of congestion, but this has not been shown to reduce mortality. The dosage of diuretics should be kept as low as possible and cessation of treatment might often be possible. In end-stage heart failure, transplant might be considered or mechanical left ventricular assist devices that can be used as destination therapy, bridge-to-decision, or bridge to transplant [1].

Lately inhibition of sodium-glucose transporter protein 2 (SGLT2i) has proved an interesting treatment modality for heart failure with reduced ejection fraction. In the EMPA-REG trial in 2015, the SGLT2i empagliflozin showed reduced cardiovascular mortality, reduction in all-cause mortality, and reduced need for hospitalization for heart failure in patients with type 2 diabetes mellitus [14]. In 2019 the results of the DAPA-HF trial showed that the SGLT2i dapagliflozin reduced cardiovascular and all-cause mortality as well as risk of worsening heart failure in patients with heart failure with reduced ejection fraction even if they did not have diabetes mellitus [15].

4.2 Arrhythmia

There is an increased risk for both brady- and tachyarrhythmia in DCM, these arrhythmias can also be a contributing factor worsening heart failure. In symptomatic sinus node disease or in high-degree atrioventricular (AV)-block without a reversible cause a pacemaker is indicated in order the relieve symptoms and/or increase survival [3]. Beta-blockers are often indicated for the treatment of symptomatic heart failure but also have antiarrhythmic properties making it useful for both rhythm and rate control. With the exception of beta-blockers currently available antiarrhythmic drugs have not consistently been shown in randomized clinical trials to improve survival in the primary management of arrhythmia. Amiodarone have shown some positive results and is highly useful to control symptoms, to terminate tachyarrhythmia and prevent recurrence [3]. In heart failure with reduced ejection fraction most other antiarrhythmic agents are contraindicated, this includes flecainide and dronedarone otherwise frequently used for rhythm control in atrial fibrillation [3].

4.3 Prevention of sudden cardiac death

An implantable cardioverter defibrillator (ICD) is an effective way to prevent sudden cardiac death in those at risk for developing ventricular tachycardia or ventricular fibrillation [3]. An ICD offers both antitachycardia pacing, rapid ventricular pacing (preferably bursts), that can terminate ventricular tachycardia, as well as cardioversion that effectively terminate ventricular tachycardia and ventricular fibrillation. In addition, an ICD also functions as a bradycardia pacemaker and in combination with a left-ventricular lead it can offer cardiac resynchronization therapy.

The ESC recommends a primary prophylactic ICD for patients with symptomatic heart failure (NYHA-class II-III), left ventricular systolic ejection fraction ≤35% despite at least three months of optimal medical therapy and a life expectancy of at least 1 year [3]. The recommendation is class I (is recommended) for both heart failure due to ischemic heart disease as well as nonischemic cardiomyopathy. The level of evidence is considered stronger for heart failure with ischemic etiology (level A) than for nonischemic etiology (level B) [3]. In the SCD-HeFT trial an ICD reduced all-cause mortality as well as sudden cardiac death in patients with reduced ejection fraction [16]. In the DEFINITE trial, with a study population of patients with heart failure due to nonischemic etiology, sudden cardiac death was reduced by 80%, however reduction in all-cause mortality did not reach statistical significance (hazard ratio 0.65, p = 0.08) [17]. In 2016, the DANISH trial randomized participants with heart failure of nonischemic origin to either an ICD or otherwise optimal medical management (both groups were eligible for cardiac resynchronization therapy), after 5 years there was a significant reduction in sudden cardiac death (HR; 0.50, p = 0.005) [18]. For the whole group no significant reduction was seen in all-cause mortality (HR; 0.87, p = 0.28), however subgroup analysis of patients younger than 68 years showed a reduction all-cause mortality (hazard ratio 0.64; p = 0.01) [18]. This caused uncertainty about whether patients with heart failure of nonischemic etiology should receive ICDs on the same indications as those with ischemic etiology. Since then, a meta-analysis of six trials, that included DANISH, has showed that ICD on primary-prevention indication in patients with heart failure of nonischemic etiology reduced all-cause mortality (hazard ratio 0.76, p = 0.001) [19]. An analysis of the Swedish Heart Failure Registry revealed a 27% relative risk reduction in all-cause mortality after 1 year, this was consistent in both the subgroup with ischemic and with nonischemic etiology [20]. We have previously published a retrospective observational study of our ICD-cohort [21]. In our study 236 patients with primary prevention ICD due to heart failure of ischemic (61.9%) or nonischemic (38.1%) etiology were included, there was no difference in cumulative risk for appropriate therapy between the groups (Mantel-Cox p = 0.985) [21]. The guidelines of the ESC recommending implantation of a primary prevention ICD should therefore be followed in patients with heart failure with both ischemic etiology as well as nonischemic DCM [3].

5. Familial dilated cardiomyopathy

5.1 Inheritance patterns

Most genetic mutations that cause familial DCM have an autosomal dominant inheritance pattern with variable penetrance [22]. However, autosomal recessive, X-linked recessive and mitochondrial inheritance patterns have been described [22]. Sometimes a mutation is found that does not occur in any of the parents, this is called a *de novo* mutation.

5.1.1 Autosomal dominant

Autosomal inheritance is related to a mutation in an autosome, i.e. any chromosome that is not a sex chromosome. Dominant inheritance pattern implies that it is enough with only one mutant allele for the disease to be expressed. This means that the effect of a mutation in a gene masks or overrides the effect of a normal variation of the same gene on the other copy of the same chromosome. Those who have only a mutation in one of their two gene copies are said to be heterozygous. Due to a complex interplay with other genes and with the environment the disease is not always expressed, this is called varying penetrance. Men and women are equally as likely to inherit a mutated gene from a parent that carries it, regardless if it is the father or mother. If one parent carries one copy of the mutated gene, the offspring has a 50% risk of inheriting it. If both parents carry one copy of the gene, the offspring has a 75% risk of inheriting at least one copy.

5.1.2 Autosomal recessive

Autosomal recessive inheritance is caused by mutation in a gene situated on an autosome but requires both the copy inherited from the father and the copy from the mother to be mutaded. For the mutation to cause the disease to be expressed the carrier needs to be homozygous for the mutation. This inheritance pattern requires both parents to carry at least one gene affected by the mutation. Men and women are equally as likely to inherit two affected gene copies from a certain pair of parents. If both parents carry one mutated gene, the offspring has a 25% risk of inheriting two mutated gene copies.

5.1.3 X-linked recessive

X-linked recessive inheritance pattern is caused by a mutation in a gene situated on the X chromosome. Since the X chromosome is a sex chromosome and females have two copies while males have only one copy, if the inheritance pattern is recessive, males will be affected, while females need to inherit a mutated gene from both their father and mother in order to be affected. Since men never inherit their X-chromosome from their father, the mutated gene can never pass to a son from his father. Daughters have always inherited one of their X-chromosomes from their father, thus an affected father will always have passed the mutated gene on to his daughters. This daughter will only be a carrier and not affected by the disease, unless she also has inherited the mutated gene from her mother. It is therefore common for X-linked recessive diseases to skip generations of daughters. A female that carry one mutated gene copy have a 50% risk of passing this on to both their sons and daughters.

5.1.4 Mitochondrial inheritance

In humans, mitochondria, and also mutations affecting mitochondrial DNA, is inherited from the mother. Both males and female can be affected by mitochondrial disease but only females can pass on the mutation to their offspring.

5.2 Family screening

5.2.1 Family screening in case of a known mutation

In many European countries including Sweden, the physician has no legal right to contact or inform first-degree relatives about the results of a genetic test. Instead the patient must be equipped with sufficient knowledge, both verbally and in written form to inform relatives about the genetic aspect of the disease, although usually there is no legal obligation for the patient to do this.

If the proband, the first identified individual with DCM in a family, has a known disease-causing mutation it is possible to screen all first-degree relatives for this single mutation [13]. If the inheritance pattern is autosomal dominant, children each have 50% risk of carrying the mutation. A simple genetic test could with certainty confirm or reject that an individual carries the mutation, this has large implications. If the individual is not a carrier of the mutated gene, no further follow-up is required, no cascade screening is needed of this individual's children, and the individual have a better chance of living a normal life.

If instead the gene test confirms that an individual carries the mutated gene, so called cascade screening should be considered of this individual's first-degree relatives. Carrying a known disease-causing mutation implies that cardiologic evaluation should be conducted consisting of at least 12-lead ECG and echocardiography. If this evaluation results in a diagnosis of DCM life-long follow-up is required. If this cardiologic evaluation is inconclusive or finds no signs of DCM continued follow-up is still required. The penetrance of familial DCM is most often age-dependent, age at diagnosis of DCM is most often seen during or after puberty up until 60 years of age [13]. Therefore, renewed assessment with at least ECG and echocardiography should be conducted every year between the ages of 10 and 20 and then every 1–3 years.

5.2.2 Family screening in case of no known mutation

In idiopathic DCM, in a setting where genetic testing is not available, negative, or inconclusive, familial DCM can still not be ruled out. All first-degree relatives of the proband should undergo cardiologic evaluation with at least 12-lead ECG and echocardiography [13]. If they are diagnosed with DCM life-long follow-up is required and all their first-degree relatives should undergo cardiologic evaluation as well. If instead the cardiologic evaluation is negative for DCM, the relative should be followed-up with repeat cardiologic evaluations; every 1–3 years for those younger than 10 years of age, every 1–2 years between the age of 10 and 20, and every 2–5 years from 20 years of age up until 50–60 years of age. The reason for this continued evaluation during life is the age-dependent penetrance. For those affected, penetrance is almost complete at 60 years of age, therefore repeated evaluation is not necessary after this [13].

6. Causative gene mutations

Many genes have been linked to DCM, some with a definite and some with a putative link. For definite DCM genes see **Table 1**, adapted from McNally et al. [22]. It is often difficult to determine if a mutation in a gene is causative of cardiomyopathy, sometimes mutations are determined to be so called variants of unknown significance. Most genes implicated in the pathogenesis of DCM are highly conserved with few *de novo* mutations occurring, making new mutations, found in a known DCM gene that alters the encoded protein, likely to be pathogenic.

Mutations that have been linked to DCM affect genes related to diverse cell structures such as; ion channels, dystrophin complexes, sarcoplasmic reticulum, nuclear lamina, desmosomes, mitochondria, cytoskeleton, z-disc, and sarcomeres. For an image visualizing different cellular structures related to definite DCM genes see **Figure 3**.

6.1 Genes associated with sudden cardiac death

The general consensus is that risk of arrhythmia in DCM scales with the degree of left ventricular systolic dysfunction. Most genotypes cannot be distinguished from each other by evaluation of the phenotype. Due to this broad gene panels are required. However, some genotypes have been shown to be prone to arrhythmia and in some

Gene	Protein	Frequency and overlapping phenotypes
Sarcomere	**Force generation/transmission**	
MYH7	Beta-myosin heavy chain	3–4% of DCM; HCM, LVNC
TPM1	Alpha-tropomyosin	1–2% of DCM; HCM, LVNC
ACTC1	Alpha cardiac actin	HCM, LVNC
TNNT2	Cardiac troponin T	3% of DCM; HCM, LVNC
TNNC1	Cardiac troponin C	HCM, LVNC
TNNI3	Cardiac troponin 1	HCM
TTN	Titin	12–25% of DCM; HCM, tibial muscle dystrophy
TNNI3K	Troponin 1 interacting kinase	Conduction defect, atrial fibrillation
Z-disc	**Mechanosensing/mechanosignaling**	
ACTN2	Alpha-actinin 2	LVNC
BAG3	BCL2 Associated Athanogene 3	Myofibrillar myopathy
CRYAB	Alpha-B-crystallin	Protein aggregation myopathy
TCAP	Titin-cap/telethonin	LGMD2G
CSRP3	Muscle LIM protein	HCM
ANKRD1	Cardiac ankyrin repeat protein	Congenital heart disease
LDB3	Cipher/ZASP	LVNC
NEBL	Nebulette	LVNC, HCM
Dystrophin complex	**Sarcolemma, structural integrity**	
DMD	Dystrophin	Duchenne/Becker muscular dystrophy
SGCA	Alpha-sarcoglycan	LGMD2D
SGCB	Beta-sarcoglycan	LGMD2E
SGCD	Delta-sarcoglycan	LGMD2F
Cytoskeleton	**Mechanotransduction/mechanosignaling/structural integrity**	
DES	Desmin	<1% of DCM; desminopathies, myofibrillar myopathy
VCL	Metavinculin	1% of DCM
FLNC	Filamin C	1% of DCM; myofibrillar myopathy, HCM, RCM
Desmosomes	**Cell–cell adhesion/mechanotransmission/mechanosignaling**	
DSP	Desmoplakin	2% of DCM; ARVC
Sarcoplasmic reticulum and cytoplasm Ca homeostasis, contractility modulation, signaling		
PLN	Phospholamban	ARVC, HCM
Nuclear envelope	**Nuclear structural integrity, mechanotransduction, mechanosignaling**	
LMNA	Lamin A/C	4–8% of DCM; multiple phenotypes, LGMD1B, EDMD, progeria
EMD	Emerin	EDMD
Nucleus	**Transcription cofactors, gene expression**	
RBM20	RNA-binding protein 20	2% of DCM; RNA-binding protein of spliceosome of TTN and other proteins
Ion channels	**Transportation of ions**	
SCN5A	Type V voltage-gated cardiac Na channel	2–3% of DCM; LQTS, Brugada, atrial fibrillation, conduction defects

Gene	Protein	Frequency and overlapping phenotypes
ABCC9	Component of ATP-sensitive potassium channel	Atrial fibrillation, osteochondrodysplasia
KCNQ1	Potassium channel	Atrial fibrillation, LQTS1, short QT1, Jervell and Lange-Nielsen syndrome
Mitochondria	**Supply and/or regulation of energy metabolism**	
DNAJC19	HSP40 homolog, C19	3-methylglutaconic aciduria type V
TAZ/G4.5	Tafazzin	LVNC, Barth syndrome, endocardial fibroelastosis 2

ARVC: arrhythmogenic right ventricular cardiomyopathy; DCM: dilated cardiomyopathy; EDMD: Emery Dreifuss muscular dystrophy; HCM: hypertrophic cardiomyopathy; LGMD: limb-girdle muscular dystrophy; LVNC: left ventricular non-compaction cardiomyopathy; LQTS: long QT-syndrome; RCM: restrictive cardiomyopathy. Adapted from McNally et al. [22].

Table 1.
Definite dilated cardiomyopathy genes.

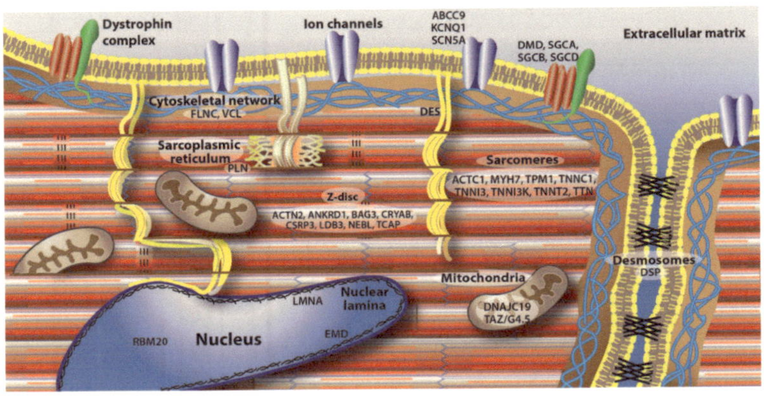

Figure 3.
Cross section of two cardiomyocytes that connect to each other with desmosomes at the intercalated disc. Definite DCM genes and important cellular structures pertaining to them are named. Image by Todd Cooper.

cases sudden cardiac death. Some genes are very rare, or only putative and not definitively linked to DCM. Out of the genes that regularly are found to cause DCM, LMNA and SCN5A stand out for their propensity to cause arrhythmia. Mutations in both of these genes can cause a phenotype with atrial fibrillation, conduction system disease or ventricular tachyarrhythmia as the presenting symptom [22]. Guidelines from the ESC give specific indications for the implantation of an ICD in patients with DCM and LMNA mutation, these are described below [3]. For SCN5A no specific guidelines are given [3]. However, it is reasonable to adapt clinical management for patients with mutation in this gene to account for the known risk for arrhythmia. This also holds true for patients with other or unknown mutations, but with a family history indicative of a high risk of arrhythmia and sudden cardiac death. Such adaptations might include more frequent ambulatory ECG-monitoring or the use of insertable cardiac monitors to screen for potentially life-threatening arrhythmias.

6.1.1 LMNA

LMNA, the gene encoding the proteins lamin A and C, is one of the most studied DCM genes. Lamin A/C form part of the nuclear lamina and have been implicated in several cellular processes, including regulation of gene expression [22]. DCM associated with mutation in LMNA tend to have age-dependent penetrance but with disease onset early in life, often dysrhythmias mainly conduction disturbances and atrial fibrillation precede the development of heart failure. The risk for sudden cardiac death is also increased, even with only moderately reduced left ventricular ejection fraction [3]. Guidelines of the ESC state that an ICD should be considered (class of recommendation IIa) for patients with DCM and a confirmed disease-causing mutation in LMNA if any of the following clinical risk factors are present; non-sustained ventricular tachycardia, left ventricular ejection fraction ≤45%, male sex, or a non-missense mutation (insertion, deletion, truncation or mutation affecting splicing) [3]. This recommendation is based upon the results of a cohort study of 269 patients with LMNA-mutation and a median follow-up time of 43 months, 48 patients (18%) reached the composite endpoint of sudden cardiac death, appropriate ICD therapy, or aborted cardiac death [23]. In a review of published cohorts of patients with LMNA-associated cardiomyopathy, in total 299 patients, some sort of dysrhythmia was reported in 92% after the age of 30 years [24]. Dysrhythmias included sinus bradycardia, first-degree AV-block, and atrial or ventricular tachyarrhythmias [24]. Notably, almost half died from sudden cardiac death [24]. This high proportion of sudden cardiac death was also noted in those patients who had a pacemaker implanted, which implies that the mode of death in LMNA-associated cardiomyopathy may be caused by ventricular tachyarrhythmias [24].

6.1.2 SCN5A

Mutations in SCN5A, the gene that encodes the sodium voltage-gated channel alpha subunit 5 involved in the main cardiac sodium channel, has been linked to several diseases including Brugada syndrome, long QT-syndrome as well as DCM and ARVC [25]. Different kinds of mutations in SCN5A have been linked to DCM and the mechanism is still uncertain. Interestingly, the phenotype varies in families with the same genotype, indicating that environmental or other confounding factors are at play [25]. Mutations in SCN5A have also been linked to progressive conduction disorder and familial atrial fibrillation. Given this, it is not surprising that DCM due to SCN5A often presents with increased risk of arrhythmia [22].

7. Future perspectives

Currently, familial DCM is likely frequently underdiagnosed, and often genetic testing is not conducted. Increased awareness and availability of genetic evaluation might provide more knowledge and gene-specific therapies and management might become available. Increased identification of affected families will mean that more at-risk individuals will come into contact with health care providers prior to developing the phenotype. This means that future studies should focus on therapies aimed to prevent the development of DCM in these individuals. Further research into the different genotypes and their burden of arrhythmia is also warranted in order to improve risk stratification for sudden cardiac death. This includes the utilization of implantable cardiac monitors in those patients who have certain high-risk genotypes but have been judged not to fulfill criteria for the implantation of an ICD.

8. Conclusion

Reduced left ventricular systolic ejection fraction is the most common indication for the implantation of an ICD regardless of type of cardiomyopathy. In DCM some genes have been linked to a propensity for arrhythmia, chief among them LMNA and SCN5A. A mutation in LMNA together with other clinical risk factors could warrant implantation of an ICD.

Acknowledgements

Thanks to Region Gävleborg, our employer, for funding this project. Thanks to Todd Cooper for providing illustrations.

Conflict of interest

Gustav Mattsson has received speaker's fee from Alnylam, MSD, and Internetmedicin. Peter Magnusson has received speaker's fees or grants from Abbott, Alnylam, Amicus Therapeutics, AstraZeneca, Bayer, Boehringer-Ingelheim, Internetmedicin, Lilly, MSD, Novo Nordisk, Octopus Medical, Orion Pharma, Pfizer, Vifor Pharma, and Zoll.

Funding

The writing of this book chapter was funded by our employer, Region Gävleborg.

Acronyms and abbreviations

ACEi: angiotensin converting enzyme inhibitor; ARVC: arrhythmogenic right ventricular cardiomyopathy; AV: atrioventricular; DCM: dilated cardiomyopathy; ESC: European Society of Cardiology; HCM: hypertrophic cardiomyopathy; ICD: implantable cardioverter defibrillator; NYHA: New York Heart Association; SGLT2i: sodium-glucose transporter protein 2.

Author details

Gustav Mattsson[1*] and Peter Magnusson[1,2]

1 Centre for Research and Development, Uppsala University/Region Gävleborg, Gävle, SE-801 87, Sweden

2 Cardiology Research Unit, Department of Medicine, Karolinska Institutet, Stockholm, SE-171 76, Sweden

*Address all correspondence to: gustav.mattsson@regiongavleborg.se

References

[1] Ponikowski P, Voors AA, Anker SD, *et al.* 2016 ESC Guidelines for the diagnosis and treatment of acute and chronic heart failure The Task Force for the diagnosis and treatment of acute and chronic heart failure of the European Society of Cardiology (ESC) Developed with the special contribution of the Heart Failure Association (HFA) of the ESC. *Eur Heart J* 2016;**37**:2129-200. doi:10.1093/eurheartj/ehw128

[2] Elliott P, Andersson B, Arbustini E, *et al.* Classification of the cardiomyopathies: a position statement from the European society of cardiology working group on myocardial and pericardial diseases. *Eur Heart J* 2008;**29**:270-6. doi:10.1093/eurheartj/ehm342

[3] Priori SG, Blomström-Lundqvist C, Mazzanti A, *et al.* 2015 ESC Guidelines for the management of patients with ventricular arrhythmias and the prevention of sudden cardiac death: The Task Force for the Management of Patients with Ventricular Arrhythmias and the Prevention of Sudden Cardiac Death of the European Society of Cardiology (ESC). Endorsed by: Association for European Paediatric and Congenital Cardiology (AEPC). *Eur Heart J* 2015;**36**:2793-867. doi:10.1093/eurheartj/ehv316

[4] Sweet M, Taylor MRG, Mestroni L. Diagnosis, prevalence, and screening of familial dilated cardiomyopathy. *Expert Opin Orphan Drugs* 2015;**3**:869-76. doi:10.1517/21678707.2015.1057498

[5] Petretta M, Pirozzi F, Sasso L, *et al.* Review and metaanalysis of the frequency of familial dilated cardiomyopathy. *Am J Cardiol* 2011;**108**:1171-6. doi:10.1016/j.amjcard.2011.06.022

[6] McNally EM, Golbus JR, Puckelwartz MJ. Genetic mutations and mechanisms in dilated cardiomyopathy. *J Clin Invest* 2013;**123**:19-26. doi:10.1172/JCI62862

[7] Maron BJ, Towbin JA, Thiene G, *et al.* Contemporary definitions and classification of the cardiomyopathies: an American Heart Association Scientific Statement from the Council on Clinical Cardiology, Heart Failure and Transplantation Committee; Quality of Care and Outcomes Research and Functional Genomics and Translational Biology Interdisciplinary Working Groups; and Council on Epidemiology and Prevention. *Circulation* 2006;**113**:1807-16. doi:10.1161/CIRCULATIONAHA.106.174287

[8] Schultheiss H-P, Fairweather D, Caforio ALP, *et al.* Dilated cardiomyopathy. *Nat Rev Dis Primer* 2019;**5**:32. doi:10.1038/s41572-019-0084-1

[9] Pinto YM, Elliott PM, Arbustini E, *et al.* Proposal for a revised definition of dilated cardiomyopathy, hypokinetic non-dilated cardiomyopathy, and its implications for clinical practice: a position statement of the ESC working group on myocardial and pericardial diseases. *Eur Heart J* 2016;**37**:1850-8. doi:10.1093/eurheartj/ehv727

[10] Mason JW. Myocarditis and dilated cardiomyopathy: an inflammatory link. *Cardiovasc Res* 2003;**60**:5-10. doi:10.1016/s0008-6363(03)00437-1

[11] Caforio ALP, Pankuweit S, Arbustini E, *et al.* Current state of knowledge on aetiology, diagnosis, management, and therapy of myocarditis: a position statement of the European Society of Cardiology Working Group on Myocardial and Pericardial Diseases. *Eur Heart J* 2013;**34**:2636-48, 2648a–2648d. doi:10.1093/eurheartj/eht210

[12] Jamil G, Abbas A, Shehab A, *et al.* Echocardiography Findings in Common Primary and Secondary Cardiomyopathies. *Cardiomyopathies* Published Online First: 12 June 2013. doi:10.5772/55036

[13] Charron P, Arad M, Arbustini E, *et al.* Genetic counselling and testing in cardiomyopathies: a position statement of the European Society of Cardiology Working Group on Myocardial and Pericardial Diseases. *Eur Heart J* 2010;**31**:2715-26. doi:10.1093/eurheartj/ehq271

[14] Zinman B, Wanner C, Lachin JM, *et al.* Empagliflozin, Cardiovascular Outcomes, and Mortality in Type 2 Diabetes. *N Engl J Med* 2015;**373**:2117-28. doi:10.1056/NEJMoa1504720

[15] McMurray JJV, Solomon SD, Inzucchi SE, *et al.* Dapagliflozin in Patients with Heart Failure and Reduced Ejection Fraction. *N Engl J Med* 2019;**381**:1995-2008. doi:10.1056/NEJMoa1911303

[16] Bardy GH, Lee KL, Mark DB, *et al.* Amiodarone or an implantable cardioverter-defibrillator for congestive heart failure. *N Engl J Med* 2005;**352**:225-37. doi:10.1056/NEJMoa043399

[17] Kadish A, Dyer A, Daubert JP, *et al.* Prophylactic defibrillator implantation in patients with nonischemic dilated cardiomyopathy. *N Engl J Med* 2004;**350**:2151-8. doi:10.1056/NEJMoa033088

[18] Køber L, Thune JJ, Nielsen JC, *et al.* Defibrillator Implantation in Patients with Nonischemic Systolic Heart Failure. *N Engl J Med* 2016;**375**:1221-30. doi:10.1056/NEJMoa1608029

[19] Shun-Shin MJ, Zheng SL, Cole GD, *et al.* Implantable cardioverter defibrillators for primary prevention of death in left ventricular dysfunction with and without ischaemic heart disease: a meta-analysis of 8567 patients in the 11 trials. *Eur Heart J* 2017;**38**:1738-46. doi:10.1093/eurheartj/ehx028

[20] Schrage B, Uijl A, Benson L, *et al.* Association Between Use of Primary-Prevention Implantable Cardioverter-Defibrillators and Mortality in Patients With Heart Failure: A Prospective Propensity Score-Matched Analysis From the Swedish Heart Failure Registry. *Circulation* 2019;**140**:1530-9. doi:10.1161/CIRCULATIONAHA.119.043012

[21] Mattsson G, Magnusson P. Long-term follow-up of implantable cardioverter defibrillator patients with regard to appropriate therapy, complications, and mortality. *Pacing Clin Electrophysiol PACE* 2020;**43**:245-53. doi:10.1111/pace.13869

[22] McNally EM, Mestroni L. Dilated Cardiomyopathy: Genetic Determinants and Mechanisms. *Circ Res* 2017;**121**:731-48. doi:10.1161/CIRCRESAHA.116.309396

[23] van Rijsingen IAW, Arbustini E, Elliott PM, *et al.* Risk factors for malignant ventricular arrhythmias in lamin a/c mutation carriers a European cohort study. *J Am Coll Cardiol* 2012;**59**:493-500. doi:10.1016/j.jacc.2011.08.078

[24] van Berlo JH, de Voogt WG, van der Kooi AJ, *et al.* Meta-analysis of clinical characteristics of 299 carriers of LMNA gene mutations: do lamin A/C mutations portend a high risk of sudden death? *J Mol Med Berl Ger* 2005;**83**:79-83. doi:10.1007/s00109-004-0589-1

[25] Veerman CC, Wilde AAM, Lodder EM. The cardiac sodium channel gene SCN5A and its gene product NaV1.5: Role in physiology and pathophysiology. *Gene* 2015;**573**:177-87. doi:10.1016/j.gene.2015.08.062